W9-DIY-504

WOMEN'S POWER TO HEAL

MOTHER OM MEDIA • CANDLER • NORTH CAROLINA • USA

WOMEN'S
POWER
TO HEAL

Through Inner Medicine

BY
SRI SWAMINI MAYATITANANDA

(MAYA TIWARI)

This publication provides authoritative information on diet and health but is sold with the understanding that the author and publisher are not rendering medical advice. It is the individual reader's obligation to evaluate her or his own medical needs, to determine for herself or himself whether specific medical advice is required and where necessary, to seek the services of a qualified health-care professional.

A Mother Om Media Book

Copyright © 2007 by Sri Swamini Mayatitananda (Maya Tiwari) and Wise Earth School of Ayurveda, Ltd.

Illustrations & Cover Art © 2007 by Sri Swamini Mayatitananda (Maya Tiwari) and Wise Earth School of Ayurveda, Ltd.

Wise Earth Ayurveda® is a unique school of Inner Medicine healing practice developed by Sri Swamini Mayatitananda (Maya Tiwari) and based on Vedic principles. The philosophy and practices set forth in this book are copyrighted by Sri Swamini Mayatitananda (Maya Tiwari) and the Wise Earth School of Ayurveda Ltd. All public presentation and/or use by unlicensed practitioners and teaching institutions of Wise Earth Ayurveda® educational programs and their content, concepts, practices, therapies creative sadhana prototypes, tables, and graphics are copyrighted worldwide and public use of them, or any part thereof, is strictly prohibited without formal written permission from the Wise Earth School of Ayurveda, Ltd.

For information about Wise Earth Ayurveda® Training for Practitioners, you may contact us at:
Wise Earth School of Ayurveda Ltd.
P.O. Box 160
Candler, North Carolina 28715-0160
Voice Mail: 828-258-9999
E-mail: info@wisearth.org
Website: www.wisearth.org

All rights reserved under International and Pan-American Copyright Conventions. Published in the United States by Mother Om Media.

Mother Om Mission and Mother Om Media are divisions of Wise Earth School of Ayurveda, Ltd.

Publisher's Cataloging-in-Publication

Tiwari, Maya.
Women's power to heal : through inner medicine / by
Maya Tiwari.
p. cm.
Includes index.
ISBN 0-9793279-0-3
LCCN 2007921572
1. Women--Diseases--Alternative treatment. 2. Women
--Health and hygiene--Alternative treatment.
3. Medicine, Ayurvedic.   I. Title.

RA778.T59 2007   615.5'38'082   QBI07-600049

Text Layout and Cover Design by Sharon Anderson, Blue Moon Design

Printed and bound in the USA

First Edition: September 2007

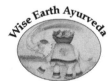

OPENING PRAYER TO THE SUPREME GODDESS LALITA MAHA TRIPURASUNDARI

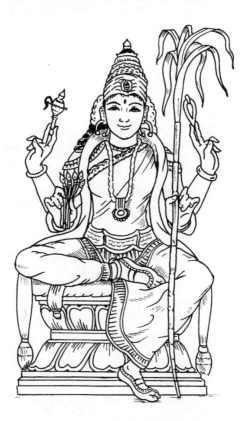

Om Ksetra-svarupayai Namah
Om Ksetr'esyai Namah
Om Ksetra-ksetrajna-palinyai Namah
Om Ksetra-pala-samarcitayai Namah.

Reverence to the Supreme Goddess who is the body of all beings
Reverence to Her who is the ruler of all bodies
Reverence to Her who protects both the soul and the body
Reverence to Her who is worshipped by the Ksetrapala
—the individual who is the keeper of the body.
—*Lalita Sahasranama*

CONTENTS

ILLUSTRATIONS

Figures

Tables

All Wise Earth Ayurveda charts, tables, and illustrations are copyrighted worldwide and public use is strictly prohibited without formal written permission from the Wise Earth School of Ayurveda, Ltd.

DEDICATION

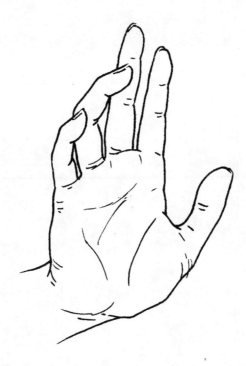

To the Mother Consciousness

And to the Mother within each and every life

May we remember:

Within each one of us, we are One

Altogether we are One

Without each other, we are One.

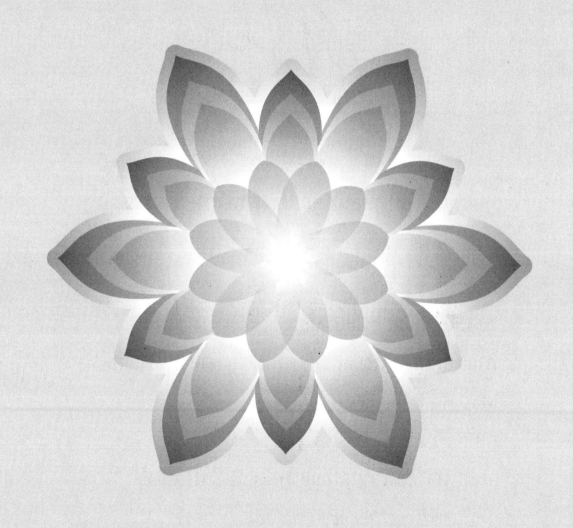

PREFACE

Introducing Wise Earth Ayurveda

More than 7,000 years ago Ayurveda established an eight-branched system of medicine—the first full-scale, documented medical system in the world—which included the most ancient predecessor to the study of Pediatrics, and the successful execution of complex surgical procedures considered to be the first reconstructive plastic surgeries.

Ayurveda's eight branches are collectively called *Ashtanga Ayurveda: Kaya Chikitsa*—Internal Medicine; *Shalya Chikitsa*—Surgery; *Bala Chikitsa*—Pediatrics; *Graha Chikitsa*—Psychiatry; *Urdhvanga Chikitsa*—treatment of eyes, ears, nose, throat, and head; *Damstra Chikitsa*—Toxicology; *Jara Chikitsa*—Gerontology, and *Vrishya Chikitsa, (Vajikarana)*—Aphrodisiacs.

Ayurveda, which literally means, "knowledge of life and longevity" came from the *Atharva Veda*, one of Hinduism's four Vedas, or spiritual record. The Vedas comprise extensive tomes of scholarly work on the sciences—such as medicine, astronomy, mathematics, physics, architecture, genealogy, and health—and also complex and detailed spiritual works—*Vedanta, Yoga, Ayurveda, Jyotisha, Vastu Vidya, Nada Vidya*, and *Tantra* to name a few—all detailing practices which reveal the knowledge of the True Self and that serve the good of humanity. According to the *Atharva Veda*, Ayurveda's timeless education of sadhana is the most effective spiritual path to awaken consciousness and enhance our Inner Medicine potential for healing ourselves.

Through the Wise Earth School and, by extension, its sadhakas—practitioners and teachers at large—it is my hope to reorder these long forgotten cyclical *sadhana* practices imperative for the sustenance of human memory. I have spent the past 25 years unearthing cosmic cyclical knowledge and reintroducing it back into the vision of Ayurveda. Some of the many practices I have restored for the preservation of the human memory, which you will find in these pages, are the lunar rhythms necessary for women's well-being; the rhythmic nature-based therapies and practices that awaken *buddhi*—our intrinsic intuition and intelligence; cosmic rites and rituals to nurture our children and heal the Whole Spirit; Uttara Vasti, the central lunar practice for women that maintains the health of the womb, which centuries ago had become defunct in Ayurveda practice; and the Vedic rites of passage for menarche. This Inner Medicine wisdom and approach contained in this book is central to the education of Wise Earth Ayurveda.

Originally, the entire broad scope of Ayurveda Medicine was practiced in the spirit of sadhana, but this original sadhana basis of Ayurveda has been profoundly eroded over the last two centuries in India. Firstly, its decline in popularity can be attributed to the progressive erosion of human connection to nature, followed by the introduction of Western Medicine, and later on by the government of India's attempts to modernize Ayurveda's medicine principles. In so doing, core principles within Ayurveda's protocols were fragmented to meet the standards of Western Medicine's clinical model. As a result, the original sadhana model of Ayurveda became perverted, and a more prescriptive and far less intuitive form of medicine ensued. As a result, the understanding of living, nourishing, and healing our bio-psychic rhythms with the cosmic elements, lunar rhythms, and the solar cycle of the seasons were lost to Ayurveda; and indeed, to the world.

This is not to suggest that the popularized clinical version of Ayurveda does not have its merits. In fact, Ayurveda's adaptation to Western Medicine principles makes it a perfect catalyst to help transform Western Medicine's treatment protocols into more effective ones for the human physiognomy. This necessary feat of integration also meets the medical dependency of the multitudes with the non-toxic approaches and medicines of Ayurveda. However, restoring Ayurveda's organic model so that its original principles of Inner Medicine healing may be preserved is also necessary.

Whatever is the inspiration or calling, each one of us has a divine right to choose healing and to be healed through myriad ways and means. The important thing is that we must be able to meet each and every person at whatever milestone they may be found in their individual journey of consciousness. To help another person, we must not only accommodate them but gleefully embrace the chance to meet them at any juncture of their journey. This is the core intention of my teachings and the writings contained in this book.

May its wisdom forever serve and bless you.

Mother Maya
Wise Earth Monastery
Candler, North Carolina
USA
January 1st, 2007

ACKNOWLEDGMENTS

Writing this book has been a blessing of joy and freedom—the Divine Mother's Grace flowing through my hands into the communal heart of wisdom. Knowing that this work serves millions of women who are ready to embrace their Shakti-packed power and discover their Inner Medicine resource for healing, I am truly swelled.

Always, my gratitude to the Mother Consciousness, who protects and guides my journey and whose work it is I serve. This project came to fruition through the help and diligent care of many people: the Wise Earth Ayurveda sadhakas, master teachers, and disciples who disseminate these precious teachings; and in particular, Linda Sarita Rocco, Nina Usha Molin, M.D., Katie Spiers Mantisas, and Theresa Ambika McGhee through their dedicated promotion of Wise Earth conferences. Gratitude to Kamala Asher and Patricia Isa Peluso whose devout service nourishes the space from which these books are born. My profound thanks to each one of Mother Om Mission's courageous coordinators, volunteers, and instructors who have opened their hearts to service—embracing the challenging work in New York's inner cities and Guyana's at-risk communities.

Firstly, I want to name those who helped with bringing this book to fruition: Catherine Elliott Escobedo for her overall support of the book's refinement and her intuitive work with proofreading, editing, styling, and the publishing process—her input to this work altogether is too numerous to list here; Nora Isaacs, whose fine editorial skills have served to hone this book; and Sharon Anderson for her excellent creative work in designing this book. I thank Marnie Mikell for her devout care and artistic skills in refining Wise Earth's drawings and illustrations.

I would be remiss if I did not acknowledge and thank publishing champion, Leslie Meredith, my spirited mentor (on *The Path of Practice*), whose knowledge of "the word" has had the greatest impact on the integrity of my writing; and to Janis Vallely, whose kindness and wisdom continue to help my work.

I wish to thank the beautiful Christiane Northrup, M.D. for her powerful book, *Women's Bodies, Women's Wisdom*, which literally broke open the ground in the medical arena, allowing women's healing freedom to enter; and for her heartfelt endorsement of my work.

Finally, I wish to acknowledge my birth mother, Kali Devi; my elder mother, Jaya Devi; and the Mother in all women. May we remember to serve the Mother Consciousness with grace and gratitude.

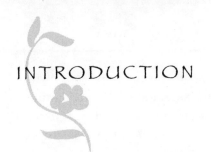

INTRODUCTION

We are all healed. We heal in life. We heal in death. We heal in rebirth. And ultimately, we heal into consciousness.

Wise Earth Ayurveda Inner Medicine healing is based in the understanding that each one of us has the ineffable ability to arouse healing powers imbued within ourselves.

THE SADHANA WAY: INNER MEDICINE EDUCATION

The primary key to remaining healthy is to maintain a life of balance. As we practice the *sadhana* way of Inner Medicine healing in our everyday lives, which I will detail in *Women's Power to Heal*, we start to develop an ongoing sense of keen awareness. As you will discover through your daily sadhanas, sacred practices, everything that appears to be external—herbs, foods, remedies, thoughts, and actions—are all melded into the fine weave of memory held in your own Inner Medicine resources. No medicine, no matter how powerful, can replace your own. Life *is* simple. We've made it complex by adding massive amounts of material appendages to it, living in a state of over-stress, exaggerating our needs, believing that "more" is better; but more options and more choices serve only to make an already packed life more weary and complex. The more consciousness you cultivate the fewer choices you need.

The principles of sadhana are steeped in the Wise Earth Ayurveda education of awareness, in other words, *awareful* practices that evoke our Inner Medicine healing potential and keep our inner rhythms in alignment with the Mother Consciousness—the indestructible maternal energy imbued in each and every person, the central support that upholds the whole universe.

Healing *is* simple. It is initiated within yourself through this awareness. Healing is a subtle thing—it is about the character of your ongoing relationship to the earth, sun, moon, sky, water, forest, animals, and children. In reality, we live in perennial initiation within the Mother Consciousness. How does this initiation work? Whatever you love or desire is automatically transferred within the subtle plane of your heart, thereby transforming the external to the internal. What you love becomes part of your vital tissues, your immunity, and your destiny.

In this book you will learn the necessity you have as a woman to realign your natural biorhythms in accord with lunar, solar, and seasonal cycles—reclaiming the Mother Consciousness within you that is your perennial right to your female cosmic anatomy and reproductive authority. In essence, you will learn the importance of restoring the Shakti-packed role of the Mother in producing and sustaining life. This must be honored as most sacred if we are to maintain the sacred in human intelligence and action.

WE ARE ALL HEALED

Each one of us has the capacity to enter the vast cosmos within ourselves and become infinitely more conscious. We are all healed. We heal in life. We heal in death. We heal in rebirth. And ultimately, we heal into consciousness. Indeed, Mother Nature provides us with many opportunities for healing. Realizing these self-truths will help us to live in health, harmony, and prosperity. Healing is the result of lives that are in harmony with Mother Nature. Good health will not be found outside of us. It is a natural state of being in the form of the True Self. Once we realize the True Self to be a conscious entity that is intrinsically whole, we may eliminate any sense of separation, which is the cause of all suffering and unhappiness.

You hold in your hands a key to connecting with this state of health. *Women's Power to Heal* is packed with healing secrets, insights, and practices that will set you on the path to true radiance and a lifetime of health. You will learn the Wise Earth Ayurveda® Inner Medicine—teachings I have spent the last 30 years developing and honing. These are simple Inner Medicine practices that will knit you back into the rhythmic weave of nature and help you to understand nature and self as one continual harmonious vibration. *Women's Power to Heal* provides you with the tools you need to practice the Inner Medicine to revive the sleeping potential in all women and includes specific practices for female conditions such as: difficult menstruation, menopause, fertility issues, hormonal imbalance, PMS, herpes, miscarriage, HIV/AIDS, osteoporosis, and yeast infections with simple, safe, and proven techniques to try at home. You'll learn about the lunar phases and why it's important to bring back your cycle to coincide with the lunar cycle, and then how to apply practices during both the full moon and the new moon.

And for those of you in good health, this book provides the ultimate in preventative medicine: guidelines for maintaining optimal health and well-being through herbal baths, compresses, internal cleansing, food choices, and rituals. Ultimately, the book takes a modern look at centuries-old wisdom, gleaning the most useful information and empowering women of all ages.

The healing wisdom and energy you will gain from this book comes from two primary tributaries: wisdom gleaned from a life of rich experiences rooted in the ancient ancestral heritage of my Hindu tradition and knowledge substantiated by the Vedas and Ayurvedas. Both streams emerge from and return to the continuum of direct transmission I am blessed to have received from the Divine Mother. I will draw from this timeless and ancient source of the Mother Consciousness to help you gain the fresh vision necessary to restore your own Shakti energies.

THE COSMIC JOURNEY

Our journey begins 12 billion years ago, with a tradition whose wisdom seers reflected the cosmic light—the light that still shines today. Because of this light, we have the power to think, reflect, contemplate, and know. We see this light not as an external force, but as the inner radiance through which we are able to see, hear, smell, feel, and remember. Our capacity for awareness is a reflection of this light. Through this consciousness we are able to light up every object and therefore experience the world, making it visible, audible, and familiar. This universal wisdom is promulgated by the Vedas in the Hindu culture, which as you will see, has informed all of my teachings.

Thirty-two years ago, I recovered from ovarian cancer. Since then, I have been able to neutralize my karmas and assume my legacy as a Spiritual Mother for thousands of women, men, and children, primarily through my work as the founder of the Wise Earth School of Ayurveda in Asheville, North Carolina, and Mother Om Mission (MOM), a charitable organization that teaches Ayurveda to at-risk communities around the world. As you will see, Ayurveda, the incomparable system of health and healing that was developed eons ago by Hindu seers in India—and the path to which I have devoted my life's work—gives us extensive information and knowledge about health and its relation to the predictable and unpredictable principles of nature.

According to Ayurveda, each person bears a unique constitution, composed of the five elements, which can be fortified by specific wholesome intentions and activities that serve individual needs. Throughout this book, you will see that once you learn your metabolic constitution, you can support your body, mind, and spirit to heal, excel, and thrive. Wise Earth Ayurveda Inner Medicine teaches you to garner physical, emotional, and spiritual well-being while embracing a continual state of joy, balance, and abundance. All illness comes from imbalances in your constitutional essence, or sense of being.

I hope that the wisdom of this work resonates within you, helps you ease physical, mental, and emotional pressures, and trust that the continuum of Mother's vibration, rhythm, intuition, and grace will rise to take their place. Throughout these pages, you will find joyful Shakti practices to help you evoke the memory of your own Inner Medicine, created by nature, so that you may "return" to your

True Self. Wise Earth Ayurveda Inner Medicine is based in the understanding that each one of us has the ineffable ability to arouse healing powers imbued within ourselves. As you will learn, to reorder these powers it is imperative that we explore our inner universe of desire, intuition, and intention. Each one of us has an internal stock of a trillion energy medicines, with the aid of a trillion more remedies provided by Mother Nature. Inner Medicine is the palpable energy and power we carry within us so that we may access and draw upon it to heal ourselves. According to my tradition, each one of us is the Whole Consciousness (*Aham Brahmasmi*) and altogether we are the Whole. Consciousness saturates each one of our births, lives, deaths, rebirths, and the final completion of each of our journeys into pure consciousness.

We should not underestimate the profound potency of our Inner Medicine for wellness. A woman at one of my workshops revealed that as a result of reciting a *bija*, seed mantra of the Goddess Durga, for two days, she was free from migraine headaches for the first time in 13 years. At another venue, a woman who was diagnosed with fibromyalgia and experienced crippling pain throughout her body found that after just one week of mudra practice she could sit on the floor in the classroom for hours without a trace of pain.

DISCOVERING THE MOTHER CONSCIOUSNESS

You will find a great deal of insight about the Mother Consciousness and her immense Shakti power in this work. To know the whole, we must know the material Shakti energy that created the universe. This primordial energy exists in its most manifested form in the female of all species and resides in its most evolved state in women.

Evidenced by millions of Hindu Goddess temples still thriving in India, this culture has stoically preserved the Great Mother tradition. The ancient Shakta and Tantra traditions which focus on worshipping the Mother Consciousness emerged from the vast pantheon that is the mind of Hinduism. Here, Lalita Maha Tripurasundari is the central goddess to the *Sri Vidya* tradition, (or Auspicious Wisdom tradition). The Sri Vidya is a branch of Shakta Tantrism that considers Lalita as the supreme form of the Great Goddess, or manifestation of Parashakti. Within the Sri Vidya tradition, meditation, prayer, and ritual practice to the Great Goddess play an important role in helping women to "see" the mirrored selves of wholeness, beauty, and wisdom—the Great Goddess reflecting in our true nature.

According to Shakta Tantric philosophy, Shakti is the feminine aspect of cosmic energy and considered by many to be Lalita. She is the primeval creative energy through whose womb the universe was delivered. The goddess endowed her power of Shakti into the womb of every female, willing her with her most potent Inner Medicine to nurture, nourish, and heal. A woman's Shakti has the power to give life, create art, nourish, nurture, and keep life in a state of equanimity. This phenomenal force is the axial power of a woman. Once known, it teaches you how to care for your body, nourish your sexuality, respect your emotions and intuition, and honor your spirit. Your Shakti is the luminous energy that gives rise to your maternal authority—reproducing life, nourishing nature's food, and inspiring the universe's continually changing rhythms. This feminine energy controls the musical throb of the heartbeat and sustains the ultimate nectar of life carried in the womb. The Shakti provides the necessary generation of energy for the ongoing cycles of life to continue. In Vedic thought, the woman's *yoni*, vagina, is the cosmic gateway through which the universe's rhythm and memory exchange with human life. Similarly, a woman's breasts replicate the Goddess Aditi's nourishment for the earth's survival. Women are the primary link that keeps human beings in touch with nourishing energies of nature. In essence, your Shakti energy is the Mother Consciousness on Planet Earth. You will find the viable means to reconnect to the Mother Consciousness when you realize that the pathway to your female wellness comes through your Shakti.

SHAKTI POWER AT WORK

Over the years I've been peppered with questions from my Western students about what they view as "subservient" roles of the women in native cultures. For example, they would ask why in Vedic tradition a young woman's coming of age invariably is linked to the rites of her marriage, or why women retreat into a state of seclusion and contemplation during their menses. The answer to these inquiries may be found in one central source of understanding. We must relearn the content of our subtle and pervasive powers as women before we are able to distinguish what our precious organic reality truly is. You'll learn about these innate powers through your relationships. You will see the magnificent munificence you have in your natural relationship to your mother, father, husband, and children. Your fulfillment as a woman will help you to recognize the true purpose of the Shiva energy—masculine cosmic energy—in your life. In so doing, the urge to compete with the male and his karmic and societal roles will dissolve.

Unfortunately, Western culture has relegated the Shakti education to the shadows wherein women's profound power has become a hidden nature to be peered at only through a masked kaleidoscope. This is why Western women are largely unaware of their fundamental power. In the present world culture we inadvertently define communal and maternal values along linear and dualistic lines of thinking. In so doing, we often miss the essential spiritual meaning of life's manifold maternal passages and transitions. Almost every aspect of living today is seen from a dualistic perspective; high and low, good and bad, right and wrong, black and white, masculine and feminine, and so on.

In the Vedic purview of life, we see the constant as ever changing, perpetually morphing into new shapes and forms, birthing the necessary rites and rituals that support the manifested reality, and thereby progressing each toward its limitless transformative destiny. Specific and perceivable, and yet the unpredictable pure consciousness, *Brahman*, is that which supports the transcending realities of time and space, the moment to moment-ness of each person's past, present, and future. Indeed, this is the way that the rishis experienced the universe cognizing that our innate power of Shakti emulates the patterns of this universal experience. When we recognize the true nature of our Shakti energy, we realize that our anatomy as women is cosmically programmed to perform in the same transcendental dynamic way. As you'll see in later pages, we have several natural transitions in our lives—for example, menarche and menopause are two of the most significant junctures in the collective life of the female. You will learn how to protect the sanctity of your sexuality, and in turn, safeguard the Shakti potential of your daughters and other young women. You will also comprehend the importance of protecting and preserving your Shakti power—preserving its cosmically creative rhythms, and staying connected to the Mother Consciousness—while embracing the divine interplay of feminine *and* masculine energies embodied by Shiva and Shakti, dispelling imbalanced ideas about the role of the opposite sex.

In order to fully own the lunar essence of our feminine powers and walk the path to wellness which comes through Shakti, we must relearn the ancestral traditions of the solar masculine energy, or Shiva force. To attain absolute harmony we must know the intertwining energies of Shiva and Shakti as inseparable—each one playing a pivotal role in the power of the whole self. Together, as content and container, they form the one firm foundation of our transcendent universe within and without. In discovering your true relationship to the solar-powered Shiva energies in your life, you'll find happiness in your marriage, home, children, and work.

Over the past 32 years, I've traveled around the globe, taught workshops, trained teachers, and guided thousands of women along the way. I see that women everywhere are eager to realize and unearth their crucial connection to the mother source of energy called Shakti. In reclaiming our wondrous birthright, women are on the forefront of retooling a whole new identity. Our ways of thinking, living, loving, caring, and being are all in the process of massive transformation. However, there is nothing new about the ideas, visions, and truths that we are rebirthing. You will find every curve and nuance of Shakti's cosmic blueprint impressed within you from the timeless journey we share.

Using Wise Earth Ayurveda to help thousands of women heal from the ravages of cancer into good health, I can say that the single most significant factor in their healing had to do with simplifying their lives. Thirty-two years following my own personal experience of healing from ovarian cancer, I continue to simplify my life. In so doing, I continue to rediscover that we possess the intrinsic power to heal ourselves. I have witnessed this power at work numerous times.

Diagnosed with ovarian cancer at the age of 23, I was given two months to live. Instead, I connected to the Mother Consciousness through the ancient circuitry of my ancestors, and a vast vista of memory opened. I witnessed the subtle planes of my timeless existence through visions and dreams. It has now been 32 years since my recovery and I have since worked with literally thousands of women to help them heal their diseases.

The wisdom of this work teaches you to recover, refresh, and refine the innate knowledge of who you really are—not as healer or the healing—but as one who is healed. It is a question of remembering: unlocking and unfolding your ancient memory of being the healer, experiencing the healing, and being healed all at once. Each one of us emerges from a journey that touches the light and the lucidness of time and space. We carry this cosmic imprint of memory within us. Recovering these memories and the sadhana that keeps us remembering who we are is well within the scope of this book. The wisdom in this work comes through direct transmission from the Divine Mother—substantiated by my erudite Hindu forebears, the knowledge of the Vedas, and a wealth of informed experience.

By writing this book, I hope to share with you some of my knowledge so that you can embark on a path of discovery of how Inner Medicine can help you heal. Learning who you are as a sentient being, power packed with Shakti, you will see that healing is a natural and ongoing process, the simple feat of which will help you garner confidence in who you are—a woman on a powerful journey.

Throughout this book, you'll hear poignant stories of healing from women like you who want to stop hurting and recover their magnificent endowment and feminine history. You will also hear many trenchant stories of the attempts by medical science to erode and destroy the Mother Consciousness. For those of you who want to get back your personal truth and Shakti power, these accounts bear crucial significance to the understanding of who you are.

Within these pages, as you awaken to your Shakti energy you will discover your personal karma, truth, intuition, and self-purpose. The power to awaken these rudimentary internal energies will bring you closer to understanding the greater force of the Mother Consciousness.

Part One

WOMEN'S SHAKTI: PRIMORDIAL FEMININE POWER TO NOURISH, NURTURE & HEAL

Chapter One

THE JOURNEY OF SHAKTI: PRESERVING THE FEMININE

*Ultimately, we women are divinely equipped to rediscover the
Mother Consciousness by cooperating with one another and
applying our shared vision of harmony to shattering the harmful
rhythms that run counter to the maternally peaceful lifeways.*

HARMONIZING WITH NATURE

Health is more than the absence of disease; it is our individual undoing and continual unfolding as we strive to awaken the heart of consciousness. The ancient science of Ayurveda recognizes that we are held in the ever continuum energy of healing. It traces our most profound links with the whole cosmos and the influences of its greater energies to what is within us. According to the principles of Ayurveda, we exist in a state of ever-generating consciousness, and our health, well-being, relationships, and work are all shaped by how we respond to internal and external conditions. No one exists in isolation. In Ayurveda, the body, mind, and spirit are interconnected and this triad impacts everything we learn, think, and do. While conventional Western medicine treats a disease in relative isolation, Ayurveda examines the whole person and traces the roots of disorder to how we respond to life.

Ayurveda explains that each of us inherits a unique metabolic composition that shapes specific mental and physical characteristics, and emotional tendencies. The three principles called *doshas*—Vata, Pitta, and Kapha—blend together to determine our *prakriti*, or metabolic type. Understanding which foods, desires, and activities support or abate each dosha can help us to make appropriate choices that sustain our ongoing state of balance.

According to Ayurveda, an imbalance with the maternal energies of nature is the primary cause for disease. These internal energies can go out of kilter when we flow against our biorhythms, which are greatly influenced by Mother Nature and her daily and seasonal cycles. As you will see, there are certain times of the year when the body, mind, and psyche naturally become vulnerable—more so when we are not in sync with nature's cycles. For instance, disease can easily take hold in the body during one of the seasonal junctures when nature's elements become more erratic. Likewise, when a woman's cycle is out of balance with the appropriate phase of the moon, reproductive disorder is certain to follow. These powerful truths suggest that the preservation of good health is entirely within our grasp. We are formed from Nature's memories and rhythms. To reclaim health and healing, we must strive to find our connection to her elements, seasons, and rhythms. Ultimately, health is about the wisdom to cultivate our inner Shakti powers to heal through understanding nature's cycles and rhythms. As I wrote in my previous book *The Path of Practice*: We are wellness. We are consciousness. Disease is an imposter. This is the vision of Ayurveda in the Wise Earth tradition that I teach.

Wise Earth teachings restore grassroots wisdom of living in *sadhana*, the ancient bedrock of nature's seasons, cycles, rhythms, and sustenance from which Ayurveda sprung. These teachings say that nature's most potent medicine is *Inner Medicine*—simple everyday routines transformed into sacred rituals that awaken our intrinsic forces of healing within and without.

Health, harmony, joy, and longevity are intertwined with the energy of Shakti. As women, we have the power of Shakti not only to heal ourselves, but to nourish, nurture, and heal everything around us. Unfortunately, our modern lifestyles tend to pull us away from our true nature. In the overwhelmingly busy world we have created for ourselves, we strive for good health, peace, and prosperity, but these goals often elude us. We devalue the very source of what heals us—Mother Nature and her moon, sun, seasons, forests, sky, water, and food. Every day, in big and small ways, we each disregard the essence of our True Self. The state of our individual and collective well-being tells the whole story of the myths of medicine that we've perpetuated.

SONIA'S STORY

An annual report to Congress showed that health expenditures in America climbed 10 percent in 2005 to 1.9 trillion dollars. More than 90 percent of our senior citizens are on medication, with half of them taking three or more prescription drugs. Ten percent of women over the age of 18 take antidepressants, with the consumption of these dangerous drugs doubling every year. This grievous trend of our collective drug habit, cultivated over the last 50 years, has become the acceptable norm in society.

Take the example of Sonia. Two months ago, a woman in desperate need of assistance brought her teenage daughter, Sonia, to a Mother Om Mission (MOM) in New York. Sonia had recently attempted suicide by taking an overdose of her mother's sleeping pills. Three years prior, she was diagnosed with Attention Deficit Disorder (ADD) and her female doctor put her on heavy doses of Ritalin. Sonia's condition gradually worsened to the point where she was experiencing multiple symptoms of insomnia, rage, and depression, to the extent that she was forced to take a leave of absence from school. Her physician then put her on a popular anti-depressant drug. About a month after Sonia began taking the antidepressant, her mother noticed that she was retreating deeper into a funk. Six months later, her condition deteriorated to the point where she would lock herself in her room for days without eating or speaking. During this period, her mother called the physician several times and confided her fears for Sonia's well-being. She suggested that the drugs may be responsible for the deterioration of her daughter's health and that she thought she should be taken off of them. The doctor assured her that would be the worst thing to do and that Sonia was simply "going through a bad phase which most teenagers experience." One week after her mother's last desperate plea to the doctor, Sonia almost lost her life.

Not knowing where else to turn, Sonia's mother brought her to see me. MOM has been counseling Sonia since and has helped to wean her off all the medicines she had been taking. She is now on the mend and free from medications, back in school, and attending regular yoga classes. She also attends a teenage group counseling program at the local community center.

MEDICINE MAN

You might think that the rise of herbs, homeopathy, and alternative therapies indicates a positive change in our collective behavior, but ironically, the rapidly growing holistic health industry is also contributing to the obsessive dependency in our culture on prescription drugs. This industry is also doing its share of massive spending to broadcast and sell its products to the consumer. According to *World Health Statistics* (WHO) published in 2002, American consumers are spending more than 500 million dollars per year on herbal-based medicines and products. In fact, nearly one-third of Americans use herbs, and it is estimated that in the year 2002 alone 4.5 billion dollars were spent on herbal products in this country. Unfortunately, a recent study in the *New England Journal of Medicine* indicated that nearly 70 percent of individuals taking herbal medicines (the majority of which were well-educated and had higher than average incomes) were reluctant to reveal their use of complementary and alternative medicine to their doctors.

While this news may be seen as a quantum leap in consumer confidence in herbal products, few recognize that this reality speaks to a dependency on medicine and a desperate need to find the magic remedy outside of ourselves. Although we all agree that natural medicines are far less toxic in their effects on our body and mind than synthetic ones, in the long run it doesn't really matter if the pill we take every day comes from a synthetic derivative or a natural one.

The rapid rise of herbal sales is forcing herbal medicine producers to wreak the same kinds of havoc on the good earth and her creatures as conventional medical corporations have been doing for the last century. In the last decade, the demand for holistic health products has quadrupled. To meet the popular demand, prominent herbal manufacturers in America are now using mono-cropping to cultivate thousands of acres of once pristine lands. Because this method of farming ultimately deteriorates the life energy of the land and heralds a host of pest invasion and infestation, herbal manufacturers are using pesticides and fungicides to spray their crops. This begs the question, what is holistic about these products?

Whether they are natural or synthetic, medicines do not heal us. We do not heal from herbs, teas, pills, powders, pellets, tinctures, and patches. Healing arises from within. Thousands of years ago, the *rishis* knew that we were immersed in an ocean of remedial sound energy and vibration. Every day at the Wise Earth School, we prove that we can attune our rhythms to those of nature, the universe, the primordial sound wave, or to the Pure Consciousness.

In the final analysis, those of us who allow ourselves to become dependent on herbal medicines have not changed our thinking on health and healing. We are still addicted to the pill and the pill pusher, thinking they will help us to heal. Unless we shift our thinking, change our attitude, and step off the mythical medicine trail in hot pursuit of the illusive magic balm, mega corporations—both conventional and holistic—will continue to assume patent rights on our mind, body, and memory while we contribute to the demise of nature.

Each of us contributes to the hurtfulness and violence in our societies—whether by omission, oversight, ignorance, or direct commission. For instance, when we go to a grocery store or health food store to shop, we may purchase a nicely wrapped, sterilized package of meat for dinner. For most people, the thought that their dinner is coming from a dead animal never enters their minds, and it certainly doesn't matter that the poor animal was most likely subjected to unimaginable torture to fatten up its meat, and then painfully slaughtered without its consent. In the past 20 years numerous research studies conducted by credible animal rights organizations concluded that animal farming in America is one of the most egregious crimes, and yet it continues to go on unchecked. Unfortunately, the majority of people are not willing to shift their awareness or change their unwholesome habits even if they are aware that they may be perpetrating the collective hurt. In fact, when Oprah Winfrey broadcast some of the findings for Mad Cow Disease on her television talk show, she was sued by the major meat cartel—a modern day witch hunt.

MAD HUMAN DISEASE

Five thousand years after the peaceful Neolithic culture rooted in the sacred feminine was destroyed in Europe, women are still struggling every day with the imprint of the atrocious memory of violence, inequality, and fear. But 50 centuries later something significant has changed; the picture we see is no longer black and white, and no longer that of the male perpetrator versus the female victim. Our societal evolution has provided us with many more shades of violence against the spirit. Sadly, the desanctification of the maternal energies are no longer caused solely by the acts of men. Although it may not be as obvious as it was millennia ago when women healers in Europe were hunted down and burned at the stake by men, today's witch hunt is now perpetuated by both genders.

Both men and women are spurred on by greed, as was the case of the meat lobby afraid of losing commercial profits. In India, there are as many women genetic engineers and biochemists tampering with sacred life as men. Every day, more women are joining the forces behind the medical drug cartel in both the southern and northern hemispheres.

The quandary in which we find ourselves is less about patriarchal control or the violence against self and nature enabled by conventional sciences. It is about perpetuating the "mad human" disease to which we all contribute by recklessly squandering the feminine energies we all possess. To take back control of our health and stop these egregious crimes, we have got to reclaim the primordial feminine force. Only the Shakti power that creates the universe can move the mountains.

To reclaim the astounding reality where each and every one of us is already healed, we must take the appropriate steps to honor and preserve the maternal energy known as Mother Consciousness. This energy is being fractured every moment. This hurt reflects deep into the womb of the female of every species. Mother's womb of life exists far beyond the uterus of her female species; it is stretched to the forest, oceans, skies, and into the core of the earth itself.

Here's an example: the Brazilian congress has voted on a project that will reduce the Amazon rainforest to 50 percent of its size. Deep in these ancient forests, 60 percent of the plants used for cancer-fighting drugs may be found. Her basin provides one third of the world's freshwater and her prana-rich air supplies a quarter of the oxygen the planet needs to breathe. At present, almost 100,000 square miles of the rainforest that had been deforested for the purpose of agriculture and livestock farming are now abandoned and will be savagely transformed into a vast wasteland. The raping of the land in the underdeveloped countries of Asia and Africa for commercial agriculture and animal farming has been ongoing for nearly a century. Moreover, through genetic engineering and patents more land, rivers, oceans, and atmosphere are being eroded and polluted.

Even though we know the devastating effects of these actions, the First World countries, and in particular, America, continues to ravage Mother Earth by moving from one Third World country to another, consuming and destroying the potent energy of the earth's Shakti. As Carolyn Merchant points out in her book *The Death of Nature*, this transformation of nature from a living, nurturing mother to an inert, dead place where its essential nature is manipulated, was eminently suited to the exploitation necessary for capitalism.

A stark example of this is the biotech company Gen Pharm, which produced and owned the world's first transgenic dairy bull named Herman. While still an embryo, Herman was bioengineered by company scientists to carry a human gene for producing milk with a human protein to make infant formula. In defending the safety of the unsavory formula, Gen Pharm's CEO, Jonathan McQuitty said, "Human milk is the gold standard, and formula companies have added more and more (human elements) over the past 20 years." Vandana Shiva, world-renowned physicist and ecologist, sums it up this way, "From this perspective cows, women, and children are merely instruments for commodity production and pro-fit maximization."

Of course, bioengineered milk could never replace the sacred maternal memory intrinsic to mother's milk. Regardless of how far science goes in deprecating the Mother Consciousness, the maternal energy is powerful and especially imbued in women. Science may succeed in the sacrilegious destruction of the female and her reproduction on Planet Earth but the Mother Presence, which is the infinite, time-less maternal energy of Shakti, will always guard the birth, life, and death of the world. Although Mother sustains massive attacks, she will never die.

REPRODUCTIVE POWER

For thousands of years in ancient India, Asia, Africa, Egypt, Greece, and Rome, societies built their spiritual beliefs around the Goddess Tradition. As a result, these civilizations maintained a harmonious existence with each other. Her leg-ends were a repository of human experience and wisdom. This archetypal knowl-edge facilitated a shared sense of communal spirit and a gentle relation between the sexes. It established the indigenous systems of knowledge that were largely eco-logical. Miraculously, this knowledge is still available to us through the Vedas.

This is in direct contrast to the present model of scientific knowledge, which is largely characterized by fragmentation and reductionism. New reproductive tech-nologies like induction, planned C-sections, and epidurals view a woman's body as a container and the fetus as created by the man's seed, thereby severing the sacred link between a mother and her fetus. Vandana Shiva poignantly describes the present state of medical technology's takeover of women's reproductive rights, "Medical specialists, falsely believing that they produce and create babies, force their knowledge on knowing mothers. They treat their own knowledge as infal-lible, and women's knowledge as wild hysteria."

The female of every species is endowed with Shakti's reproductive power. Creatures possess the innate right to life given to them by the divine Mother

Consciousness. This inherent energy of Shakti gives only the female creatures the power to create babies. The womb, embryo, fetus, and eggs of humans and animals are sacred. Both animal and human babies assume the resemblance of their parents and bear the same vulnerabilities. The child, colt, calf, or mouse all instinctively know who their mother is, and have the maternal memory to cuddle up, nurse, and be nourished and protected by her.

For some time, conservationists and anthropologists have studied maternal behaviors that are instinctive to each creature. A study from the early 60s focused on a baby Rhesus monkey abandoned by its mother shortly after birth. Researchers placed the baby monkey in a room with two "mothers." One of the surrogate mothers was made of wire and had no distinguishing features of a mother except that it had a bottle attached to it containing milk. The second wire mother had a soft blanket and a "face" on it. Over a 24-hour period of time, the baby stayed on the soft mother the majority of the time—even though it had no food to offer. Instinctually, the baby monkey was drawn to the surrogate that could provide the tenderness it associated with a mother.

The cosmic role of the mother in producing and sustaining life must be honored as most sacred if we are to maintain human intelligence. It should never deign to become the property of science, commerce, and technology. A striking similarity exists in the way medical technocrats, scientists, and their allied lobbies approach women's reproduction and the life force rights of animals.

In a recent issue, the *Los Angeles Business Journal* describes what happens to the once-living embryos of mice used in stem cell research. Nearly all embryonic stem cell lines, and all the ones approved for federal funding, are grown in what is basically a mush of crushed mouse embryos that provide an assortment of nutrients and growth factors that are able to keep human embryonic stem cells from differentiating. The mere violence and grotesqueness of this action against the female embryo is unimaginable, no less so than the unspeakable horror the little creatures must feel before their brutal deaths. The growing plague of violence enacted against the maternal organs—womb, embryo, fetus, umbilical cord, and breasts—of the female reinforce the continued and unrelenting erosion of the archetypal mother and her maternal instinct.

ANIMAL MAGIC

Accepting that creatures big and small share the intrinsic right to live their lives to fruition and to enjoy their time on the planet is the primordial first step to recovering your Mother Consciousness. As my spiritual teacher His Holiness Swami Dayananda Saraswati once told me, 'to experience compassion is to know that the maternal wellspring within you is about to mature.' In my meditations, I have witnessed the pain and humiliation of the animals and their great suffering at the hands of the humans.

Here, in the beautiful Pisgah Mountains where I live, the field mice love to take shelter in the monastery. The *sadhakas* (spiritual aspirants) at the monastery devised a tiny box house with a trap door that lures mice in and keeps them safe inside the box until they can be returned to the forest. The first time they used it they caught one mouse. But after that not a single mouse was ever caught in it again, regardless of the dollops of fresh organic peanut butter they put in it each night to entice them in. So they decided to use a commercial, allegedly humane, glue trap to catch the mice. They quickly succeeded in catching a mouse before realizing the glue pad held the feet of the mouse so securely that it was very difficult to release the poor creature. Frustrated by the situation, they summoned my help. Knowing that the mouse would be terrified for his life, I brought over some herbal medicated sesame oil that we generally use for Shirovasti, the Ayurvedic therapy used on the head to reduce mental stress and anxiety.

As we do prior to any treatment, we chanted the fear-relieving mantra for the mouse as I proceeded to pour the oil over his little head. He was so scared, his little body shivered with anxiety. Completely drenched in oil, he glared at me through his big, awesome eyes. After he was oelated, the mouse was instantly released from the pad. To our surprise, he didn't race for the forest. Instead, he stepped off the glue, shook his body vigorously to get the oil off, took a leisurely look around as if he was scolding us, and then scooted into the forest.

I wondered what the family of mice that lived in the forest thought of this little creature returning home all drenched in oil. Did the mother mouse rush to console him, or was she amused by his unsightly appearance? Was the family embarrassed for his humiliation and did they give him the space to recover his self-dignity? The sadhakas never again use such a punishing trap. (However, I'm sure they would never be able to catch another mouse on a glue trap regardless of how much peanut butter they placed on the pad!)

For years, I have chanted and "ooomed" with the cows, meditated with and taught yoga to the deer in the forest, and spent much time closely observing animals. I realized that within a split second of his devastating experience the little mouse took to spreading the news to his clan. He probably projected his distinct vibration for many square miles around him, without uttering a single sound. The animals can do this through their heightened power of vibrational language skills by using their species' mind to broadcast their stories through nature's inaudible vibrational network.

I am confident that animals possess many deeply instinctive skills that far outweigh human dexterity in communication. Great and small, each and every creature, including microorganisms, are wired with a definitive model of maternal memory to respond to life in ways that maintain and support the universe's state of equanimity. Instead of brutalizing, hurting, punishing, and humiliating the animals, we need to protect them. By observing them in their natural habitat we may learn how to retune our maternal energy. This is one way we can be certain to regain the memory of the Mother Consciousness.

The behavior of the elephants in Thailand during the tsunami in Southeast Asia gives more examples of the amazing sensitivity of animals. On the day the waves hit, the agitated elephants at the camp ride in Khao Lak, Thailand, had been bellowing and screaming since daybreak—the approximate time the earthquake that caused the tsunami cracked open the sea bed off Indonesia's Sumatra Island. While tourists were astounded at the strange rapid processions of local birds in flight, the elephants broke loose from their chains and charged for high ground. The elephant handlers (*mahouts*) and tourists at the camp ride intuitively followed the departing pachyderms up the hill to safety. After the rush of waves subsided, the elephants were led downhill to help clear wreckage and dig for bodies among the massive debris. (In contrast to their magnificent strength and size, these pachyderms possess the subtlest of senses. With their supple trunks, they can find and retrieve a pin from a haystack.) Their poignant sense of smell helped them to sniff out and recover human remains trapped in the tsunami shards.

Elephants are nomadic, social animals that clan together and are regulated by fixed laws. A herd is usually led by the oldest cow (a female elephant); elephants have a matriarchal society consisting of mother and her offspring along with her grand-calves. It is common knowledge among the mahouts that elephants have a highly developed maternal instinct, and use this ability to communicate with each other especially during times of massive disaster or clan crisis. Time after time, they demonstrate their powerful sense of the Mother Consciousness. Elephant cows act as "midwives" assisting one another in the birth of their young and performing many duties that relieve the mother of stressful, mundane tasks. The calves are kept in kindergarten groups, which are safeguarded by different aunts and crones while others feed. They will form a protected circle around young when danger approaches.

The elephant cow intrinsically knows that to heal another, we must heal the society. Recognizing that healing is a pervasive energy that comes from the Mother Consciousness, we are pressed into safeguarding the maternal energy in all forms of life—especially in women and the animals where this force is the most vulnerable. We will not recover the innate sense of freedom and joy that are the content of our own healing if we continue to perpetrate the horrendous perishing and suffering of the mother force.

Ultimately, we women are divinely equipped to rediscover the Mother Consciousness by cooperating with one another and applying our shared vision of harmony to shattering the harmful rhythms that run counter to the maternally peaceful *lifeways*. We may regain this luminous way of being by learning how to

listen to our inner rhythm and trusting the Shakti to reclaim our feminine power
to nourish, nurture, and heal. We stand a better chance of this happening when we
recognize that residing within us is a plethora of inner resources for healing.

THE SOURCE OF HEALING

At the age of 21, Margaret was going through her first heartbreak from losing her
boyfriend to her best friend. Her mother brought her to a meditation program at
the school thinking it would help Margaret get over the sense of deep hurt and
betrayal she was feeling. Vibrant and redheaded, Margaret had all the signs of
her fire being aggravated, or what we call a Pitta condition. When she arrived her
eyes were bloodshot and her face had broken out with a bad rash. The first words
that sputtered out of her mouth like spitting fire were, "I'm so heartbroken, I don't
want to talk." So I gave her a long cooling hug and assured her that she could be
silent for as long as she needed. The next day directly after meditation, Margaret
rushed in to see me. She was stung on her little finger by a "Yellow Jacket" wasp
while taking a walk in the fields and was obviously in pain. Weeping and bewil-
dered, she kept asking, "Why me? Am I not suffering enough?" I quickly drew
the sting from her finger and rubbed it with some walnut salve I had on hand to
draw out any remaining poison. After the treatment she gave a thunderous sigh. It
was obviously not the appropriate time to explain to Margaret that Mother Nature
had just given her an acupuncture session for free. The emissary wasp had stung
her on the tip of the little finger of the right hand. According to Ayurveda's *Marma*
principle, this was the precise meridian point that would send the most energy to
the left ventricle of her heart. Evidently this was the area of the heart that was in
physical need of stimulation.

Sometimes maternal love hurts, but Mother always serves us faithfully by
knowing how and when to intervene in our healing process. The following day
after meditation practice, everyone present was shocked at how rapidly Margaret
had rediscovered her sense of lightness and joy. The greatest medicine is within
us. We should not underestimate this.

MEMORY LANGUAGE

Aditi, Hindu Goddess of Creation, fed the gods her milk and taught them the
healing secret that is carried in the seed-memory of plants, herbs, and minerals.
In turn, the gods passed down this wisdom to the Ayurvedic seers. From the days
of yore, the healing efforts that upheld life came from the feminine. She restored
joy and health to the body with her herbs, teas, ointments, poultices, foods, and

rituals. The relationship between food and medicine to the body is that we eat in order to be in dynamic exchange of memory, energy, and information with the cosmos. Foods, grains, seeds, herbs, powders, and teas can all be nature's Inner Medicine when we know how they interact and work to evoke certain dynamic and predictable responses within body and mind. When knowledgeably used, the essences of nature's foods trigger the like element within our vital tissues to spur their memories into responding.

Each tissue layer carries its own significant memory of both its cosmic and practical functions. Once this memory is awakened, the tissue itself remembers what to do and how to do it to keep the body healthy. Disease is simply a matter of forgetfulness. When the tissue memory is kept in good order, the tissue continues to thrive with its self-generating energy keeping its functional memory vibrant. The rishis were impeccable in their wisdom. They recognized the link between memory, energy, and healing. Moreover, they knew which herb spoke to which tissue, and how long the required conversation, the depth of the sound, the subtlety of the rhythm, and the necessary timing for applying nature's remedy to the appropriate condition. The remedies are intended to prod the tissue memory so that within a determined length of time (depending on the condition), the tissue will be revitalized. As a result, the self-generating intelligence within the tissue memory will take over the healing process to rectify its symptoms, and reset its internal harmonic rhythm. The remedy, then, will have served its purpose. By this means, no medicine should be taken for long periods of time.

Loss of vital tissue memory is the fundamental cause of disease. Therefore, to reclaim good health we must first repair tissue memory, whose health is controlled by the Mother Consciousness. To achieve this, we will need to remain alert to our internal conditioning, and the conditions around us. Modern living has turned the fluid, wisdom-generating Mother Consciousness into static, inflexible, and stabilized matter. However, we can unlearn these unnatural and mundane habits and remedy the harmful vibrations and sense of isolation we have created within and without. By delving into guided self-inquiry, and acquiring the necessary knowledge of the unique karmas that shape each and every one of our lives, we may regain significant memory and eradicate disease.

The Vedas provide us with numerous practices to invite, focus, and direct the profound remedial energies to come to the fore. For example, through *mantra* (incantation of sacred sounds), *mudra* (sacred hand gestures), *yantra* (sacred mandalas and drawings of energy), *dhyana* (meditation), the ritual practice of yoga, and *prayogas* (sacred ceremonies) we may prompt explicit healing energy to aid specific conditions. We will explore many of these practices within the context of feminine spiritual aims and healing requirements as we journey together in this Shakti river. Each year, I witness hundreds of women reclaiming their Inner Medicine potential. Because it is apparently hidden from the senses of sight, smell, taste, touch, and sound, it makes it easier for us to overlook the evident. This calls for a drastic change in our core understanding—the perception of who we are and how we are configured.

Imagine a vast macrocosmic network of invisible, immutable wiring that transmits charges, signals, energies, and vibrations through the microcosmic body, all of which is held in a translucent, omnipotent gel of cosmic memory empowered by the Shakti. This is the anatomy of the Mother Consciousness. Human birth has endowed each one of us with the most complex intelligence and the greatest capacity for compassion of any species. This is who we are.

Figure 1.1 Cosmic Sound

Chapter Two

THE DIVINE AUTHORITY OF WOMEN

If we are to gain the Mother Consciousness,
the love for the One must include love for all;
prosperity for all must precede prosperity
for one's self. Health for all must occur first
before health for one's self can be accomplished.
Poverty in the world must be eliminated before
we can personally harvest true abundance.
Peace for the self must be peace for all.

Karma holds the golden key to healing. Healing comes directly from continual cleansing and ridding of karma. Healing also comes through wisdom—the process of awakening *buddhi*, the higher mind that holds the power of intuition, compassion, and resolve. This invaluable intuition is created from memory that spans the depths of the evolutionary universe. As you will learn in later pages, the buddhi cannot be invoked by mere mental or physical activity. As we traverse this feminine path of Shakti together, we will explore the exposition of buddhi and the living art of sadhana as one of the viable pathways to awakening your intuitive awareness. Before we explore the vast field of intuition and memory, however, let us examine our life of karma.

KARMA HOLDS THE GOLDEN KEY

Life's sacred journey is one of continual healing, the ever-flowing wellspring of energy, ideas, creativity and fulfillment, joy, and love wherein we seek completion through both the individual and collective consciousness. We begin this journey by healing into life and end each cycle by healing into death. While in the act of living, we spin karmas—actions we perform from our free will. According to the Vedas, all of our actions bear consequences; through them, we accrue merits and/or demerits in our lives. When our karmas are aligned with the universal *dharma*—truth—we may sustain a life of balance.

Indeed, each one of us possesses a chain of karma that stretches to the profound extremities of the brink of the universe's first dawn. Unique to your karma is the entirety of your irrefutable experiences in consciousness. Generally, your karma may explain why one person might be attracted by archetypal images, people, and situations while another is repelled by them.

Most people revolve the same karma, life after life, confronting the same lessons, challenges, ambitions, desires, likes, and dislikes over and over again. This is because they do not understand that each life's sojourn is intended for the development of awareness—and in so doing to cleanse, transform, and evolve their particular largess of karma. Circumstances, environments, and the people you intimately interact with may differ from life to life, but the lesson of the karmas can remain largely unchanged when we do not recognize them. The purpose of each life is to learn the lesson of our individual karma, and to understand and assimilate these lessons. By this means, we may eradicate the lessons we have clearly learned, and thus put them to rest permanently. We can do this by the practice of Japa Meditation (See *The Practice: The Art of Taking Pause* on page 26) which involves "catching" the repetitive karmas, holding them in a kind space, and recognizing that when the time is right, the divine energy will show you the core cause for their reoccurrence.

WE CANNOT ESCAPE OUR KARMA

Thirty-five-year old Maria blamed her mother for everything that went wrong with her life. So she traveled thousands of miles from her home in San Diego to an ashram in India. There she met Jaya, a female disciple who had been living at the ashram for many years. They quickly grew close, but as the relationship grew Maria realized that she was responding to Jaya in the same defensive way she responded to her mother. Not surprisingly, their friendship quickly became contentious and strained. A month later, Maria was asked to leave the ashram because of the tension between her and Jaya. Maria called me as soon as she returned home to confide her grief. Listening to her, I realized she had superimposed her grief with her mother onto her association with Jaya. In fact, she told me that Jaya resembled her mother and "had the same annoying manner about her." She had tried to escape the difficulties she was having with her mother, only to seek out the same affiliation with someone who was symbolic of her mother. We cannot escape our karma.

To break the old habitual karmic pattern, I taught Jaya a significant meditative practice of taking pause (mentioned above). At first she struggled with her emotions and could not sit still for more than a few minutes at a time, but after a year of practice, she has developed a deeper insight of her karmas and together they are consciously fostering a new relationship built on love, kindness, and respect for each other.

THE KARMIC BANK

Consciousness involves emotional, intellectual, and spiritual growth and development. We cannot grow in the Mother Consciousness if we keep spinning the same web of karma many lifetimes over. Ultimately, we heal when we apply our precious life's journey to cleansing and wrapping up personal karmas. According to the Vedas, we accrue karmic merits and demerits in accord with our deeds and actions in each life. These scores are maintained in an individual cosmic account called *sanchitakarma*. This system may be likened to a sort of interest-bearing bank account. Positive actions bear merits. Conversely, negative actions carry demerits. However, unlike the bank account where the bigger the balance the happier you feel, you would strive to bring the balance to zero in your personal sanchitakarma account. Zero balance means that you have finished all your karmas and therefore have no more *samskaras*, imprints remaining in the soul to propagate rebirth. Look at it this way—the ultimate purpose of life is to gain pure consciousness in order to attain self-realization. But we cannot accomplish this goal without having a physical vehicle, a body through which we may express, use, and finally exhaust our individual set of karmas. According to the rishis, the physical human body is the perfect vehicle in which to live and learn life's vital lessons. As a result, you can eliminate your individual karmas while you cultivate the essential wisdom we call self-knowledge. Once this knowledge is attained you have no further need to effectuate a physical body through rebirth. Indeed, with the expenditure of all individual karmas, the body cannot subsist because all of the imprints remaining in the soul are washed away.

THE COURAGE TO PAUSE

Through incorporating a simple meditative practice into your daily routine, you can learn how to witness your thoughts and actions rather than perpetuating them. This will help you to stay present with yourself and provide ample inner space and serenity to resolve conflicts that can perpetuate karma.

Taking a 20-minute pause daily can help you to assimilate the events of each day. It takes courage to do nothing. With practice in the art of pausing, you will learn to skillfully do nothing, the best antidote for fear, anger, and other debilitating emotions. Staying present in the continuum of thought, action, and karma will reveal your karmas and transform your response to challenges. In so doing, you may learn the nature of your own karma.

Each one of us is conditioned to respond to specific situations in a certain way because of our karmas. This practice will aid you to become an objective observer of your thought process, especially when it is disturbed. As you trace thoughts and activities to your unique set of karmas, you will be able to exercise better judgment and control in situations and circumstances you may face.

When we take this critical pause in our daily lives we can avoid the more difficult times. By this means you may become conscious of your karmas and avoid more challenging "pauses," such as the difficulties we may experience while in menopause. Reclaiming the art of taking pause will help you rid many challenges and difficulties that may accompany what are meant to be natural changes in your life. It can help you avoid adding to false perceptions in your life such as, "it's someone else's fault," or, "disease and pain are inevitable as long as we live." Disorders result from being out of sync with yourselves and not knowing your karmas.

After sharing this practice with numerous women, they reported feeling lightness, courage, clarity, confidence, and even improved memory. This practice will help you build the necessary trust in the divine Mother Consciousness. You are asked to leave all concerns in the care of the buddhi while in the meditation.

THE PRACTICE: THE ART OF TAKING PAUSE

This practice is best performed in the evening before you go to bed and while facing the direction of the sun.

- Sit in a comfortable, quiet, and uncluttered space in your home.
- Allow the mind to settle.
- Listen to your thoughts. When a fearful, anxious, agitated, or otherwise troublesome thought arises, do not engage it. Simply step back from the thought and watch it.
- Become the witness observing the thought, or thoughts. Let the thoughts flow. If you find yourself fidgeting, or responding to the thoughts by recalling the incident from which they arose, recognize that you are intruding in the free-flowing process of being a pure witness. Distance yourself again from the thoughts. They will reoccur.
- As the thoughts flow, repeat the following affirmation (or some variation) silently.

> *Let me see the karma behind my thought. Unfold this karma in its*
> *own time so that I may understand my actions and why they create*
> *distress. Show me the resolve for this karma.*

- After you are done with the affirmation, sit for a few minutes longer, but do not try to recall your thoughts or concerns that arose during the meditation. Be aware that by expressing your intention, it will be held in a safe space within the Mother Consciousness. Trust that any conflict will show itself in the way of truth, and that your intention would be fulfilled.
- Retire for the evening and do nothing else.

SEVEN KEYS TO GETTING RID OF OLD KARMA

To remember the art of the natural pause and mindfully integrate it into your daily routine, you may choose to memorize the wisdom laws of karma as I see them, which I have set out below:

- Simplicity has the greatest power for healing.
- Everything you do must be an act of inner *puja*, sacred rites and rituals offered to the Mother Consciousness within you.
- Karma is swift with its joyful rewards when you live to safeguard the cosmic truth.
- Keep the center of your living space clean and open. Cuddle yourself and family in the hearth of your home.
- Home is a metaphor for Mother Nature. The living space is your Tree of Life.
- Honor the cycles of the moon to protect your womanly reproductive karma.
- Bowls and drums are symbolic of the divine womb. Play the drum to heal the food. Eat from a bowl and heal the womb.

ANATOMY OF FEAR

The most prevalent negative emotion of our time? Fear. The increase of fear karma within our present environment speaks to the rapid rate of deterioration in the greater energy field that supports life.

You may not even be aware that you are harboring energies that can hurt and devastate your life. Yet our mental and emotional space can unwittingly be held hostage by these negative emotions and you cannot take too lightly the power that these destructive energies may have in undermining your life force, health, and creative abilities.

There is a dark, insidious cloud of helplessness that is masking our joy, evidenced by the growing number of suicides, mass suicide pacts, and profound levels of depression experienced by significant numbers of people the world over. Women all over the globe are taking more medicines for debilitating depression and to reduce factors leading to cancers and heart disease than ever before—obvious symptoms of a dangerous and mounting tendency toward despair and alienation. I believe this dangerous trend is based on the heightened atmosphere of fear, caused by the internal and external harm inflicted on the Mother Consciousness. Anxiety, stress, depression, obsession, and lethargy are some of the many faces of the fear anatomy. These emotions are rooted in the psyche of women and children who tend to respond to these vibrations more profoundly than men. Fear, like all emotions, operates through the cosmos' subtle network of energy and vibration carried within the subtlest level of our existence.

Let's explore how fear actually works to perpetuate itself in our psychic anatomy. Considered the core vulnerability of all species, particularly in humans, the fear emotion is richly elucidated by the rishis who provided us extensive information on the cosmic anatomy. They explained the various command centers for emotional responses located within the brain; what we call the "emotional brain" is described by the seers as the finer workings associated with the fourth, fifth, and sixth chakras (psychic centers of consciousness within the body). These three chakras relate to the function of the mid-brain.

FEAR FACTOR

As we will see later on, fear comes from the erosion of our heightened awareness that is interconnected by an ancient circuitry of more than 70,000 *nadis*, or energy conduits in the body. Recently, a *Newsweek* article called "Anxiety and Your Brain," reported on some recent research on rats. Scientists surgically dissected and removed parts of the animal's brain in the quest to locate the structure responsible for fear conditioning. They discovered that the amygdala—a small, almond-shaped structure that lies near the center of the brain and that is intricately connected to other regions of the brain through a network of nerve fibers— acts as the brain's fear command center. Once the amygdala perceives a threat, it can trigger a body-wide emergency response within milliseconds. Through a process called fear conditioning, one can readily perceive an ordinary stimulus as a warning sign. A rat was exposed to a distinctive sound and then administered a shock. After a few repetitions, the sound alone would produce a paralyzing effect on the rodent. Lacking an amygdala, however, the rodent would not freeze at the sound of a tone.

On a physiological level, prompted by impulses from the amygdala, the hypothalamus produces a hormone called corticotrophin releasing factor (CRP). This signals the pituitary and adrenal glands to flood the bloodstream with epinephrine, norepinephrine, and cortisol, or what we call stress hormones.

At the brain level, the thalamus receives information from direct sensory perceptions and posts it to the amygdala, which elicits the body's instinctive defensive responses—attack, defend, avoid, submit, or escape—thereby placing the organism on high alert. In turn, the hippocampus accesses the threat by drawing memory information from previous experiences. The sensory cortex, located in the rear of the upper hemisphere of the brain, discerns the threat to distinguish genuine danger from a false alarm. If the threat is inconsequential, the entire brain response is reset by the prefrontal cortex, which suppresses the amygdala response. So, we can see from the scientific viewpoint how the brain responds to the memory of fear.

But this isn't the only point of view. I like to look at the workings of the brain from the Vedic perspective. In my ongoing work on cosmic memory, I explain the process in the following way: memory, impulse, and ego functions are stored in the *ahamkara*, which, according to Vedic anatomy, is located at the base of brain. Receiving the impulses of a threat, ahamkara sounds an urgent message throughout the memory-based organism. The ahamkara is sustained by *prana*, the kinetic life force of the universe that affects our memory function when impaired. As a result, the aggravated prana sends a fright signal throughout the organism causing the production of abundant supply of *ojas* (immunological buffer) in the body. Then ample glucose is released into the bloodstream to counteract the debilitating shortage of prana. At such times, the heart begins pumping erratically while muscles tense and body temperature drops. In short, the body's routine immunological functions temporarily shut down and direct their instincts to combating or escaping the threat. The entire sequence of response triggered by the amygdala to its closure in the prefrontal cortex depends on ahamkara to provide stored memory to guide the entire chain of operation. Ultimately, the resolve of fight or flight response occurs in the buddhi, which controls the activity of the cerebral cortex, as you will see.

While the fear response is necessary for the organism to gather and safeguard itself in times of potential or grave danger, a constant barrage of low impact adrenaline surges, as well as overstimulation of the subtle nerve circuitry within ahamkara, can cause a severe erosion of memory. Loss of memory triggers increased susceptibility in our fear response to perceived danger. Moreover, it creates a great sense of internal confusion and trepidation since we are subconsciously aware that our protective response shield had been damaged. Simply put, the more memory we lose, the more vulnerable we become.

Once an emotion saturates the network, it impacts the collective mind, and often-dominant emotions and perceptions have a tenacious grip on the mind. Propelled by the vibratory force, entire masses of the population can begin to think and sound alike. Have you ever wondered why politicians, socio-religious leaders, or cult leaders can influence vast numbers of people with ideologies that to the clear-minded person are irrational and destructive? Never underestimate the force of vibration.

MANY FACES OF FEAR

As women whose inherent karma upholds the most active maternal force, we are profoundly impacted by fear, the most powerful collective emotion of our time.

For this reason, the entire world has been in an inadvertent state of anxiety and mourning from the horrific events that we hear about: the tsunami in Indonesia; the World Trade Center attack; and the wars in Iraq. But lesser-known events also have a subtle yet significant impact on our psyches. For example, the 1994 genocide of the Tutsi people in Sudan where the Hutu-led Rwandan government massacred between 800,000 and 1.1 million people, or the floods in Guyana, South America that incapacitated the whole country leaving more than 400,000 people homeless and at risk of critical diseases. And we can't disregard the ongoing disharmony in our communities caused by abuse, violence, terrorism, harshness, and unkindness. As a result of the mounting aggression within our internal and external worlds, fear globules, which I can visibly detect around those who are experiencing fear, have been dominantly saturating the global environment of the mind. In short, primal fear is literally in the air.

The fear emotion assumes different guises as it interacts with each element; vulnerability in the earth element creates physical instability with a sense of uncertainty and lack of confidence in the Self. At its extreme, it accounts for lethargy, depression, and deep attachment. In the water element, fear generates and reinforces a sense of greediness and deprivation of food, family ties, and material wealth. It also accounts for maternal suffering and the depletion of the maternal energy and instinct such as the grave difficulties young women face bringing their first-born child safely into the world. In the fire element, fear manifests as emotional and mental instability, anxiety, anger, volatility, and aggressiveness. At its heightened state, it may also produce a sense of ruthlessness, extreme obsessiveness, and distrust of others. Fear processed through the air element patents itself as indecisiveness, isolation, and loneliness. Acute impairment of this element produces paranoia and some forms of phobia. Vulnerability in the space element attracts fear in the form of severe mental and emotional disorders such as bipolar depression, multiple personality syndrome, extreme phobias, and homicidal or suicidal tendencies. Thankfully, positive emotions and thoughts are also promoted by the vibratory network, which we will discuss later on.

PROTECTION FROM FEAR KARMA

The current time of fear domination was known to the Vedic seers as a critical period on earth called *Kali Yuga*. To prepare, they provided humanity with an elaborate record of sadhana, Inner Medicine healing practices, to help strengthen both the personal and cosmic anatomy. Sadhana practice goes far beyond the reach of its actual physical components of rites, ceremonies, prayers, mantras, meditation, and yoga. Practicing sadhana is a profound way of connecting the Self and every living being to the Mother Consciousness so that we may acquire wisdom. Following is a universal affirmation you may continually use to foster energy of peacefulness and maternal awareness:

> Within each one of us, we are One
> Altogether we are One
> Without each other, we are One.

If we are to gain the Mother Consciousness, the love for the One must include love for all; prosperity for all must precede prosperity for one's self. Health for all must occur before health for one's self can be accomplished. Poverty in the world must be eliminated before we can personally harvest true abundance. Peace for the self must be peace for all. In exploring inner harmony through the timeless pathways set out in this book you may "reach" the One within and begin to recognize the natural resonant rhythm of your psyche. Recognizing that each one of us is the cosmic vessel of the Mother Consciousness, we may see ourselves in every living being, indeed, in every grain of sand.

CONQUERING FEAR

As emissaries of the Mother Consciousness, women have the power to dissolve fear both collectively and individually to regain a sense of freedom, harmony, and security. We may lead the way in recovering the fundamental principles and practices necessary for the support and stability of all beings, beginning with reclaiming a life of non-hurting. We must change our individual relationship to violence before we can eliminate fear from our universe. For this, we must start to restore the Mother Consciousness to her full creative resplendence. By emulating the Supreme Goddess Lalita and doing the Inner Medicine work that will rid universal fear, we may once more reclaim our essential state of fearlessness, courage, and joy.

RECLAIMING A LIFE OF NON-HURTING

The emotions of pain and hurt are felt by every creature. Judging by the billion or more untimely deaths in the world every day—including the lives of the animals and other species we drive into extinction—we are forced to consider the collective reality of violence and hurtfulness we share. Violence breeds fear. Through habitual response we have been conditioned to contribute to the effect of hurtfulness, harm, damage, and injury in our personal lives, families, and communities. We need to learn that obstacles and challenges may always prevail in our lives, but we do not have to hurt.

Caroline, a 31-year old yoga instructor, had been diagnosed with breast cancer. Her oncologist had advised her that her tumor was not responding well to the radiation therapy. When I met her, she was emotionally desperate. She told me that she had been shadowed by painful family memories as long as she could remember: at the delicate age of 20, her paternal uncle had accidentally shot her grandfather during a deer-hunting trip. This single inadvertent yet fatal act had haunted her family for generations. Then at 16, she lost her father to liver cancer, and Caroline grew up witnessing her mother's arduous struggles to support her family.

Two months later, Caroline's tumor had shrunk to more than half of its original size—the first time since the onset of her treatment that there was any noticeable change. Caroline wrote to me:

> Directly after leaving the Ancestors' Conference, I sensed that a great load had been lifted from my psyche. I felt lighthearted and clear minded for the first time in my life as you guided me with the Vedic ancestral food offering to my father and paternal ancestors. Somehow, I was able to put the memory of my father's agony into clear perspective and trace the roots of my illness and misery to the shooting incident...I have no doubt that the shrinking of my tumor was directly connected to the healing ancestral experience I allowed at the conference.

The bottom line is that we can't feel peace of mind until we eradicate the mentality of violence. For this we have got to stop the killing. It is said in the *Chandogya Upanishad*, "A person is what her desire is. It is our deepest desire in this life that shapes the life to come." So let us direct our deepest desires to change the habit of violence into one of peace. Once we learn new habits, we can control how we respond to hurtful situations and people. By letting the heart speak to the mind (as you will learn in the practices of Pranava Upasana and Bhramari Breath & Sound Meditation in Chapter Three) you can renegotiate the most injurious of situations and respond in a way that keeps you and others from getting hurt. To accomplish this, we have to change our responses to aggression, hurt, harmfulness, pain, and anger.

To alleviate fear and anxiety try doing these simple practices at the end of your day: avoid feeding your imagination with angry, violent, scary, or untoward images. Sit for about 20 minutes and collect yourself at the end of each day. Remove the television, DVD, and so on from your bedroom. The room you sleep in needs to be calm, full of sweetness and comfort. A small altar with a bell, *dipa*, or bees wax candle and gentle music adds the element of tranquility to your space of reprieve and rest. You may do a brief self massage of your scalp and soles of feet with *brahmi* or *bhringaraja* oil. If fear or anxiety persists, take the mild remedy described on the following page about an hour or so before bedtime.

CALMING TEA

Combine the powders in warm milk and drink.

1/2 cup almond milk
1/2 teaspoon jatamansi powder
1/4 teaspoon brahmi powder
1/8 teaspoon nutmeg powder
1/8 teaspoon licorice powder (optional)

TRANSFORMING VIOLENCE INTO COMPASSION

To live a life of non-hurtfulness, we have to cultivate the discipline of living in non-violent, non-aggressive ways. For example, yesterday I found myself stifling back an irritated response to an apprentice who I felt was being aggressive and unreasonable with her demands toward an instructor at the school. Immediately, I retreated from the situation and entered my inner silence to help reconcile my response and transform it into compassion.

Every day, we have to choose not to contribute to the toxicity that permeates our mental and physical environment. The biggest injury comes from our own personal habits of harboring unconscious anger and disregard for self and the feelings of others. I teach my students and disciples to stay present in themselves at all times and to recognize when they are trespassing the law of kindness. I remind them that the most heroic thing they can do is to find the strength to meet their challenges and grow from them.

So how do we do this? To stop the violence you have to start from within. We have to make the commitment to inner tranquility our first priority. When you strive to cultivate inner harmony you will find peace everywhere; this is the most profound way we can effectively rid the horrific toxicity of violence that surrounds us. We might even be able to shift the unspeakable violence that occurs right here in the underbelly of our culture into a space of healing.

We must strive to create the simplest possible ways to live and let live. Mahatma Gandhi puts it beautifully, "live simply so that others may simply live." In remaining ever present with your thoughts and responses, you may identify and remove negative vibrations and energies that internally rise. Taking timely pauses every day will help you to reconcile your mental process with your impulses and responses. This is not always an easy thing to do unless we are willing to step away from anger, fear, prejudice, shame, guilt, and other negative emotions that hold us back from the pure spirit of love and warmth that exists in the core nature of each person.

STOPPING THE VIOLENCE

In the United States, 1.5 million women are raped annually. One out of six women has experienced an attempted or completed rape; almost two million women suffer some form of physical abuse every year. An average of 30,000 deaths occurs annually from the use of guns—regardless of the more than 20,000 laws on handguns already on the books. Annual suicide rates in the world exceed one million and growing. Men and boys comprise close to 80 percent of suicide victims.

Sixteen million animals are butchered every day to satiate our citizens' appetites for meat and flesh. With the worsening of violence comes the progressive wearing away of the Mother Consciousness and its profound vibratory force that buffers us from harm. When you make the commitment to a life of non-hurting your first priority—such as becoming a *sakahari*, or vegetarian—you will find yourself returning to your maternal Shakti power. As women, we must safeguard life by transforming our speech, thoughts, and actions into positive instruments for harmony.

CULTIVATING SHAKTI AWARENESS THROUGH MUDRA

Vedic knowledge says that each one of the 15 *nityas*—goddess emanations of the Supreme Mother of the universe Lalita—is depicted with the sacred hand gesture for releasing and conquering fear, the Abhaya Mudra, (See *The Practice: Abhaya Mudra* on pages 35-36). Mudras are Vedic hand gestures infused with cosmic prana specifically designed to shift negative energy into positive vibration. The phenomenal inner energy practice of mudra is one of the means we will be using time and time again to awaken the Mother Consciousness. Mudra is considered one of the most highly developed forms of yoga. Mudra Vijnanam is the knowledge of sacred hand practices developed by the Vedic seers to quickly move and purify energy in the body while they connect us to our origin in cosmic consciousness. Mudra, derived from the Sanskrit root *mud* ("to bring joy"), is a powerful means of attracting the universe's primary energies within body, mind, and spirit and seal them within us.

Mudra practice may be traced back to the most ancient Vedic rituals for the goddess. The gods and goddesses of the Hindu pantheon are depicted with their hands in various mudra positions, said to evoke tremendous powers. The mudra positions connect us with our hidden powers within and bring awareness to the subtle body. It is an exact yogic science by which we may develop our internal and external dispositions and help to reverse degeneration within the body. Mudras enhance breath and inner vibration. They bring light through our hands, converting them into cosmic conduits for healing. They also make us aware of the cosmic five elements coursing through our fingers, connecting our hands (symbolizing our actions of dharma) to the universe. Like the practice of mantra, mudra is used as a meditation tool to redirect prana, strengthen the life force, and stabilize the body's energy and heighten its immunity. At a more profound level of healing, mudra practice helps us to seal our sacred intentions and realize them almost immediately. In this healing continuum, we may seize the chance to cleanse and rid old karmas as we emblazon Shakti energy within.

ABHAYA MUDRA: PRACTICE FOR RECEIVING PROTECTION & RELIEVING FEAR

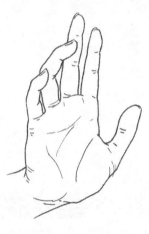

Figure 2.1 Abhaya Mudra

The Abhaya Mudra practice that follows is a powerful Inner Medicine practice to enhance courage and fearlessness. In practicing this mudra, you are saturating the vibrational airwaves with the energy of peace. In these highly-charged gestures, you will experience an immediate transformation of awareness. Mudra practice, once developed, invokes a sense of limitless space and inner leisure. Vast matter of the mind quickly shifts to find alignment with the greater energies. These ancient practices are intertwined with the energy of the five elements, which we will delve into more deeply as we move along.

According to the Vedas, this particular mudra has been practiced by the gods, goddesses, and sages to induce the state of absolute valor and fearlessness. The fear of death, considered the deepest trepidation of the human being, may be removed through dedicated practice of this sacred hand gesture. Through Abhaya Mudra practice, you may strengthen your inner resolve, rid conflicts, and paralyze the fear globules. If you know the emotional faces through which fear shows itself in your life, you may keep these in clear view as you invoke this practice. It is a significant practice to clear the conscience and gain serenity.

THE PRACTICE: ABHAYA MUDRA

- Sit in a comfortable position, facing east.
- Raise your right hand to chest level with the palm facing forward.
- Loosen the wrist and let the fingers separate gently.
- Hold the mudra for 10 minutes or so.
- You may perform this practice with your eyes open and softly focused on a fixed area, or you may opt to keep your eyes shut.
- You may engage this practice anywhere, at any time that you experience fear.

Chapter Three

RECLAIMING FEMININE INTELLIGENCE & INTUITION

Nama avyadhinibhyo vividhyantibhyasca vo namah.

Reverence to the Divine in the form of the Female Power
(Shakti) that defends the entire world in various forms.

—*Rig Veda*

From a young age, I was fortunate to have lived simply and in sync with nature's rhythms in a village where every member contributed to the greater family. This reality, along with the infinite largess of my cosmic memory, has certainly shaped my intuition. Through providential grace I also have an earthly mother who is the quintessential example of innate wisdom, and has a sense of knowing about each of her children.

My mother's intuition has never failed. The day before Hurricane Ivan hit, my mother left an urgent message for the school's administrator to cancel the September course because there would be flooding at the school. Incredibly, Hurricane Ivan charged in with full force at 4 a.m. the next morning. Bridges, barns, fences, and shards floated out to meet us on the pathway to the school that morning. My mother's profound gift of intuition has had an indeterminable impact in shaping my own response to life. Her simplicity, nobility, and wholesome regard for Mother Nature has preserved her instinctual, commonsensical wisdom to this day. We can all take a valuable lesson from my mother's example. By slowing down and reclaiming the necessary pauses in our everyday lives, we are given the chance to strengthen our powerful maternal intuition and ultimately make choices that render our lives simpler, rather than more complex.

When the power of intuition is at work, healing is inevitable. During the healing process, our body, mind, and spirit become the ever-flowing river that resolves itself into the Mother Consciousness—the ocean of simplicity. This is why we must strive to rouse the buddhi—the higher mind that holds the power of intuition, compassion, and resolve—so that our thoughts may thrive beyond the senses.

RECLAIMING THE GREATER MIND

The Vedic seers, the greatest quantum physicists that ever lived, mastered the art of perfect communion with the Mother Consciousness. Theirs was the language of intuition, complete awareness stepping down directly from the cosmic vibration and arising in their buddhi. They recognized the cognitive potential of the greater mind is within every human. Rather than depending on direct or indirect experience, inference and sensory perception, they knew that intuition emerges from the accumulation of knowledge existing in your karma. Given that each one of us has a karma that probably spans billions of light years, there is much credence to the buddhi. Indeed, buddhi transcends the function of the brain and goes far beyond the boundaries of rebirth.

To comprehend the buddhi, we must understand how the mind functions. Our phenomenal ability to learn, assimilate, perceive, comprehend, and remember comes from the mind and its mental faculty, or *manas* as it is referred to in Sanskrit. Recent scientific research in the filed of neurobiology is continually shedding light on the physical dimension of the mind. They are discovering what the Vedic seers knew for millennia: that the mind is not isolated just to the activity of the brain located in the skull. Through its intricate network of 100 billion neurons located in the brain, the mind travels on its wave of neural patterns throughout the body. Thoughts, feelings, ideas, viewpoints, beliefs, and attitudes arise from the neural activities in the brain.

The scientific principle of neuroplasticity tells us that the brain responds to our subjective experiences, which are capable of changing the function and structure of the brain itself. In the present culture of healing and human development, we wrongly attribute functions that belong to the buddhi to that of the mind. For example, psychotherapists define the word psyche as "soul, spirit, intellect, and mind." The psyche may be influenced by all of these components of the subtle and physical anatomy, but it is not equivalent to any one of them. In fact, the basis of the psyche is in the *pranamaya kosha*, pranic body, or second sheath of the human anatomy that is largely pervaded by prana, or life force of the body. Similarly, "mindsight" one of the newer terms in the field of psychotherapy attributed to the function of mind, translated as "insight and empathy," does, in fact, describe the function of the buddhi.

The rishis recognized that the cultivation of intuition lies in opening to the cosmos. When awakened, the buddhi can reveal knowledge of the cosmic reality by allowing us to transcend the mind and the various strata of the manifested world. Entry and ascension into the buddhi can occur only through the transcendence of awareness. For this to happen, we must first enter the sanctuary of buddhi through self-knowledge—the kind of knowledge that is beyond the boundaries of fact and information. In other words, we need to be spiritually educated.

AWAKENING INTUITION

There is a difference between knowledge and education. Knowledge is a natural evolving process that is within the knowing potential of everyone. It is based in the immutable reality of the universe. Education, which is what academicians, professors, teachers, lecturers, scientists, physicists, researchers, and educators are called on to do, is generally an external manifestation of information. Such information intends on shaping, developing, and influencing the mind. This form of education does contribute to the growth and well-being of our mental faculties, and to some extent our emotional and cognitive abilities. And although academic education is desirable, it does not necessarily inform our wisdom. The primary reason? The normal means of education are based in the dominant perception influenced by the mind's association with what we hear, see, feel, smell, and taste. Such education alone is not sufficient to awaken our intuitive ability. For this, we require the use of the buddhi.

Herein lies the paradox: it is impossible to reach the buddhi through any practice or mind-borne activity. We first need to transcend our mental faculty and sensory perceptions, which includes personal experiences since these may or may not contribute to the truth. Most practices that use the thinking process defeat the objective in reaching the buddhi. For this reason, seeking out mind-based therapies or finding new diagnoses for your disorders can serve only to enhance the inundation of mental, emotional, and sensory overload. Luckily, the sages designed sadhana practices like mudra, mantra, meditation, pranayama, yoga, yantra, chanting, and Vedic rituals to help you transcend the mind. As you will see, these priceless practices give us the chance to renegotiate karma, dissolve unwholesome habits, and help us move toward a profound sense of resolve within.

Once you transcend your mental plane and awaken your intuitive prowess, you'll experience an immense sense of inner freedom. For this, you need to summon the courage to know who you are and be true to yourself. In other words, put down your masks and present to the world your genuine, unpolished face. I learned this lesson under the most extreme circumstances with cancer, and I fully understand how very painful and difficult it is to embrace authenticity.

In the more than quarter of a century since I first began practicing meditation to arouse the buddhi, I have experienced numerous and distinct leaps of consciousness. The whole network of cosmic memory revealed itself to me. Frequently, I see events before they occur. The deities come alive in my inner universe, and often times, I dialogue with them.

As you move deeper into your buddhi meditation practice, you too will discover that your consciousness takes on a life of its own. You will begin to eagerly anticipate the time you have set aside for meditation. You will experience long periods of lucidity and clarity. You will override challenges before they manifest and recognize that you are forever healed. Your energy will attract the butterfly, hummingbird, breezes, spring and blue skies, and everything you require to soothe spirit. On the mundane plane, you will know who is calling you before you pick up the phone—and when the unexpected happens you will not be as surprised.

The beauty of intuitive education is that you do not need a Ph.D. or any kind of degree to awaken your primordial, commonsensical intelligence. But you do need to practice sadhana. In these pages, we will together explore the inner universe, probe your buddhi's potential, and bask in the sheer joy of doing so. Now, let us walk the path of the wise crone.

FOLLOWING THE WISDOM PATH OF THE MATERNAL

My grandmothers and elderly aunts never used a timer, alarm clock, or beeper in their lives to keep them on schedule. Yet they were always punctual in tending to their everyday tasks. They perfectly coordinated taking care of their homes and farms, nursing the young children, cooking three meals a day on wood stoves, fetching water from the well, caring for the milking cows, serving their families, helping us with our homework, and giving oil massages to all the children before their bedtimes. On occasion, they even found the time to pitch in and aid the aging midwife—the one and only midwife in my childhood village—to bring new life into the world.

Although the village elders all carried a palpable sorrow hidden under their sweat—harboring under the vicious ancestral memory of being plundered by their British colonizers—they remained vibrant and healthy. Not once do I recall any member of the community having any of the disorders common in modern societies such as the flu, cold, headaches, yeast infections, ulcers, allergies, obesity, high cholesterol, osteoporosis, stroke, heart disease, depression, or HIV/AIDS. (There were a few cases of deaths from cancer, which were kept secret due to the taboos that persisted in spite of communal wisdom.)

I remember the women gathering their forces in hallowed communal events for the villagers. The only medicine they used were castor oil, rubbing oils for bodily pains, neem powder, black sage powder for brushing teeth, herbal cough syrup, clove oil, red lavender oil, and several homemade ointments. Poultices, plaster, rubs, and compresses were the general treatment and application for a host of conditions. Life was simple. We have the power to make it simple again by reclaiming the commonsensical way of the native people, many of whom had no formal education but excelled in the sweet ways and magical vocabulary of Inner Medicine healing.

To start practicing the wisdom of the crone, there are a few simple steps we may take in everyday life so that we are prepared to receive the exquisite experience of living from the heart. Awakening the intuitive self comes easily when we make the act of kindness our first priority. For this, we have got to take a break from our habitual, mundane activities and re-examine our individual purpose as women.

ABOVE ALL, BE KIND

The smallest act of kindness is worth more than the greatest intention.
—Kahlil Gibran

When you work from your intuition, kindness overflows as compassion and care. When you work from kindness it strengthens intuition.

Transforming our personal reality of fatigue, pain, and overwhelm requires cultivating the mind of kindness. Kindness is a universal form of communion that increases support, love, and care, thereby transcending race, color, religion, gender, and social status. Everyone responds to kindness. At Mother Om Mission (MOM) in New York's inner cities of North Bronx and the South Bronx where we use Wise Earth Ayurveda's remarkable work with many teenagers from at-risk communities, we see how the simple act of kindness has helped these children to improve their self-esteem. Many have turned away from destructive paths due to their improved sense of self and our instructors' positive involvement in their daily lives. They come to MOM because of kindness, they feel safe, and they know how it feels to be nurtured and cared for.

These are kids who practically grew up outdoors in the inner city streets amid the lure of gang violence, domestic abuse, drugs, and guns. Yet, once they become connected to each other in an environment of kindness, they choose to invest their time in their studies and becoming part of a close-knit group. Through meditation, they learn how to witness their thoughts and actions. As a result, they become responsible for them. They learn that a simple act of kindness may yield the most profound healing within, whether it's keeping a mantra in mind, helping a frail person cross the street, giving a seat to the weary, or lending a helping hand, a kind word, or a big smile.

Shepherded by the greater energy of empathy, each person helps bring the miracle of healing to each day. We receive so much more than we give when the gift comes from the mind of kindness. Making kindness our first priority helps to rid the barnacle of suffering and unhappiness we unwittingly attach to the underbelly of our lives.

WE ARE ALL CONNECTED

We are all connected through the profound field of vibration and therefore share a common responsibility for the well-being of our world, one that is entirely shaped by our collective karma. When we help somebody with kindness, we serve the maternal spirit of self and connect to the ever-flowing energy of grace and humanitarianism in our world. It becomes a more loving space with an increased vibration of consciousness, which is necessary if we are to grow our intuition. Ultimately, the greatest kindness is to recognize the One Consciousness that lives within each of us. Practicing the sadhanas that awaken buddhi (see *The Practice: Pranava Upasana* and *The Practice: Bhramari Breath & Sound Meditation* at the end of this chapter) is a profound way of connecting to the Mother Consciousness.

Whether it's love, prosperity, or health, we must have these things for *all* before we have them for ourselves. In exploring the path of kindness set out for us by the rishis, we can "reach" the One within and begin to recognize the natural rhythm of our intuitive psyche. In so doing, we may recover the idea that every person is a cosmic vessel—*nimitta karana*—of the Divine.

Knowing this, you can start to garner the ancient and crucial wisdom of kindness as your constant companion. Take the example of Cynthia, a professor of theology with three impressive degrees to her name. At one of my workshops, she sat next to Jeanne, a young, unstable woman who fidgeted throughout the program and rose several times from her seat during the meditation, creating unwanted disturbance. Cynthia was so aggravated by her that she told me that she had to restrain herself from physically removing Jeanne from the session. When she told me this, Jeanne happened to overhear her. Jeanne angrily confronted Cynthia, and a heated argument erupted. An elderly participant who had been sitting in the back of the room quickly approached both women and quietly uttered a few words, "You are sisters on this beautiful day, standing in the loving presence of the Mother, what can be so wrong that you would want to fight with each other?"

Immediately, they both calmed down. She then proceeded to embrace both ladies in a three-way hug. The spirit of kindness and reconciliation was so powerful that everyone on line waiting to see me began hugging each other. The intuitive wisdom of the crone was at work; she had managed to diffuse a potentially volatile situation within a split second by using her emotional intelligence. She realized that both women were suffering; one from instability and the other from impatience.

After the dust had settled and everyone left the hall, the crone remained and told me her story. She was once an executive in a major multinational company. During the prime of her career, her husband suddenly died from a massive heart attack. She took a year's sabbatical from her job and went to an ashram in India where she learned of a new and gentle way of living. By the time we met, she had been practicing meditation for 20 years.

From her personal karma, she understood about pain, anger, fear, and hurt. To really understand these things is the beginning of wisdom at work. Therefore, be kind to yourself. Be kind to your karma. Be kind to the children. Be kind to the men. Be kind to each other. Be kind to the animals. Be kind to the memory of your ancestors. Be kind to the life force in whatever form it assumes. Above all, be kind. We all need to strengthen our positive connection to each other. Kindness brings us closer and provides the warmth of support we need while casting off the mind's hurtful habits that do not serve us well.

TAKE PAUSE AND PAUSE AGAIN

It is not enough to be busy. So are the ants.
The question is; what are we busy about?
—Henry David Thoreau

Imagine a life with no stress: awakening to the day with a pause and meditation; going to work at a job you love; having a calm pace throughout your day so you can appreciate all that you are doing, and coming home to prepare a scrumptious, healthful dinner and sharing it with your loved ones. Visualize a life where during a leisurely stroll you notice the breeze in your hair, feel the sunlight permeate the pores of your skin, open your arms wide and take a deep and cleansing breath. Imagine going to sleep every night with a prayer. This doesn't have to be a mere fantasy. These things are possible when you live in the Mother Consciousness.

So many women walk around in a stupor, keeping busy, pursuing material objects while feeling drained and empty within. We need to slow down and take pause, especially if we are in the menopausal years when hormonally-propelled emotions can dredge up old hurts, fears, and grief from unfulfilled desires. We do not want to be caught unprepared in the spiraling emotions of mid-life crisis. At whatever juncture of life we find ourselves, we must begin to address our deepest desires and authentic needs.

The way to find our purpose is not through material possessions, fanciful dreams, stressful ambitions, or by simply giving up. Only through harvesting the space of kindness within and having a sense of shared responsibility for each other's well-being can we grow into the richness of our intuitive ability. For this, we must create the inner space. To fully resolve our unfulfilled desires or inner conflicts, we need to first recreate our living spaces to generate calmness.

You can start by clearing the clutter out from one room and dedicating this space to being your temple, your space of sanity. Once the space around you becomes light and serene it will affect your mind. Wholesome thoughts will start to flow. Put aside a specific time every day to catch up with yourself, whether it's getting out in nature, sitting in your quiet temple space, or taking a bath with essential oils like lavender or rose.

RECLAIMING YOUR LIFE

After reading the various practices (sadhanas) in the pages of this book, my editor called me on the phone. "No one is going to have the time to incorporate all of these sadhana practices in their busy lives," she told me. That is precisely the problem. If we are to achieve any degree of consciousness, we need to take the quantum pause, slacken our pace, and slow down so that we may create the inner space and time to reassess our priorities. We have got to recast our schedules and reinvent our perceptions of what we actually consider necessary to meet our real human feminine needs. We cannot hope to squeeze in the life-generating practices set out in these pages in an overloaded, tense, and stressed environment and expect them to work for us.

When Liana first arrived at the monastery to see me, she was stressed to the breaking point. She complained of forgetfulness, insomnia, fatigue, nervousness, anxiety, loss of appetite, and disorientation. In addition to being a single mother to a 7-year old daughter, she was writing her Ph.D. thesis; attending an early morning yoga class; working as a full time college administrator; visiting a psychotherapist three times a week; and attending Alcoholic Anonymous meetings twice a week. She ate most of her meals on the run.

She also employed a part-time nanny and lived in a palatial home in the suburbs of New York, for which she had to meet her monthly mortgage payment of more than $3, 500. She wanted to learn a meditation practice to ease her conditions that she could fit into her schedule before bed. What is wrong with this picture? It doesn't matter how many self-help practices we do if we don't reprioritize what is important to us to sustain health, kindness, and awareness. We could spend an entire lifetime being "successful" women without finding time for our greater gifts from the Mother Consciousness. We must shift our "dreams" and "ambitions" to fulfill what is truly our greater feminine purpose.

My advice to Liana was to cut back her working schedule by 20 percent, secure an extension to complete her dissertation, and move to a less expensive home closer to her work—all of which would give her more time to care for herself and her daughter. Slowing down and taking pause are the fundamental first steps if we are to benefit from the profound Inner Medicine of healing sadhanas set out in this book to help you develop your intuition.

Remember, this sacred work has little to do with medicine, conventional or otherwise. I have provided you many healthful recommendations such as herbal remedies to help you immediately relieve your tensions and address full-blown disorders you may be experiencing. These short-term remedies come with ample instructions on how to use your own energy to prepare them to arouse your Inner Medicine healing powers. In doing so, I hope that your own profound instinct for healing will begin to override the actual medicinal remedy.

WHAT IS INNER MEDICINE?

The idea that most ailments can be cured by shifting the mind is nothing new. According to the *New England Journal of Medicine*, scientists report that 75 percent of all diseases can be remedied by our mental functions. Deep illnesses like cancer and heart disease have strong psychological and spiritual components. In using Inner Medicine healing, we not only explore the inner world of our mind, but go beyond its boundaries into the vibratory sanctum of the buddhi. Inner Medicine healing is earthed in the understanding that each one of us has the ineffable ability to arouse healing powers imbued within ourselves. To reorder these powers it is imperative that we explore our inner universe of desire, intuition, and intention.

My teachings do not mesh with the concepts and implications of modern medicine as we know it. In fact, they do not deal with any form of medicine that prescribes medication, confers dependency, and trains the mind/body to expect wellness to come from a pill, a remedy (natural or unnatural), or from any external agent. Once you learn this way of living, you will find your dependency on medicines decreasing until you no longer require them. We must get away from the burgeoning ideology of becoming a *permanent* health seeker.

Existing in the present culture are too many drugs, too many therapies, too many healing modalities, too many archetypal concepts, and too many individualized health practices. Because of this overkill, you may easily find yourself stuck in a holding pattern of co-dependency and crises that has little or nothing to do with the process of healing. Even though you think you are healing yourself through these methods, you might be doing more harm. No wonder we are exhausted. While mentally, emotionally, physically, and spiritually inundated with a continually growing number of disorders, we often mistake these conditions and illnesses for our ineffable nature. In continually identifying with our diseases, illnesses, and disorders, we lose sight of our invincible force of wellness within and our profound ability to heal ourselves.

People, conditions, behaviors, and circumstances are ever changing. In a split second our vibratory field can be energized by the grace of a sage, a passing breeze, a gurgling brook, or the silent musings of an ancestor. Our passing concerns and conditions should never be escalated to the status of permanency. This type of thinking only serves to deepen personal fear and the collective obsessive, and render so many people into the unconscious state of being a perennial health victim!

Martina was a 42-year old dancer who had a successful career in film. Unfortunately, she was unable to embrace her success. She walked through life feeling fat, malnourished, and unloved. When I first met her, she was obsessed with her weight even though she had the perfect body mass for being a Kapha-Pitta metabolic type, and appeared to be fit. But she was obviously unhappy. She told me that she frequently skipped meals and ran 10 or more miles a day. She complained of aches, pains, and sadness and confided that she had been jumping from one health fad to another to "lose" unwanted weight. Over the last decade she has been on the treadmill of 12 different types of "holistic health" diets, a myriad of dietary supplements, two cosmetic surgeries, and failed silicone breast implants. Obviously, her obsession about her weight and physical appearance masked the deeper problem of unhappiness with herself, one which was never going to be solved with diet, pills, cosmetic surgery, or exercise.

When I saw her, she was on a raw foods diet and was having immense pains in her stomach. Apparently, her system wasn't assimilating the raw foods properly and consequently she was unable to move her bowels without taking a large quantity of laxatives every night. I encouraged her to talk to me about her feelings and routines for the past few years. In her frankness, I realized Martina was probably willing to begin facing the underlying issues for her discontent and misery, most of which may be traced back to the poor and abusive environment of her childhood. So I recommended the best Inner Medicine healing of all—a life of sadhana. Since her time and busy career did not permit her to do on-site studies, I recommended that she begin her healing by studying our Distance Learning Course on Wise Earth Ayurveda Nutrition.

After completing the course a year later, Martina came to Wise Earth for a weekend workshop. She looked happy and healthy. She was free from medication, pills, cosmetic surgeries, and supplements, and had adjusted her exercise schedule to three times a week. She told me how much she now enjoys cooking for herself and her friends.

PROPERLY APPLY THE CONCEPTS

When I first began teaching Wise Earth Ayurveda in the United States in 1980, I introduced the concept of the chakras and doshas and their influence on our psychospiritual nature. Many holistic practitioners and writers have since exploited these concepts, but this may actually do the present culture more harm than good. Unlike the intention of the rishis and sages, modern practitioners tend to use these concepts to label people with fixed categories for their transient conditions.

Philosophical concepts need to be understood properly if they are to be positively applied. For these archetypal concepts of human nature to be grasped, we need to be awakened to our innate resource of the buddhi's consciousness. In the last two decades or so, we have added many more ancient archetypal concepts of behavior to our healing-oriented vocabulary such as *kundalini, tribal, reptilian, shadow self,* and *lower chakra,* to name a few. While these words may give insights into our cosmic anatomy, excessive and misdirected use of them only serves to propagate human judgments and obsessions.

Mind you, there is nothing wrong with being fascinated about cosmic concepts and their relevance to your greater nature. When used in a positive way, these concepts may reveal valuable insights into your nature. Take the concept of Ayurveda's unique metabolic type, for instance. It is a marvel to see people grasping the knowledge of their unique metabolic type, having fun while learning about their metabolic composition, and then putting that new knowledge to good use: for example, Vata type is airy and rough; Pitta type is fiery and quick; and Kapha type is heavy and stable. Understanding your individual body type allows you to positively guide your health and behavior. However, we must be careful not to become too obsessive about our body types. When you begin to solely identify with your body type, and worst yet with your conditions, you lose sight of your marvelous gift of humanity. The Sanskrit word "dosha" from which the body types are derived actually means "fault." In identifying or typecasting yourself solely as a Pitta, or Vata, or Kapha person, or becoming fanatical about choices that support each type, you are limiting your True Self and infinite joy to the mere mundane. You are more than bodily fluids, tissues, and diseased conditions. You are the ever generating, ever changing infinite consciousness. It is wise to remember that you are a whole entity with body, mind, and spirit, each with your own incredible karma.

FINDING YOUR PERSONAL FREEDOM

The wisdom of intuition is easily accessed once you recover your feminine authority. To give prana to your self-expression you will need to take a commonsensical approach and begin converting your present education into awareness. The modern culture has left little room for personal awareness to bloom into concrete wisdom. Culled from long years of experience, awareness is crucial to your progress. Because we have lost so much of our ability to recognize what is happening within our own sphere of awareness, we have forgotten the relevance of the body's innate rhythms as they relate to the cosmic cycles. In our everyday activities we experience a growing sense of disharmony and disconnect, largely due to the mechanized and sanitized approaches around us.

To reclaim our feminine authority, we must first regain personal freedom. Intrinsic in this freedom is the ability to shout for joy, hear the sweet magical sounds within and without, and speak your truth as earth guardian of the maternal divinity.

The critical obstacle is simply the lack of understanding of what personal freedom means. Personal freedom has nothing to do with being able to do whatever we want, whenever we want. In trying to regain our full feminine powers, we tend to go overboard and do reckless things. This approach can only deter our quest for personal freedom. First, we must break free from all impediments such as outdated taboos—the pervasive guilt complex of the First World culture—patriarchal suppression of the feminine, and horrendous biomedical acts that are usurping women's reproductive power and incapacitating their buddhi.

We must ponder what is to become of our maternal freedom to think, know, and express who we really are—divine beings carved out by sacred hands of the Divine Mother. This pondering has everything to do with your healing. To rid the grief and guilt, you must heal the rift with your ancestral memory. Reclaiming your sonic, vocal authority is a primal means of doing so. Thankfully, in the law of Mother Nature every challenge comes with a solution. Light must erase every period of darkness, and invariably we find our light when we are able to target the core of the shadow that surrounds us. Marnie's triumph from lung cancer shows how we can all recover our inner light.

Marnie first visited Wise Earth three years ago, after she had been diagnosed with lung cancer. Her oncologist recommended a course of radiation treatment, along with chemotherapy. She was single, a confessed workaholic, and a smoker whose aunt and grandmother had both died from lung disease. And she was scared. After her diagnosis she left her job, stopped smoking, but flatly refused conventional medical treatment.

As I always do, I began by encouraging Marnie to tell me about her life, desires, aspirations, and disappointments. She shared with me that she was not close to her family and had not visited her mother for more than three years. She was unhappy with her work, did not have any close friends, and had been increasingly despondent for the past 10 years. In addition, she had unfulfilled dreams about becoming a musician. As a teenager, her music teacher told her that she had the gift to become a concert pianist but her parents felt she would not be able to make a proper living as a musician.

The most poignant energy about Marnie was her grief, which was etched in her face, the depressed lines around her mouth tending to pull her lips downward aging her appearance beyond her years. Even before she told me about her rift with her mother, and her aunt and grandmother's demise from cancer, I had noticed that the lines on her left side of her face were more pronounced. According to Wise Earth Ayurveda diagnosis, the left side of our body reflects our lunar or maternal characteristics, the right side our paternal. Marnie's core problem appeared to be hinged to ancestral maternal grief. It was not surprising that she had a problem with her lungs, not only because she was an avid smoker, but because of the genetic vulnerability in her lungs passed down from her mother and grandmother. Most likely her addiction to cigarettes arose from that susceptibility.

Having closely observed thousands of people over the years, I have come to understand that each organ holds a specific set of memories that produces disease when impaired. Not only are lungs important to our life force, prana, and respiration, they sustain the organism's *prinana*, sense of joy. In Marnie's case, she had arrived into the world with an overload of ancestral grief. Now, in the grasp of a potentially fatal disease she had no choice but to convert her grief into joy so she could heal her "bout" with lung cancer. From what I see, the collective grief of our female population is rapidly increasing. Last year alone in the United States, 82,000 women suffered from lung cancer, 90 percent of whom died from the disease.

As a primary course for Marnie, I introduced her to a form of meditation we call Pranava Upasana (see pages 52-55), where we use specific primordial sounds of the Vedas to enhance tissue memory. Marnie had begun to master the practice over the period of the 10 days she spent at Wise Earth. Moreover, every morning she volunteered to drum for all the Vedic chanting sessions we performed, dedicating her efforts to the sound healing practices of Vedic chanting, drumming, and meditation. She became visibly transformed right before our eyes. Many of the students noticed that Marnie was now laughing, looking visibly younger, and that both her hair and complexion were glowing. Marnie had obviously started to harvest her sense of joy. In so doing she has begun to shift the grief that was feeding her illness. After she retuned home, she continued the Pranava Upasana practice and resumed playing the piano as an accompaniment to her chanting. She also began working closely with a holistic practitioner/herbalist in her area and, along with her practice of Wise Earth sadhanas, she journeyed for two more years into full recovery. She has since reconciled the rift with her mother and family and has started her own work as a musical coach and consultant to talented children.

Like Marnie, each one of you has at your disposal the necessary resources for healing grief. Her story reaffirms that you have the power to heal at the deepest level of your being. Many women give up hope, thinking that it would take a massive amount of personal work to make a difference. This is not true. For more than 25 years, I have witnessed the incredible power of these simple practices applied to everyday life. Granted, given the continuously swelling numbers of ailments, diseases, and distresses women experience today, we have a ways to go to fortify our natural rhythm necessary to blossom intuition.

Happily, you have access to the ancient Vedic wisdom in this book that will help you to regain your feminine splendor. And, thankfully, in the past few decades there has been the proliferation of holistic practitioners and healers who are striving to reconnect to the greater energies of the cosmos. These healers recognize that the source of healing is within. We call their practice New Age, when ironically their knowledge is based in ancient wisdom! We also refer to holistic medicine practice as "complementary," an expression that is true only by contrast to the "uncomplimentary" way conventional medicine has strong-armed itself into the global healing field. We tend to forget that Western Medicine and its dominant credence have been around only for a few centuries.

It's also a comfort to know that more and more people *within* the present medical system are driving forces for change. In fact, some of the most popular tomes of work on holistic health and wellness come from conventionally trained medical physicians and scientists who are now some of the best-known energy healers in America such as Deepak Chopra, Dean Ornish, Andrew Weil, Carolyn Myss, and Tracey Gaudet. Since the majority of people are programmed to put their faith in the word of the medical status quo, this budding trend may actually prove helpful to many more people. This is a very important development in our time especially since much of the developed world's population will need to overcome and cure their worst malady—dependency on medicine. The medical establishment in America is responsible for more than 100,000 people dying from medical mistakes every year. It spends 21 billion dollars annually to market pharmaceuticals to the medical professionals and incorrectly fills 26 out of every 100 prescriptions (five of which are usually fatal).

TAKING BACK REPRODUCTIVE RIGHTS

As a profound means of repossessing feminine authority and retrieving Shakti power, women must take back their reproductive rights from the hierocracy of medicine and science.

Firstly, women must awaken to the power of their buddhi to strengthen their organic ability of intuition, sensitivity, and introspection. Once you evoke your buddhi force, you will start to recognize and discard the onslaught of medical misinformation, and find instead the Inner Medicine means to resolve your health challenges. The present deluge of medical misinformation relative to women's conditions is staggering. In 1982, the *New England Journal of Medicine* published its research findings on fibrocystic breast disease citing what they had discovered: that 70 percent or more of what is diagnosed fibrocystic breast disease is, in fact, normal developmental changes in the fatty and the connective tissues of the breast.

Radhika's story illustrates the unnecessary angst and hurt these medical misdiagnoses can cause. In the early 80s, Radhika, a 43-year old woman from New Delhi came to me for help. Her female gynecologist had just informed her that she had a 90 percent chance of having breast cancer because of an existing condition called fibrocystic breast disease, and she was scared.

Frankly, I had never heard of such a condition, but was not overly concerned because I could tell from Radhika's appearance and energy field that she was not exhibiting any pre-cancerous signs. To double check my intuitive assessment, I read her pulse in the Ayurvedic way of *nadi-pariksha*. Her only "condition" was that her Vata (bodily air humor) was being restricted by an excess of Kapha (bodily water humor), causing her breast tissue to be somewhat dense and swollen. In Radhika's case these symptoms had emerged as a result of her perimenopausal state. Once she knew her condition was not cancerous, but in fact, easily corrected by doing the practices that will bring her menstrual rhythm in harmony with the lunar cycles, she was literally jumping for joy.

Wise Earth Ayurveda unearths and re-introduces exhaustive information on the power of women's reproductive health linked to the cosmic cycles. It tells us that when a woman's ovulation cycle is in harmony with the full moon it increases her chances of optimal health. When surgery is performed in the waning cycle of the moon, especially those relating to a woman's reproductive health, her chances of recovery and survival are greatly increased. One explanation for this is that naturally ovulating during the full moon cycle strengthens ojas, cellular immunity. Remarkably, the findings of William Hrushesky, M.D., an oncologist at Dorn Veterans Affairs Medical Center in South Carolina who has studied the effects of the lunar cycle on a woman's health, concurs with Ayurveda's teachings.

According to his research, deaths from breast cancer are far less common when surgery is performed on or around the 10th day following ovulation rather than around the time of menstruation. Dr. Hrushesky says that as many as 12,000 American lives and a quarter million lives worldwide could be saved if women were operated on at this time. Imagine unearthing this knowledge through science when the rishis had established it many thousands of years ago!

Dr. Hrushesky also found that a woman's cellular immune function waxes and wanes during her menstrual cycle—yet another fact that Ayurveda has been propagating for more than 7,000 years. Taking into account both fertility and menstrual cycles and realigning them with their appropriate lunar phase could literally save millions of lives. Unfortunately, Dr. Hrushesky's remarkable findings have not prompted significant changes in current medical practices. One reason for this is the massive distance modern science has put between itself and the reality of the Mother Nature; not surprising since the multibillion dollar medical industry would have to shift the mind-set of its entire global medical conglomerate and reverse the status quo.

Western Medicine has a massive battle ahead when and if it chooses to regain a holistic vision. We only need to look at Hormonal Replacement Therapy (HRT) for a prime example of Western Medicine's lack of holistic vision. The ancients would consider HRT, an approach that deals with the symptoms of a disease rather than its cyclical cause, a tragic turn in the lives of women. A 1995 report monitored the health of over 100,000 nurses since the mid-70s; results showed that those who took HRT for five years or more had a significantly higher rate of breast cancer. It's true that many studies do show that HRT can help women to increase bone density and reduce the risk of bone fractures. But why endure the ugly side effects of HRT like breast tenderness, cramps, nausea, blood spotting, and water retention, along with physical and emotional disorientation when you can easily reclaim the natural intelligence of your hormonal rhythms and heal without medicine?

Lauren is a 60-year old woman with a great sense of humor who came from Chicago to attend the Ayurveda & Women's Health Care workshop at the school. She was put on HRT for five years after complaining about mild menopausal symptoms such as irritability, occasional hot flashes, and night sweats. After a bone scan X-ray showed significant bone loss, her doctor immediately placed her on HRT. Lauren said she began feeling nauseous from the first week and felt constantly disoriented. She experienced memory loss, breakthrough bleeding and spotting, had tender, swollen breasts, and ballooned four dress sizes larger due to water retention. In short, Lauren was miserable. As Lauren puts it, she felt that her treatment with HRT felt more like HURT: hormones undergoing replacement therapy.

After coming to the class, Lauren learned about the Uttara Vasti home therapy, healing food preparations, and lifestyle practices for menopause and osteoporosis. I advised her to spend six months weaning herself off HRT by using the Uttara Vasti therapy in accord with the new moon cycle. In addition, I recommended healthful foods that were unrefined, organic and natural estrogen replenishers like nuts and fruits, pineapple juice, mung and soya beans, and whole grains such as brown rice, hulled barley, and millet. Within three months of doing this, Lauren completely weaned herself off HRT. After her first application of Uttara Vasti, she had no more disorientation or menopausal symptoms. Two years of practice later, Lauren enjoys vibrant health. Her recent annual checkup also revealed an astounding improvement in her bone density. She disclosed that she was also experiencing a wonderful sense of serenity for the first time in her life in which her sense of trusting and knowing was growing. Lauren now devotes her time to instructing Wise Earth Ayurveda and has gathered a thriving community of women who meet regularly to support each other with their sadhana practice.

PRANAVA UPASANA: MEDITATING ON OM

Western doctors and thinkers are starting to recognize what the rishis saw many centuries ago, that nature is a unified whole, and that the human mind and body are irretrievably linked to it, as well as inseparable from each other. The age-old practices of yoga, meditation, and primordial sound healing are now being used to explore the fields of the mind, and we are discovering what the Vedic seers have always understood—that meditation gives way to knowing, intuiting, and healing. Patanjali, the third-century scholar and author of *Yoga Sutras*, the earliest and classic text on yoga and meditation, wrote: "Through absorption and concentration, the processes of meditation, we may go beyond sensory perceptions."

For eons, the Vedic people have been cultivating a meditative life, which has helped them to secure the pathway to intuition and inner freedom. You, too, may eventually journey to the summit of your mind and transcend it. At the very least, you may reach a point where you can observe the way it works. For beginners, a successful meditation is one that leaves you feeling tranquil and rested. As your mind empties itself of distractions, thought and action start to flow in harmony with each other. You take away from your period of sitting in meditation the freedom to focus completely on the activity in which you are next engaged.

At Wise Earth School, we teach various forms of primordial sound meditations (see the practices: Pranava Upasana and Bhramari Breath & Sound Meditation described in detail at the end of this chapter). As noted earlier, primordial sound meditation practices have proven to be profoundly effective in awakening buddhi. The goal of all buddhi meditations is to sit and stay present within the self; these potent practices pave the way by making the mind as calm as the surface of a lake on a windless day. Your thoughts may move lightly on the surface of the mind without disturbing it. Once you are able to move past perceptions, thoughts, desires, and imaginings, you have entered your buddhi. As you enter the sanctuary of the buddhi, you move away from common perceptions of sights and sounds. Ultimately, you must get beyond dreams and visions, beyond even the grasp of intelligence, into the realm of pure consciousness, what the rishis call *anandam*, "the abiding joy and complete fullness." That is your true nature. Your mind and senses cannot lead you into this inner universe.

Reflecting on the sacred syllable OM is a direct means of accessing buddhi. According to the rishis, OM is the cosmic seed sound from which the universe is produced, by which it is sustained, and to which it returns. Through the transformation of this primordial sound, the entire universe emerged, constantly revolving into other shapes and forms. When we incant OM, we use the entire spectrum of vocal range from throat to lips. By doing so, we recall the most ancient phenomenon—the cosmic sound of the Mother Consciousness. Reciting OM helps to calm the mind and opens the gateway to the vast inner realm of silence that lies in the buddhi. This sound meditation makes you more sensitive to the movement of your breath. The practice is also very useful whenever you feel anxious, angry, or are experiencing any other kind of emotional distress. The Pranava Upasana practice that follows is an excellent preparation for meditation, because it helps you to develop your inner silence through sweet, harmonious sounds resonating through your own voice. The beauty of this practice is in its simplicity. You can do it anywhere, at any time, to promote relaxation and/or ready your mind and body for meditation. Remember—whatever your condition, wherever you are, you can always breathe, and explore your inner primordial sound.

THE PRACTICE: PRANAVA UPASANA

Start the day with 10 minutes of Pranava Upasana. As your focus on quieting the mind improves, you may wish to extend the meditation to 30 minutes.

- Sit in lotus posture on the floor or sit with a flat back in an upright chair with your feet firmly planted on the ground.
- Close your eyes and breathe until your breathing is even and gentle.
- Take a deep inhalation and feel your breath flowing into your belly and circulating into your womb to stimulate Shakti prana.
- On your next exhalation chant *OM*, unleashing your voice like the pouring of golden honey.
- Hold the cosmic sound for as long as you can.
- Reduce the volume of your sound incrementally until it ends in silence.
- Repeat this for 5 to 10 minutes.
- When you are finished, continue to sit, breathe, and observe the deep inner silence you have created.

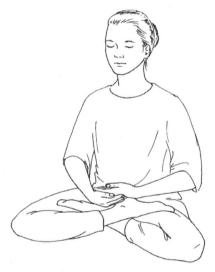

Figure 3.1 Meditation Sitting Posture

Having calmed the mind and allayed thoughts in the bosom of the cosmic sound, you might want to go deeper into your Shakti energy to build a strong foundational support for the buddhi. The powerful practice of Bhramari Breath & Sound

Meditation has proven to be a profound experience for women. Considering its source in the actual breath of the Goddess Bhramari, this practice awakens intuition and reconnects you to the Mother Consciousness.

BHRAMARI BREATH MEDITATION: THE INNER BUZZING OF THE GODDESS

Bhramari Breath & Sound Meditation is a potent primordial sound meditation derived from the Goddess Bhramari. The Sanskrit verbal root *bhram* literally means "bees" and refers to the resonant hum of inner consciousness, reminiscent of the sound of buzzing bees. As Bhramari-Devi, the Mother took the form of the precocious queen bee. Surrounded by her bevy of bees, Bhramari-Devi is symbolic of the rise of consciousness from the root chakra to the summit of consciousness. The name of this practice also comes from a classical Indian dance wherein the Bhramari Mudra is used to represent the bee. The internal buzzing sound central to this practice penetrates deep within the invisible network that supports the *ajna chakra*, the sixth chakra located in the mid-brow, the point where mind merges into buddhi. This exquisite sound practice also fortifies your cosmic memories and exercises tenacity in holding the mind in a state of balance.

Apart from the ultimate goal of self-awareness, Bhramari Breath & Sound Meditation has numerous other benefits. It balances the immunological and nervous systems; strengthens prana breath that flows to the heart and brain; and resonates in the ajna chakra. In this age-old meditation practice, the vibration activates the nervous system and brain, bringing the mind into a state of balance. The buzzing process also purifies the Shakti prana and helps to raise its energy from the base of the spine up into ajna chakra thereby heightening intuition.

THE PRACTICE: BHRAMARI BREATH & SOUND MEDITATION

- Sit in a comfortable meditative posture in a quiet place.
- Release the stale breath from your body with a forceful exhalation through the nostrils.
- Take a deep, leisurely breath and lock all the apertures of the face by using the fingers of both hands to close your eyes, nostrils, ears, and the mouth, as shown in the diagram on the next page.
- Begin to vibrate the vocal cords by making an audible humming sound until you run out of breath.
- You will feel this buzzing sound penetrating throughout your entire inner universe, linking you to Goddess Bhramari.

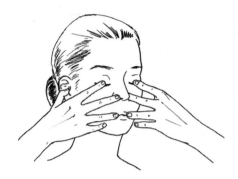

Figure 3.2 Mudra Hand Pose for Bhramari Breath & Sound Meditation

Part Two

COSMIC ANATOMY
OF WOMEN

Chapter Four

FEMININE HEALTH
& LUNAR CYCLES

According to the Bhavana Upanishad, the human
body and the cosmic universe that subsist in time
and space are both conceived in the subtle formation
of the Sri Chakra—abode of the Goddess Lalita Maha
Tripurasundari. Human sustenance and well-being
are tied to the turn of the lunar wheel, and women
are the cosmic keepers of the moon time.

A life of balance means that we must reclaim the ancient memory that empowers our health and consciousness. It means that we must adhere to the cyclical rhythms of the body, mind, and spirit. It means we must learn how to read the eternal pulse of nature, striving to know the rhythmic signs, signals, and symbols as they materialize with the circling of the lunar wheel and movement of the seasons. This calls for a definitive shift in thinking in the way we view ourselves in relation to the world. A leap of faith must happen if we are to reorient and instigate quantum change in our everyday routine habits. How we respond to the momentum of each day, week, month, and season has much to do with our willingness to relearn our biorhythms and understand their vital interconnectiveness with both nature's knowable and unpredictable cadence.

We can overcome unconscious damaging behavior in our everyday lives; I see this happening every day in my work around the world. On Mother's Day, 1998, we had just opened the doors to MOM in Queens, New York where we serve a community of predominantly Asian and African descent. My assistants asked the women who were experiencing life-threatening diseases to stay on for the evening satsanga to meet with me. Thirty-six women stayed on, seven of whom had cancer. Most of them were in their 40s to mid-50s, could not afford medical insurance, and were therefore not taking any form of treatment for their diseases. I opened the satsanga with the usual Vedic darshana, where I see and bless each person. When asked what their primary wish would be, each one responded with almost the same answer: "My health so I can take care of my children," "My health so I can take care of my husband," or "My health so I can work and earn the money to send my two children to college." Each woman also expressed deep fear of dying from her disease.

In these deeply sacred moments, I always call on prayer and my inner guide to help me charter the way and ask that the deeply seated fears and obstacles be removed. I invoke the essence of profound faith and trust in the Mother Consciousness and ask each participant to do the same. When asked if they would participate in their own healing, they all answered "yes." When asked how many were prepared to pare down their present activity and pay attention to their healing process, they replied affirmatively. When asked how many were committed to attending the teachings that would help them to change their lifestyles and habits, there was a slight show of hands. When asked how many would sign up that evening for the ongoing free, self-help community classes, two people reluctantly raised their hands. Most of the participants appeared embarrassed and a palpable murmur of random and cohesive mutterings that sounded like, "I can't because I need to take care of . . ." flooded the vibrational space. When asked who would like to have the Ayurveda remedies and quick fix, everyone brightened up. The vote for this "solution" to healing was unanimous.

Picking up on the routine clue, my aides rapidly began to package *vibhuti*—sacred ash from our ashram in India. I gave each woman a package of ash with specific instruction on how to apply it on the forehead and provided each with a short mantra for healing. Finally, I informed them that the magic of immediate healing from the holy ash would be awakened when they began to attend and participate in MOM programs, and that this healing would grow in steady increments as they become more attuned to the program. (The vibhuti is much more than a placebo. Prepared with the ingredients of prayer, mantra, yantra, and sacred fire, and used by the Vedic monks from the time of yore, it does possess spiritual powers. But like all *siddhis*, special spiritual powers, it must be co-mingled with a person's awakening of consciousness before its magic can take effect.)

Seven years later, 23 of 36 women from this group have incorporated MOM's wisdom into their lives. What happened for this massive transformation to come about? Although most of the women were reluctant to make any major changes at the time of the initial meeting, something significant shifted in the mind and heart of each and every woman at that satsanga—more than the concern for their physical or mental health. These women had grown accustomed to living with hardship and grief, which had became an intrinsic part of their vital tissue and memory. As often happens in the gatherings, I bring forth the voice of truth which is projected and heard, and stirs something deep inside of each person—Shakti arising within that moves in ways that often surprises us. Gradually, the women began to attend MOM's classes and became greater advocates of the work as their health and family's well-being began to show noticeable signs of improvement.

All of them are now completely free from disease without having taken any form of conventional medicine or treatment. Jen, a young woman with HIV, is now totally healthy. Four years ago, she was absolutely asymptomatic, and there was no longer any sign of the virus in her bloodstream. Three of the women, including Jen, have since joined MOM's Instructorship Team and go about the community teaching other women how to realize the power of the sacred ash, although mostly they use it as a symbolic metaphor.

What is the secret of healing that these women discovered at MOM?
• Knowing how to safeguard personal freedom
• Knowledge of their inner rhythms
• Recognizing their innate power to self-heal
• Learning to nourish and nurture themselves

These are the gems of wisdom that all women need to seek to unearth their Inner Medicine healing potential. Through MOM's practice, they learned how to reprogram their mental, physical, and emotional patterns of habitual behavior into the wisdom of caring for themselves.

As a whole, women carry the instinct and natural impulse to feed, nourish, and nurture. Unfortunately, through centuries of society's perversion of a woman's natural life-generating force and characteristics, her own understanding of these innate maternal qualities has become distorted and misplaced. As a result, women tend to be more susceptible to the emotion of fear. We spend a good deal of time feeling inadequate and worrying about myriad of things we fear.

When asked about their primary worry, all of the women in the group expressed concerns for others and what would happen to their family, children, husbands, parents, and work if they were to become further disabled. Although a deep anxiety, fear of dying was their *secondary* concern. Blissfully, we can change all the fear globules around us into the energy of primal security as we put into practice the inner rituals of the nityas and strive to live in alignment with their moon cycles.

A WOMAN'S TIME WITH THE MOON

The ancients claimed that all substance of life is created from the dust of Mother Moon, the cosmic source. The moon's perpetual cycle determines all rhythms, desires, and possibilities on the earth. Its luminous and visibly shifting shape keeps our heads craning upwards to the magical skies and heavens. The moon significantly influences a woman's biorhythms and her body, mind, and spirit are intricately connected to her cycles. Her ovum is *artava*, from the Sanskrit root *rtu* meaning season. Rtu also implies "ritual," suggesting that the rhythm of life comes from the ritual dance of the seasons and, in particular, the lunar season. In her Shakti, a woman also carries the healing and regenerative powers of the cycles within her.

What we know about our internal rhythms and their relationship to the greater energies of the cosmos can literally save our lives. We can learn the healing secrets of the cosmic pulse by paying attention to our own cycles and rhythms. Human sustenance and well-being are tied to the turn of the lunar wheel, and women are the cosmic keepers of the moon time. Throughout time, native traditions honored the moon and her manifold phases recognizing the prosperity and nurturance that she brings with each subtle turn and change: the Moon of Popping Trees, Silver Salmon Moon, Garlic Harvest Moon, Moon of the Serving of the Rice, Moon of the Great Heat, Moon of the Cold Dew, Moon of the Falcon, Moon of the Bat, Moon of the Deer, Moon of the Frog, Moon of the Turtle, Moon of the Buffalo Bull Hunt, Moon of the Deer's Antler-Shedding, Moon of the Falling Leaves, Moon of the Lotus, Jasmine Moon, Snow Moon, Strawberry Moon, Raspberry Moon, Sandalwood Moon, Peacock Moon, Swan Moon, Crow Moon, Hare Moon, Cow Moon, and so on.

Less than a century ago, the names given to the moon told the whole story of a people's rhythmic way of life. Living in accord with the lunar calendar maintained the ancestral memory of the crones. This way of being, of honoring the cyclical, circular movement of time kept their vibrant memory alive. People had an intimate relationship with nature and the earth as they moved from day to day in rhythm with the lunar wheel.

Indigenous life kept a constant momentum. Foraging and gathering food, digging into the black earth, chasing animals, cutting wood, feeding fire, and performing daily rituals were the activities that maintained a limber body and healthy spirit. After such arduous physical exercise, no one suffered from Chronic Fatigue Syndrome. Women did not experience breast and uterine cancer, osteoporosis, endometriosis, obesity, and food disorders. No one died of a degenerative disease. On the contrary, the well-being and intuitive power of the individual, family, and community flourished.

When this natural movement within nature ended because of the trend toward immobilized agriculture, we lost our rhythm with Mother Moon. This loss of knowledge of the moon cycles has resulted in the loss of the precious human gift of intuition. In later pages, you will find how our intuitive ability is maintained by the rhythmic breath of living in harmony with Mother Moon.

KEEPING THE RHYTHM ALIVE

In the farming village on the coast of the Atlantic Ocean in South America where I grew up, the sadhana of living was maintained in harmony with nature's rhythms with rituals passed down from the memory of the Motherland. Separated from the traditional soil of India, my people dedicated their energies to the preservation of the old ways. The fields, waters, skies, forests, animals, and earth were sacred, and they were stewarded by the timing wisdom of the lunar calendar.

The morning meal was the most important meal of the day. It represented the end of the daily moon cycle and the beginning of the sun cycle. Yellow mung dhal and whole wheat chapati was the usual feast. The meal began with my mother offering the first bite to the goddess in the fire in her wood stove. My father then led the grace for the bounty of the meal. We ate with our hands, a mudra custom that goes back to ancient times, as you will discover. (The fingers represent the five elements, and in using the hands to touch the food we are able to evoke these elements within ourselves). Because we ate from our hands, the taste of the food was transformed into a magical feast of shifting sights, sounds, and flavors. I continue to grow most of my foods by the wisdom of the lunar wheel, eat from my own hands, and honor the magic of my ancient roots. I am never far away from the bosom of Mother.

VEDIC WHEEL OF TIME: MANDALA OF THE MOON

For our female ancestors, the counting of each month began with the minute sterling sliver of a moon, the first sign of light in the dark sky. A disappearing moon marked the end of the month. Ancient cultures referred to the dark days of the moon as the "Sleeping Moon," "Resting Moon," "Woman's Moon," "the days of lying down," or "the marked days," intuiting that the Supreme Goddess was skillfully working as she retreated with her *nityas* into the womb of her moon to replenish its vitality for the next cycle. Mother's first rising from below the vast depths of the western horizon was always hailed with joy, a celebration of the Supreme Goddess's act of resurrection.

The silver crescent of the new moon heralded a new month, a fresh new beginning of time. The crescent moon is displayed on the flags of many Middle Eastern and North African countries, including Nepal, Pakistan, Turkey, Algeria, Libya, Singapore, and Tunisia. In C.E. 631, Muhammad sent two devout Muslims to the top of a mountain to observe the first crescent moon. This observance marked the beginning of the 12 lunar months of the Islamic calendar. Seventeenth century Japanese poet Basho puts it best, "Burn the house down to see the rising moon." When we consider that every moment of time is created by the moon herself, this recommendation may not be so rash! Early natives celebrated the first sighting of the new moon. Vedic tradition declared the new moon as a crucially auspicious time called *amavasya* because it signifies the goddess's emanation of rebirth that was destined to grow bolder in awesome splendor into the full moon, *purnima*. The full moon is also a crucial time for celebration. Even today, devout Hindus celebrate the significant moon cycles with prayers, worship, fasting, feasting, vows, and offerings to the deities. Ultimately, the moon is an intoxicating symbol of rhythm and the most ancient way of marking time.

The Vedic astronomers plotted out our vast history by the cycles of the moon. This calendar—known as the Wheel of Time, *kalachakra*—comes from their vast knowledge of the cosmos and its relation to the greater energies. The Vedic calendar is determined by the lunar cycles, divided into two fortnightly periods, *pakshas*, and 30 lunar days, *tithis*. These 30 days are equivalent to 29.53 solar days. The first fortnight, *shukla paksha*, is the bright cycle of the waxing phase that begins at the new moon. The dark fortnight, *krishna paksha*, or the waning phase, begins at the full moon.

The Vedas say that the kalachakra represents the history of eternity as it evolved from Lalita, Supreme Goddess of Eternity, whose peerless beauty is praised by the gods and goddesses. It reveals that there are 16 major phases in life (explained in detail in Chapter Sixteen) each of which is represented by a notch in the lunar wheel, which keeps time and bears its significant record in time and space. Fifteen rays of light emanating from the moon called nityas, forms of Lalita, mark the same number of lunar days of the waxing moon, not counting the full moon. In other words, nityas are the changing projections of Lalita who represents the full circle of time.

Although we can perceive her altering shapes and forms, the moon reflects the unchanging nature of Lalita's eternity. The full moon, which falls on the 16th day of the waxing moon, is referred to as *Sadakhya*. This is considered the 16th phase of the moon, represented by Tripurasundari, full moon personified as Lalita. The nityas are considered lunar deities named after their individual Shakti power emanating from their Supreme Source, Lalita, and each has their own sacred mantra, yantra, and rituals. These sacred practices, found on the following pages, bring abundant health, wealth, and well-being to humanity when performed in accord with the appropriate tithi, or lunar day.

The crones knew that consciousness is set in motion by the vibration, rhythm, and cyclical circle of time, marked by the moon's shifting shape. Among the oldest discoveries of a 16-notched moon cycle is that of a 30,000-year old piece of bone unearthed in the Dordogne region of France; the 16 notches are thought to mark the lunar cycle. Another ancient bone with 16 notches was discovered in equatorial Africa, as well.

The critical moon phases and their potent energies influence our lives in more ways than we can imagine. Although we are aware of it, each day in the circle of living we experience these 16 lunar transitions in subtle ways—four lunar transitions occur in each phase of the day between dawn to midday to dusk to midnight and back to dawn. For example, in the first phase that occurs from dawn to midday we experience awakening, lightness, mobility, and pause.

Reclaiming our biorhythms means recognizing the impact of the lunar junctures on our personal healing and transformation. Before we journey with the nityas to discover their nature and meaning in our lives, let us examine the two significant junctures of the moon's waxing and waning cycles.

FOLLOWING THE MOON

The moon's transition from one phase to the next is known as the lunation cycle. During the waxing moon, shukla paksha, the lunar cycle moves from new moon to full as the Eternal Lalita projects her stupendous power through the changing shapes of the nitya deities in the night sky. The waxing moon begins to gather strength and brings with it the energy of potency, regeneration, and rejuvenation. A harbinger of rest, reprieve, and strength gathering, the waxing moon offers a natural period for women to absorb and retain their health, wealth, and creativity.

During the roughly 14 days of the waning cycle, krishna paksha (when the moon is in transit from full to new), there is a dominant force of cleansing and reorientation. The waning cycle offers ample opportunity to expend energy, complete tasks, strengthen our breath power and life force, detoxify and cleanse the organism, and bring the fruits of our labor to completion.

NEW MOON: SEASON OF RETREAT

The Menstrual Cycle

The moon cycles reflect the five natural progressions of creation: birth, growth, fruition, dissolution, and death. The new moon marks the time of rebirth and renewal. Women naturally seek their rebirth at every new moon by releasing their profound life-making material back to the earth. Describing the women folk traditions in India, author and activist Pupul Jayakar states, "Blood fecundates the earth and through a magical process of alchemy transforms it into rain and food." As you will see, the new moon is the natural time in the lunar circuit to menstruate. Menstruation is caused by the sun absorbing energies from the earth, which in turn draws the womb's lining from the body in accord with its cyclical need for renewal and replenishment. Ancient women honored the menstrual blood as the essential life-generating material willed by Mother Moon to cleanse and purify their inherent Shakti energy so that new and fragrant life can blossom. A woman's monthly blood comes from the red bindu, or "cosmic seed" of Goddess Shakti, located in the root chakra where kundalini lies.

The ancient Sumerian city of Uruk arose between 4000 B.C.E. and 3000 B.C.E. in the alluvial plains between the Tigris and Euphrates rivers. In the Uruk record, it is stated that the reigning queen of the Third Dynasty of Ur took to ritual offerings to the moon in the final days of her dark cycle, or new moon phase. This culture believed that a drumming ritual would resurrect and return the moon from the underworld. Describing the ancient tradition of the Uruk, Layne Redmond states, "This monthly ritual drumming may also have facilitated the flow of menstrual blood. Menstrual cycles and lunar cycles retained their ancient association; references from the ancient world suggest that women normally menstruated en masse at the dark of the moon."

The cosmic genesis of a woman's magical anatomy can be traced to the ancient Sanskrit names referring to her procreative anatomy. The vagina is known as *chandra-mukha*, moon-faced; a particular blood vessel in the vulva is called *chandra-mauli*, moon crested, and, as you'll see, her ovulation and menstrual powers are strengthened by the lunar rhythms.

Ancient Ayurveda sages recognized that the moon significantly influences a woman's biorhythms and that her body, mind, and spirit were intricately connected to her cycles. When the cycle is in a state of balance and not impaired by the use of contraceptive pills, birth control devices, disruptive sexual activities, and harmful foods and medicines, the natural ebb and flow of a woman's monthly cycle remains in harmony with the cycles of the moon.

During the period of menstruation, activities need to be reduced to the essentials so that the body, mind, and spirit may flow in accord with the natural rhythms of the new moon. Retreating from the normal routine and everyday intrusions is necessary so that you may remain mindful of the great transformational experience of shedding the lining of the uterus (endometrium) so that it can be renewed once more.

THE WISDOM OF THE ANCIENTS

There are many contra-indications associated with the menstrual cycle. Many of these are based in the wisdom of the cosmic rhythms and have been handed down from the Vedic tradition. However, modern interpretations of these have often been misconstrued, as many of the dharmas (universal truths) have been when they are perverted to meet the standard of colonization and neo-Christian religious and political motivation of Western civilization. Instead of looking at it through this lens, let's explore the authentic and logical basis for these contra-indications from the Vedic perspective.

Caution: No bathing during the menstrual cycle/new moon.
Vedic Explanation: Vata dosha is prevalent during this time. Vata is the air principle whose nature is erratic, dark, cold, and ungrounded. At the purely physi-

ological level, the body needs to be kept cosseted, protected, and stabilized with the least degree of intrusion so that the necessary discharge can be pulled by its own rhythm and completed without interruption.

Caution: No swimming or washing the hair during the menstrual cycle.
Vedic Explanation: At the psycho-energetic level, we need to safeguard the body against the persuasive rhythm of the water element. Water is one of five powerful elements used to bless, cure, heal, nourish, nurture, and revive the body, mind, and spirit—liquid moonlight that folds us back into the memory of the Goddess. Every day in India millions of Hindus pay homage to Ganga Mata, Goddess of the River, honoring the Mother with specific ritual ceremonies. When driven by the tune of an adverse rhythm, the same blessing can turn into a tsunami, glacier, avalanche, hurricane, or storm that takes to fracturing the balance of the earth. Unlike the mundane understanding of cleansing we have, the ancients knew that water is sacred and powerful, and like all the elements has its own cosmic energy and memory. Water, guided by its cosmic memory, can influence the flow of the menstrual cycle to its own strong beat—exactly what we do not want to have happen during menses. Conversely, we want the fire element, which is the dominant memory of the blood, to flow in tempo with its own rhythm and tune.

Caution: Avoid gardening, cooking, and being near the preparation of food during our cycle.
Vedic Explanation: This is not due to the irrational thinking that our menstrual blood is unclean, unhygienic, or toxic. The cosmic memory of food—that which is derived only from plant life according to the Vedas—is imbued with prana, a rising energy flowing up from the earth toward the sun and sky. Conversely, our menstrual blood is instilled with apana vayu, the downward-flowing, bodily air pulled down from the body by the magnetic forces of the earth. These two powerful sadhanas do not go hand in hand. Plant-derived food is also Kapha in nature, full of youth-giving energy that nourishes the body; menstrual blood is dominated by Pitta and Vata, which fosters the cleansing of the spirit. It is most unwise to introduce the rising, energizing nature of our food into our blood, or to mix the downward-flowing, cleansing energy of blood into our sustenance, either by preparing food during our menstrual cycles or by slaughtering animals and eating them.

Even if your cycles don't coincide with the moon's rhythms, you can observe the Vata nourishing practices during the new moon in order to eventually restore your natural cycle. You will find these practices, along with the Kapha-nourishing sadhanas to be used during the time that follows menstruation, to continue building your inner wisdom. Details on these wondrous practices are set out in Chapter Fourteen.

THE INTELLIGENCE OF THE FEMININE

Each phase of life has its own intelligence shaped from eternal memory, and each has its own rhythm, which calls for its own set of conditions. The period of the menstrual cycle prepares cosmic matter for reproducing life; planting, cooking, and preparing food nourishes and sustains this life. Once you gain this understanding, you may practice the sadhanas that help support each awesome moment. It is a matter of awareness. Learn how to let these significant junctures support and help you build your wisdom—just as Naomi did.

Naomi, who was attending a program on Ayurveda & Women's Health at Wise Earth School, came to see me after class. She appeared listless, her skin sallow and drawn. She told me that it was her 36th birthday. For five years, she had been living with anorexia, a serious food disorder that had grown progressively worse. She was also suffering from a psychogenic amenorrhea, which is temporary cessation of the menstrual cycle generally caused by malnutrition, stress, tension, fatigue, low body weight, or exertion. Before her period stopped, her menstrual cycle was erratic and had shifted toward the full moon, a sign that her biorhythms were seriously out of balance. Ironically, Naomi was a board certified OB/GYN and a very bright woman. She confessed that she had been pushing herself to exhaustion in an effort to build her private practice in Los Angeles where she had been treating female patients for the past three years.

It was quite obvious to me that Naomi was extremely stressed and needed to pause, step back, and take stock of her life and its priorities so she may discover her joy. As with all individuals who experience food disorders and/or amenorrhea, joy is the crucial element to resolving their distressed condition. I advised her to do the Uttara Vasti therapy (detailed in Chapter Five) with the new moon until her cycle returned. I also told her that even though she did not have her menses, she shouldn't bathe on the new moon or the day after. When I told her this, she got angry and told me that she didn't see the point. I told her to please humor me. I also instructed her on crucial changes in her daily activities such as waking up in the morning with the sun, sitting in an early morning meditation, preparing a healing pot of *kichadi* (basmati rice with split mung bean) every day, and taking a daily walk after dinner while doing a simple breathing practice so she could relearn her relationship to food and nurturing through the daily and seasonal rhythms.

She eagerly took to the Uttara Vasti, but accommodating the food sadhana practice was altogether another matter. She did everything she could to resist having a direct relationship with her food and nourishment. As Naomi continued her studies at Wise Earth, I began to learn more about her. Her father and mother had divorced when she was 14 years old. Shortly afterwards, she began her menarche. When she started college she moved in with her father, the successful owner of a business that exported American beef all over the world. As far back as she could remember, the smell of raw meat and blood made her nauseous and caused her to vomit. She became a vegetarian at the age of 16, but had retained the memory of meat, blood, and gore, and its association with food, causing her to be repelled by any form of nourishment.

As she slowly worked her way into the kitchen, refurbishing it into a sadhana shrine designed after Wise Earth School's kitchen, she put the knowledge of the food sadhanas she had learned to use. The sadhana practice of rhythmically grinding aromatic spices in a *suribachi* was an irresistible attraction for Naomi. She ground and ground the spice seeds until she had successfully replaced the stench of raw animal blood and flesh, a deep sense memory of death that she had retained throughout her earlier years, with the healthful, fragrant scent of wholesome life. One year later, her menstrual cycle arrived.

Like clockwork, it came on her birthday, which was also the anniversary of the day she first saw me when she came to Wise Earth. She was so overjoyed that her confidence began to swell in leaps as she invested more time exploring the pure magic of sadhana. She is now deeply involved in the healthy preparations of her meals and teaches Wise Earth work at her medical office. Without a trace of anger or resistance remaining about the universal protocols of to bathe or not to bathe, Naomi now instructs her students on the fine art of honoring their feminine cycles during menses. Naomi still experiences some challenging moments with the dynamic approach of Wise Earth Ayurveda. While she is fascinated by the depth and rapidity of her own healing as proof of Wise Earth Ayurveda's effectiveness, she needs time to transition from a decade-long period of training with conventional medicine. (I've noticed that conventional scientists, physicians, and educators have great difficulty grasping and dealing with following a spiritual path that can't be backed by conventional science. Perhaps, due to the strong development of their mental faculties, they take longer to develop their spiritual largess.)

In a recent letter to me she wrote, "Wise Earth Ayurveda's paradigm does not have sufficient scientific documentation or proof of its healing concepts." Having heard this opinion from many of my students who are physicians and nurses, I had to smile. I wrote back and informed her that, indeed, we do need to document Ayurveda's incredible resurgence and age-old success in treating diseases. However, we must also consider that the Vedic seers were some of the greatest scientists and physicists that ever lived. Compared to modern scientists who research, investigate, and analyze the sciences to learn what they do not know while they create massive havoc within nature's blueprint, the ancient seers gently explored, developed, and disseminated the cosmic sciences from a wealth of knowledge of what they already had discovered about the universe. Moreover, they deeply respected the universe's intelligence, always honoring—never competing or battling with—the source of its genius.

FULL MOON: SEASON OF NURTURANCE

The Ovulation Cycle

The lunar phases were observed by the ancient people to ensure the nourishment and protection of sacred life. The rituals and ceremonies performed during the various aspects of the moon cycle kept the human memory alive and thriving. Native women faithfully observed seasonal rhythms to ensure the earth's sustenance and nourishment, and recognized that the cycles of the seasons, like the rhythms of the womb, were created from the moon's phases.

At the opposite spectrum of the dark days of the new moon is the light period of hope and rejuvenation celebrated at the time of the full moon. The full moon marks the time of beautification, abundance, and fertility, the result of transformation and purification of the primordial blood into the translucent essence of ojas. True to the feminine form, the moon is seen as the matriarch of all planets, herbs, sacrifices, austerities, rituals, arts, music, festivities, and dance.

The beginning period of the full moon is the natural cycle for ovulation and the most potent time of nurturance for women. During ovulation, Pitta dosha is most dominant. I will elaborate on the full moon practices that support Pitta in Chapter Fourteen.

Blessed with increasing moonlight and the powerful energy thrust from Goddess Lalita and her divine emanations during the waxing phase, a woman's ojas naturally increases. Her sexual vitality is once more replenished. During this time, healing sadhana practices such as oil massage, aromatherapy, warm baths, moonlight dips in water, and the use of healing gems appropriate to your metabolic type, are appropriate.

From the menstrual cycle to ovulation and back again, a woman's anatomy of consciousness is revealed. Primordial matter once cleansed and revived during menses is renewed once more for the making of life. Controlled by the energy of the lunar deities, eggs grow and develop in the womb during the moon's waxing cycle between menses and ovulation. Studies show that the immune system cells known as lymphoid aggregates also begin to develop in the wall of the uterus during this time. At the physiological level, this may explain why you may experience an abundant surge of creative and sensual energies, vibrantly growing in tandem with the moon as she becomes brighter and brighter.

At the full moon when ovulation is at its natural peak, neuropeptides FSH (follicle stimulating hormone) and LH (luteinizing hormone) cause the rise of estrogen levels in the body. On the other hand, our emotional need to withdraw from the world of activity and retreat into a time of introspection happens almost immediately after the full moon. During the waning cycle following the full moon, the body, mind, and spirit also wane. A woman naturally yearns for quietude and resolve. At this time, you can do serene practices such as meditation, journaling, drawing, painting, fasting, and other heart-opening activities that build and strengthen your inner harmony. You will find wonderful sadhana practices for the waning lunar cycle to draw from in Chapter Fourteen.

To honor the goddess and mark the auspicious cycles of her lunar wheel, Hindus perform elaborate sacred rituals with yantra, mantra, tantra, and prayogas. On the eve of the full moon of Ashvini (September-October), the harvest festival of Kojagara is celebrated with a night vigil of prayers and festivities. As legend has it, Goddess Lakshmi descends to the earth on this auspicious night to bless us with wealth and prosperity. The village women tell the ancient story of a queen whose husband's wealth was lost and then regained due to her night vigil and profound devotion to the Goddess Lakshmi. In his magnificent ode to the feminine beauty of the full moon, Kalidasa (India's poet laureate) tells it best:

A diadem adorns the night of multitudinous stars
Her silken robe is white moonlight
Set free from cloudy bars
And on her face the radiant moon
Bewitching smiles are shown.

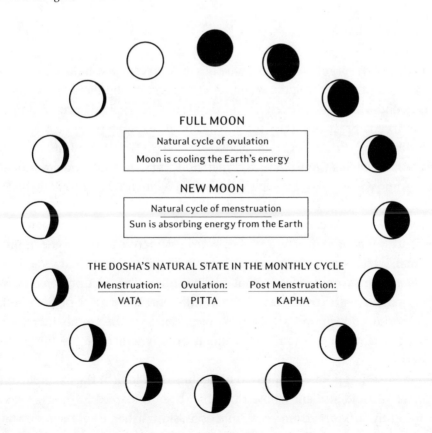

FULL MOON

Natural cycle of ovulation
Moon is cooling the Earth's energy

NEW MOON

Natural cycle of menstruation
Sun is absorbing energy from the Earth

THE DOSHA'S NATURAL STATE IN THE MONTHLY CYCLE

Menstruation:	Ovulation:	Post Menstruation:
VATA	PITTA	KAPHA

Chart 4.1 Moon Chart: Menstruation and Ovulation Phases

Chapter Five

CARE OF THE WOMB: INTRODUCTION TO UTTARA VASTI

Sharanagata dinarta paritrana parayane
Sarvasyarti hare Devi Narayani namo'stu te.

Salutations are to you, O Narayani
O you who are intent on saving the distressed
and the dejected that takes refuge under you
O you, Divine Mother, who remove the
sufferings of all!

WHAT IS UTTARA VASTI?

Among the many forgotten gems of wisdom in Ayurveda is Uttara Vasti, a practice of cleansing and nourishing the womb. A warm and loving therapeutic treatment, its effectiveness has been proven by thousands of women who have used this Wise Earth Ayurveda practice successfully to heal and realign a plethora of conditions. Unlike douching, this practice is guided by your internal rhythms and specific conditions, as well as time, place, age, metabolic type, mental, and emotional conditions. Almost every day, I receive letters from women who are astonished at the speed and profundity of its healing repair.

In Ayurveda's galaxy of effective therapies, Uttara Vasti is the single most essential practice for a woman. The Sanskrit word *vasti* refers to the stomach lining of the animal, which was used in ancient times to create the first Uttara Vasti therapy bag. *Uttara* means womb, cosmos, that which is filled. The wise perceive the womb as uttara—filled with contentment and fulfillment, the carrier of life itself. The main reason we do Uttara Vasti is to restore balance to the womb, thereby bringing back our female cycle to the new moon from wherever in the lunar wheel it has strayed.

Uttara Vasti is a powerful method of healing. Just look at the example of Katherine, a 42-year old student whose cycle had been impaired for many years. She was constantly suffering from yeast infections, skin rashes, depression, irritability, lethargy, and insomnia. Within three months of practicing Uttara Vasti, she was a transformed person. Her cycle had shifted to the new moon where it needed to be, the rash was gone, her skin looked great, and she was sleeping soundly for the first time in a decade! She had rediscovered her vitality and virility. Katherine tells her story in her own words.

> *What I love about Uttara Vasti is that I feel 10 years younger, full of life, and now I can embrace the idea of taking time for myself. The first time I did UV I couldn't believe how nourished I felt, the warmth of the tea inside of me. Then I took a bath with the left over decoction and oiled myself with sesame oil afterward and just meditated and went to bed. I feel like it is a time I take to really love myself.*

WOMEN'S HEALTH—REDEFINED

Modern, sanitized society sees menstruation as an unclean, mundane, and inconvenient happening that may as well be pushed back into oblivion with sanitized pads or tampons and disinfected with antiseptic douching formulas. It is important that we understand that Uttara Vasti has no relationship to "douching" as we know it. Unlike Uttara Vasti, douching has nothing to do with healing; most modern women use douching for hygienic and cosmetics reasons—more like a cleansing detergent rather than a treatment for specific conditions.

Commercial, over-the-counter douching products as well as those prescribed by doctors have been proven harmful to the health of women. A current medical advisory warns that frequent and excessive douching can increase the risk of infections, such as pelvic inflammatory disease, bacterial vaginosis, chlamydial infection, premature birth, sexually transmitted diseases, and cervical cancer. The Ness study conducted in 2002 by a team of gynecologists and obstetricians indicated that 87 percent of the 1,200 women interviewed who were using popular commercial brands of douching products reported incidents of bacterial vaginosis after use. When these commercial douches were tested in vitro, it was discovered that they inhibited natural vaginal microorganisms, thereby disturbing the eco-balance of vaginal flora. One popular commercial brand contains everything from D&C red #28 to diazolidinyl urea.

This was the brand Pamela has started using when she first reported a recurring problem with vaginal yeast infections, erratic cycles, and a nasty vaginal rash. A 40-year old nurse practitioner who came to study at Wise Earth School, Pamela was willing to "try anything" to get rid of her problem. Jenny, a Wise Earth instructor whose classes Pamela was attending, recommended that she stopped using the commercial douching formula and use instead the Uttara Vasti therapy with the Triphala-Aloe Decoction (see page 83). Jenny also advised Pamela that the safest and most potent time to do the practice was for two days on the next new moon cycle. In this way, she would both treat the condition and bring her cycle back in consonance with the new moon. Eager to try the practice, Jenny started to do the Uttara Vasti bath with the recommended decoction. The next time she came to class about three months later, Pamela appeared joyful. She reported that after only two bath applications her infection and vaginal rash were both gone.

Pamela is now a dedicated student of Wise Earth Ayurveda and is attempting to bring these teachings to the nurses in the hospital where she works. I always find it interesting to find women who are seeking holistic approaches to heal their disease when they have been firmly indoctrinated to embrace the prescriptive, medical model of healing. Not at all reconciled to the natural approach, many attend my workshops out of sheer desperation. In all cases, I sense in them a hunger, an inexplicable yearning to return to their natural roots. Like Pamela, many such women work patiently to learn how to shift their trained perspectives and habits to embrace their natural rhythms.

JOANNE'S STORY

This reorientation is not always an easy process to accomplish. I can always expect to be interrupted and/or confronted with sheer, unmitigated fire afterward, sometimes even in the midst of my presentation. But nothing could have prepared me, or my assistants, or the hundreds of attendees at a conference in San Francisco in 1992 for the incomparable Joanne. While the students were receiving my transmission on Shakti energy and learning of the infinite value of Uttara Vasti, Joanne, who sat right in front of me in the first row, was obviously agitated. By the time the assistants began demonstrating the making of the Uttara Vasti decoction, and showing the Ayurveda therapy bag, Joanne was beet red in the face with fury. Finally, the poor woman could bear no more. She jumped up with lightning rapidity, pulled the Uttara Vasti therapy bag from my assistant, and started to strike her with the bag! The participants quickly rose to the assistant's aid and peeled Joanne away from her.

The class took a break as the women gently escorted Joanne outdoors in the courtyard. I went out to see Joanne to try to calm her and to find out why she went ballistic. I instructed the assistants to make her some raspberry tea, excellent for soothing Joanne and her liver, anger being a response from the impairment of this organ. She was so tense that I sensed her body was held harder than the board we sat on. As my voice became gentler, Joanne jumped up and started to shout at me in indecipherable syllables that sounded like choked and painful squeals. Once more, the women stepped in to cajole her, and served her the tea. I returned to finish the class, and left my home address with her, asking her to write to me and let me know why this education has stirred such a deeply disturbing response. I felt sad to see her lose her self-control to such a profound extent. Perhaps, it was my voice that struck the wrong cord—or the right cord depending on which perspective you take.

Although I have encountered only a few unhappy campers in a quarter century of teaching Wise Earth Ayurveda's Inner Medicine healing ways, I understood that, for many people, this education isn't easy to follow. Obviously, the ancient knowledge of self and nature reaches a deep place within and stirs old, unresolved beliefs and dogmas. I kept Joanne in my meditation and knew that she would write to me when she was ready.

Joanne's letter arrived in the spring of 1995—exactly three years after her amazing outburst. I had since moved to another address, but somehow her letter found me. My book, *Ayurveda: A Life of Balance*, had just been published and Joanne had purchased a copy for herself. She apologized for her behavior, and set out to tell me her story in a 20-page tome. Joanne told me that her husband had physically and emotionally abused her for more than a decade before she finally had the courage to up and leave him shortly before she stumbled into my class. She was angry at her mother, also abused by her husband, an alcoholic for as long as Joanne could remember. At the time Joanne came to class, she was beaten up, frightened, lonely, angry, jobless, and childless. She had a fibroid the size of a breadfruit which she has since had surgically removed. She said my role as a Spiritual Mother rubbed her the wrong way, and that the power of my voice wrenched at her gut. At that moment, she felt a violent hatred toward me.

Not surprising, since many women who have problematic relationships with their earthly mother often transfer this anger toward the Spiritual Mother. Something touched her so deeply that she was offended and terrified to the core. Joanne's intense response was actually hatred toward herself. She saw a woman who was seen as a Spiritual Mother, one who was physically, and emotionally free from the tethers of life and in complete control, a reality which served only to heighten Joanne's sense of fragility and helplessness in that particular moment. As she wisely pointed out in her missive, her intense reaction forced her to open the gateway to her journey of healing. No coincidence that Joanne chose my book as the pivotal tool for her healing.

According to Joanne, that solemn day when she lost her face in public marked the first of many days of her conscious effort to find herself. She felt inclined to begin her holistic approach to life with a change of diet and nutrition. She informed me that she was fond of the Wise Earth Ayurvedic way of cooking and that the menus in my book were a blessing for her. Although she still has some resistance, she is imbibing in nurturing Uttara Vasti baths from time to time.

For me, Joanne represents millions of women who respond with frustration and angst at any approach that strays from the western medical model that looks at a woman's fertility as a "crisis" rather than as a result of natural changes in a women's female cycle. Because the intrusive and negative solutions for feminine care such as tampons, antiseptic douching agents, hormone patches, and HRTs have become the norm, another approach can be frightening for many women.

Others like Alice have discovered how easy it is to honor their feminine rhythms and heal. Unfortunately, it took a devastating sexually transmitted disease for Alice to come to this work. Since she was a teenager, Alice had been plagued with uncontrollable rage. After five years of conventional psychological therapy and two divorces, she turned to spiritual practices such as yoga and meditation to heal her anger. Her anger was subsiding and she appeared to be on the mend with her temper. Then she met Ray, a middle-aged man 10 years older than her, at a yoga class, fell head over heels in love with him, and moved into his flat two months later.

Her mother, Jeanne, a Wise Earth senior practitioner, was very unhappy about the relationship and the rapidity with which Alice was moving into a sexual relationship with a virtual stranger. She confided in me that she did not trust Ray and that he had a reputation as a carouser. Although he appeared to be a gentle and quiet person, Alice's mother told me that Ray's ex-wife had divorced him citing irreconcilable differences due to emotional cruelty and infidelity on Ray's part.

As it turns out, Jeanne had good reason for being distrustful of Ray. Only three months after the nuptials, Jeanne brought Alice to the school to attend a meditation program. After the class, Alice asked to see me in private about a health problem. Before I could close the door to the satsanga hall where I would meet with people, Alice started to weep bitterly. She had gone to see her gynecologist a few weeks ago because she was feeling listless and feverish and was experiencing terrible burning in her vaginal passage. The day before she came to the school, she had received a phone call from her doctor informing her that the test indicated that she had contracted gonorrhea. Alice was devastated. At once, she was facing disillusionment with the man she had given her love, trust, and body to, and feeling strong anger about her impulsiveness and this betrayal.

I consoled Alice, advising her to take some time to herself to heal by putting distance between herself and Ray while she re-evaluated her physical and emotional needs. I gave Alice a regimen of Uttara Vasti on the new moon to be taken with the Triphala-Aloe Decoction and recommended a few Ayurvedic herbs and healthful foods (which are detailed in Chapter Six). I instructed her to follow my instructions for three months under her mother's expert guidance.

Alice called a month later. Her voice was light and cheerful. She had good news. She had been using Uttara Vasti and the food recommendations and felt more vibrant and composed than ever. She had just returned from visiting with her gynecologist and her doctor was shocked to discover that she exhibited no trace of symptoms, and tested free and clear of gonorrhea. (He wanted to learn more about Uttara Vasti and the Wise Earth program, and has since attended two of the practitioner training programs.) Alice left Ray, and has now begun a new life in close connection to her mother as she strives to learn more about herself, recognizing how to care for and respect her Shakti power.

THE COSMIC NATURE OF WOMAN

In order to fully comprehend the importance of Uttara Vasti, we should understand the meaning of Shakti. Long before modern science learned how to control a woman's sacred reproductive function and manipulate her intrinsic rhythms, the Vedic seers recognized that a woman's fertility, abundance, and splendor were tied to the movement of Shakti prana. This is the primordial feminine power of the Shakti that moves within the body and psyche of every female through a specific prana that circulates within the two lower chakras, located around the perineum and sacrum. Manifested as the procreative energy, Shakti prana flows within the genitals, womb, and belly of a woman.

Ancient *vaidyas* (Ayurvedic physicians) noted that women naturally possess a delicate and fragile balance within the body due to their Shakti prana and its extensive powers. When this equanimity is disturbed, they recognized that it would have long-term effects on the maternal strength and prowess of the woman, negatively influencing the maternal bedrock of all aspects of life. The ancients protected what we have neglected to preserve—a woman's creative primordial energy. Indeed, the health of the entire earth lies in honoring the female energy and its interconnection to nature's rhythms.

According to Wise Earth Ayurveda, a woman's natural rhythms are kept and preserved by her monthly menstrual cycle (ideally occurring with the new moon). At this time, menstruation is set in motion by the sun absorbing energies from the earth, which in turn draw the menstrual waste from the body. When the use of contraceptive pills and other birth control devices, harmful foods and activities, and disruptive sexual activities do not tamper with a woman's monthly cycle, it remains in harmony with the new moon.

Linda, a Wise Earth practitioner, tells the story of Martha, a 50-year old woman whose breast cancer disappeared after six months of Uttara Vasti. Martha did not want to take the conventional therapy recommended by her physician so Linda guided her into the Uttara Vasti therapy every month on the new moon. She cooked Wise Earth's healthful food and played my Vedic chanting CD for Martha during the six months of her therapy and now her cancer is completely gone. She has now continued the practice on her own. The last time they spoke, Martha said that she could now feel the Shakti in her belly—like a soft glow getting brighter with every practice. She told Linda she feels like she is walking on air, and that she was stunned by how quickly her cancer disappeared after taking the Uttara Vasti treatment. She called Uttara Vasti 'a loving therapy that is more than nourishing, it's nurturing.'

"I have since helped numerous women whose cycles were impaired and I am continually amazed at how quickly their cycles revert back to the new moon," says Linda. "In most cases, it happened after only one application of Uttara Vasti." Many of these women have told me the same thing that Martha said. They felt like they had a glow in their belly.

A WOMAN'S MOON

To understand Martha's remarkable recovery, we can examine the wisdom of the ancients. According to Wise Earth Ayurveda, a woman's magic is irretrievably linked to the moon. The ancients called the dark days of the moon "Woman's Moon," and "Resting Moon," linking a woman's physical, emotional, and spiritual state to the lunar wheel. The dark moon provides a cozy climate for a woman's sadhana of rest, reprieve, and replenishment. Mother Moon takes to recharging her Shakti during this time. Likewise, a woman is advised to create a gentle space to conserve her feminine powers and inculcate her creative potential during this time. At its first sighting from below the depths of the horizon, the rising moon was once hailed with joy and celebration. It stood for the Divine Mother's act of resurrection—a metaphor for the woman's menstrual cycle. A woman's menses greatly affects her Shakti prana; her monthly cycle is the primary means through which this prana is revitalized, cleansed, and restored.

The Vedic culture recognizes that a woman's blood preserves her Shakti and that this blood carries the Divine Mother's potential for new life and rebirth. This phenomenon may be attributed to the workings of the red bindu, located within the root chakra, as noted earlier. When Shakti prana is strong, the bindu acts as a magnetic lodestone, drawing in the energy of the moon to revitalize the womb. For this reason, the blood vessels within a woman's vulva carry the magnetic energies of the moon. The woman's womb is moon-shaped; her vagina, moon-crested; her menses, moon-blood; her juices, moon-nectar; her tears, pearl drops of moonlight; her hair is moon-mane; and her eyes are the light and dark moons. How strongly is a woman affected by the constantly changing rhythm of the moon? Lady Ise, a 10th century Japanese poetess, said it best, "When I have sad thoughts, even the moon's face embroidered on my sleeve is wet with tears."

The rhythm of the red bindu also causes a woman to discharge her uterine lining at the appropriate cyclical time during the new moon phase. As a result, her hormone levels are naturally reset. The process we call menses does not encompass the far-reaching magic and miracle of a woman's blood.

Native cultures of various faith traditions revered a woman's sacred connection to the lunar wheel. German peasants called the menstrual blood, *die Mond*, "the moon." The French called the monthly blood, *le moment de la lune*, "the movement of the moon." In China, the menstrual blood is said to be the yin principle, the primordial essence of Mother Earth that gives life to all things. The cycle of the moon is even suggested in the commonplace metaphor, "a woman's period." "Period" comes from the Greek term for "going round," the cycle of life.

In the past, a woman marked the passing of the months by her monthly cycle, and the number of children to whom she gave birth roughly marked the annual cycles. Native cultures guided their daily affairs by the appearance of the moon. Individuals, families, and communities marked their calendars by the crescent moon and then, again, by the full moon. The visibly changing shape of the luminary in the night sky was their sole calendar, and each culture named its nocturnal turn with names that sustained memory of their sacred relation to Mother Earth.

The time of the menstrual cycle is a very sacred and yet vulnerable period for a woman. Women who are menstruating are required to go at a slower pace and to allow the body to cleanse itself; they are also advised to pare down activities to the bare essentials so that body, mind, and spirit may experience the least degree of intrusion. Wise Earth Ayurveda recommends a minimum of bodily cleansing at this time. Quick, cool showers or wiping down the body will do. Refrain from sexual activities, as well as from all cooking activities. The latter measure is to prevent the energies from the powerful menstrual blood from pervading foods. Maintain a light wholesome diet of salads, fresh juices, light grains (basmati rice, millet, couscous, amaranth), pasta, tofu, leafy greens, and fresh fruits. Herbal teas such as raspberry, organic rose flower, peppermint, ginger, lemon balm, hops, and chamomile are also revitalizing during this time.

LEARNING FROM THE ANCIENTS

Wise husbands of yore recognized the heightened energy field within a woman's body, mind, and psyche during her menstrual time. They would plot out a piece of land in the forest and surround it with a stone wall, high enough so that the potent menstrual energy could not permeate beyond it. Women convened there to share their living stories while squatting to let their menses go back to the earth. Through their menstrual blood, they were putting the Shakti energy that had been transformed through their own bodies back into Mother Earth to continue the cycle of replenishment and regeneration. Nowadays, we have lost touch with this necessary continuum of fertilization—giving back to the earth the riches of our bodies as we evacuate so that the ongoing cycle of the earth's memory may be preserved.

Ancient women did not wear pads and tampons and all the other horrific products that now invade and desanctify the sacred yoni, vaginal passage. Amazing as it seems, they knew their personal rhythms. They knew exactly what time of day and month they would need to retreat to their bleeding sanctuary. Traditionally, during the menstrual time, women were served meals by the elder women. Children and young people were kept at a distance from the menstrual ground and lodge. Instinctively, the animals retreated deeper into the forest and away from the lodges. In fact, the ancient texts inform that the animals were terrified of the potency of the menstrual blood. They recognized that the lining of our inner moon was evacuating the procreative material of Shakti, which would be poisonous if imbibed by them.

THE PRACTICE: UTTARA VASTI

ALIGNMENT OF A WOMAN'S CYCLE WITH LUNAR RHYTHMS

When we lose our relationship with the lunar wheel we just go around and around "spinning our wheels" in a way that is undirected and unfocused. Even if your cycles no longer coincide with the moon rhythms, you may use the Uttara Vasti practice to restore your natural biorhythm. For those whose monthly cycle has ceased, continue to practice this sadhana for a few days during the new moon cycle until you are 60 years of age. It will help to maintain healthy hormonal levels, recall the natural rhythms of your Shakti prana, and revitalize your spirit.

Monthly application of Uttara Vasti in alignment with the new moon cycle is recommended. However, in the case of vaginal infections, and/or malodor, you may use the Uttara Vasti Bath as necessary at any time during the moon cycle for no more than three consecutive days. Use the Triphala-Aloe Decoction presented below for these conditions.

Get a calendar of the moon cycles. It provides you with information on the timing of the full moon and the new moon. You may learn the various notches of the lunar wheel and their significance to your daily lives. (See *Moon Chart: Menstruation and Ovulation Phases* on page 71.) Try to keep an eye up in the sky to view the changing moon. It wanes on the right side and waxes on the left. How do we remember that? You may memorize the word "wane-right." The waning moon is considered the time of the moon after the full moon. The waxing moon is the moon that comes after the new moon. We need to know this because the moon works with the exact rhythm and timing of our womb. *Dhara*, a Sanskrit word referring to both "bowl" and "womb" infers that we carry the moon inside the bowl of the womb.

WHEN TO PRACTICE:

In the event of a hysterectomy, it is still necessary to do the practice since there is now a void, a vacancy, or a feeling of loneliness inside the space that used to hold the womb. The practice should be done for some years after menopause to keep the energy of the womb and mind refreshed. Refrain from doing Uttara Vasti from 65 years of age and older; this is when the elderly want their Shakti to be left undisturbed so that they may wind up its mystery and wrap up their karmas.

CONDITIONS:

Practice Uttara Vasti under these circumstances: sexually active (16 years and older); vaginal infections, malodor, dryness, or soreness of vaginal passage; PMS; irregular or excess menstrual flow; venereal disease; infertility; hormonal imbalance; menopause; disorders of the uterus; breast cancer; directly after sexual intercourse; or as a birth control measure. For ovarian and uterine cancers, supervision by a qualified Ayurvedic physician is mandatory.

CONTRA-INDICATIONS:

Do not practice: during or right after menstruation, vaginal bleeding, or hemorrhaging; in extreme hot or cold weather; directly after eating; during diarrhea; after emesis, purgation, or enema; if emaciated; at certain daily junctures (sunrise, noon, sunset, midnight); if a woman or girl not yet sexually active (see bath instructions on pages 85-86); if pregnant (wait four months after delivery of child) or breast-feeding (wait one year then begin); directly after miscarriage (wait three months); directly before menses; during fibroid treatments or bleeding fibroids; and if a child under 12 years old.

APPROPRIATE TIMES FOR APPLICATION:

7:00-8:00 (morning and evening)

INAPPROPRIATE TIMES FOR APPLICATION:

Sundays and holy days; death anniversary of parents, spouse or children; dawn; dusk; noon; midnight; during dark moon cycle; or at full moon; *Yama Damstra** (November 20th-December 9th).

    *Yama Damstra occurs while the earth is reversing its course around the sun, from a southerly to northerly direction. At this time, it is said that Yama, Lord of Death, ventures out in earnest to collect the souls of the deceased. Because it is considered to be a time of heightened fear and disturbance for a human being, all cleansing and depleting practices are not advised during this period.

UTTARA VASTI SCHEDULES FOR MONTHLY USE:

Cycles in Harmony with the New Moon

Perfect Cycle: Menstruating on the new moon. Always wait two or three days after your cycle ends to do UV. For example, if your period occurs in the new moon cycle and ends on a Friday, do the UV on Monday, Wednesday, and Friday. In detail, if menstruating on the new moon, and your period ends on the 3rd, 4th, or 5th day after the new moon, then wait two days after your period has ended (6th and 7th day) and do the UV on the 8th or 9th day. If your cycle ends on the 8th or 9th day after the new moon, refrain from doing UV.

- The 1st through the 8th days of the new moon are appropriate.
- UV is most potent the 1st and 2nd days after the new moon.
- Never start UV on the night of the new moon, always begin one or two days after.

Cycles Out of Harmony with the New Moon

Impaired Cycle: Menstruating on the full moon. Always wait one day after the new moon begins to do UV. For example, if your period occurs in the full moon cycle, you would do the UV on the onset of the new moon. For example, if the new moon begins on Monday, do the UV on Tuesday, Thursday, and Saturday.

- The 1st through the 8th days of the new moon are appropriate.
- UV is most potent the 1st and 2nd days after the new moon.
- Never start UV on the night of the new moon, always begin one or two days after.

Menopausal Cycle

When the menstrual cycle stops, continue UV for five to seven years to help fortify your hormones and sensuality. If the cessation of period is premature and/or due to medical intervention, begin the use of UV following cessation and continue the practice until you are 60 years of age.

- The 1st through the 8th days of the new moon are appropriate.
- UV is most potent the 1st and 2nd days after the new moon.
- Never start UV on the night of the new moon, always begin one or two days after.

PREPARING UTTARA VASTI DECOCTIONS:

Use a double boiler when preparing the decoctions because they need a warm and gentle quality for introduction into the womb space. You don't want to introduce direct heat to the decoction, since it would have to be introduced through the lower pathways of the body. The lower pathways do not have the power of *agni*, digestive fire, to counteract direct heat. We want the treatment to be gentle.

INGREDIENTS:

red raspberry leaves

pink or red rose petals (organic)

aloe vera gel

triphala powder

1 large jug of water

UTENSILS AND EQUIPMENT:

One double boiler or, alternately, one large pot and one small bowl which fits loosely in the pot, two small stainless-steel pots, one metal strainer (4 to 5 inches in diameter); one reusable UV bag with douching nozzle; and two bath towels.

UTTARA VASTI FORMULAS:

Use a double boiler to prepare all douching solutions. All formulas listed yield one application each. Use only organically grown ingredients.

TRIPHALA-ALOE DECOCTION | ONE APPLICATION

Conditions: PMS, painful menstruation, premenstrual cramps, sterility, stagnation, venereal disease, prolapsed rectum, breast cancer, osteoporosis, and endometriosis.

2 cups water
1 teaspoon triphala powder
1 tablespoon aloe vera gel

Bring water to a boil in a double boiler. Add triphala powder, then cover and allow to simmer for approximately three minutes. Remove the container from heat and allow the solution to steep for 15 minutes. Strain through a fine sieve, retaining the sediment. Pour the aloe vera gel into the solution and pour the decoction into the UV bag. (You may add the sediment to your bath water following the treatment). Follow the directions on pages 84-85 for administering the treatment while it's still warm.

ROSE-RASPBERRY DECOCTION | ONE APPLICATION

Conditions: scanty menstrual flow, irregular or excessive menstrual flow, vaginal dryness, uterine disorders, vaginal malodor, soreness or dryness of the vaginal passage, and breast cancer.

2 cups water
1 tablespoon dried red rose buds
1 tablespoon dried raspberry leaves

Bring water to a boil in a double boiler. Add the dried leaves and buds, then cover and simmer on low heat for approximately five minutes. Remove the container from heat and allow the solution to steep for 15 minutes. Strain through a fine sieve, retaining the herbal roughage to add to your bath water following the treatment. Pour the decoction into the UV bag. (You may add the sediment to your bath water following the treatment). Follow the directions on pages 84-85 for administering the treatment while it's still warm.

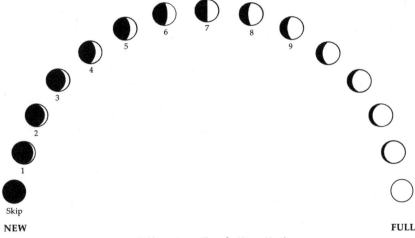

Table 5.1 Lunar Chart for Uttara Vasti

GATHERING HARMONY WITHIN

Keep in mind that healing is a sacred thing. It is a goddess-like quality. Always keep the spirit of quietude with and around you. Offer a prayer of gratitude before you apply your therapy, such as the following mantra of gratitude to the greater energies:

Brahmarpanam Brahma havih
Brahmagnau Brahmana hutam
Brahmaiva tena gantavyam
Brahmakarma samadhina
Om Shantih Shantih Shantih.

Brahman is the offering
Brahman is the oblation
Poured out by Brahman into the fire of Brahman
Brahman is to be attained by the one who recognizes
Everything as Brahman.

(Brahman refers to the Absolute One, Pure Consciousness)

Directions for Applying Uttara Vasti
- An oil massage or self massage is recommended before therapy.
- Observe a light diet on the UV therapy days.
- Spread a clean towel in the bathtub.
- Attach the nozzle to the UV bag and close the shut-off clip.

- Smear the nozzle with an ample amount of sesame oil or cocoa butter.
- Hang the UV bag containing the solution approximately three feet above where you will be lying.
- Undress and rest comfortably on your back with legs apart and knees bent.
- Take a few deep breaths.
- Close your eyes and feel every limb in your body relaxing.
- Insert the nozzle into the vaginal passage.
- Squeeze your buttocks firmly together and lift the hips slightly off the ground. (Some solution will spill in the process.)
- As soon as the UV bag is empty, relax the hips, release the nozzle from the vaginal passage, and allow the decoction to flow out gradually.
- Gently get up and remove the wet towel from the tub.
- Since the retention of decoction is so brief, you may immediately repeat the process.
- Afterwards, take rest in a warm and cozy space for a few hours.

UTTARA VASTI BATH

Many women in their 20s to 60s who are sexually active would not consider doing the Uttara Vasti therapy I've outlined in the preceding pages because they are fearful of a nozzle being inserted into the vagina. For these women, I have developed the Uttara Vasti Bath as an acceptable alternative, which I have found to be profoundly effective.

Appropriate Conditions:
Young girls; virgins; sexually inactive or celibate; aged or post-menopausal; victims of sexual abuse; women with fear of vaginal intrusion; women with miscarriage or abortion (to be performed four to six weeks after incident).

Exception: In the case of vaginal infections, and/or malodor, and sexual abuse you may use the Uttara Vasti bath at any time during the moon cycles as necessary for no more than three consecutive days. Use the Triphala-Aloe Decoction presented earlier for these conditions.

THE PRACTICE: UTTARA VASTI BATH

Fill the bathtub to about a quarter of the way up, adding one gallon of UV decoction to the warm water. (Choose the appropriate decoction for your condition.)
- Assume the squatting posture in the tub. Invite the water into the vaginal channel by

squeezing your buttocks firmly. Hold the extracted decoction in the vaginal channel
for about two minutes before releasing the buttocks muscles.
- Repeat this procedure three times.
- Dry yourself with the bath towel and gently massage your belly for a few minutes.
- Rest for a few hours after the therapy in a warm and cozy space.

Simply by sitting in a hip bath laced with decoction and contracting the vaginal muscles to absorb the healing water into the uterus, a wealth of healing can occur. Many women, both old and young, have shared the sense of happiness and lightness they experience after this gentle practice, like Seema.

Seema is a 14-year old girl who had migrated to America with her parents from a small village near Ahmenabad in Gujarat, India. Her menstrual cycle began at the tender age of 11, and since then she had been suffering from excessive bleeding with terrible cramps that would last almost 10 days of the month. Her period was obviously vitiated, as she was menstruating in the full moon cycle. By the time her mother, Savitri, brought Seema to see me she was frantic and scared about Seema's well-being. The girl approached me slowly with downcast eyes, slightly hunched over, and was obviously mortified to discuss her problem. She was a mere slip of a girl weighing only 85 pounds. Not surprisingly, I could see that Seema was extremely anemic. Savitri informed me that Seema had been isolating herself in her room since her menstrual cycle began, and was embarrassed to let her friends know about her cycle, since none of them had yet had theirs. I sensed that Seema was going through a period of shame and confusion, clearly not knowing what was happening with her and why.

I asked her mother to leave me alone with Seema. I talked to her about another young girl, Meegan, who had her cycle at an even earlier age than Seema, and explained how I helped Meegan to overcome her challenges by embracing her female nature. As my storytelling continued to unfurl, Seema appeared more and more alert, shifting into an upright position on her knees on the floor where she was sitting. I told her that, like Meegan, menstruation is a natural goddess-like rite that all girls must eventually go through to become a woman.

Noticing her visible relief, I asked Seema to go and bring her mother back into the room. As she arose she came over and gave me a hug and began weeping. I consoled her and asked her why she was crying. As I held her in my lap, she confided a startling secret. She thought that her bleeding was a horrendous act of punishment for leaving her sick maternal grandmother, who she calls "Nannie," behind in Ahmedabad. She was very close to her grandmother who had lived with her family and had helped to raise her since she was born. Doubtless, the grief Seema bore for the three years since she had left her Nannie had somehow contributed to the premature and heavy flow of her cycle.

I informed Savitri of her daughter's sadness and concerns about her grand-mother and asked her to continue the dialogue with her child when they returned home. I also gave Seema specific instructions on how to do the Uttara Vasti bath during the new moon phase and instructed her mother to follow the mineral rich food sadhana plan for Pitta type, set out in Appendix Two. I asked Savitri to assist Seema in the process. It was clear that, like many parents who love their chil-dren, Savitri did not recognize the necessity of taking her girl into her confidence, inquiring about her trauma, and walking her through the stories and pathways of the gift and awesome glory of what it is to become a young woman. To read more about a young girl's coming of age, see the Kala Ritu Menarchial Rites set out in detail in Chapter Fifteen.

Two months later, Savitri wrote me a note informing me that Seema's cramps were gone after the very first bath and that after the second new moon treatment, her period shortened to five days with regular flow. Six months later, Seema has continued with the practices. One of her friends has since begun her cycles and Seema was only too glad to be a guide to her. She is now doing exceedingly well, putting on weight, and integrating with her many friends. She told me that she will be returning with her family to Ahmenabad to visit with her Nannie during her summer break from school.

Like Seema, numerous young women have successfully reversed conditions such as premenstrual syndrome, menorrhagia, dysmenorrhea, amenorrhea, and leucorrhea, simply by using the Uttara Vasti Bath. (Read more about these condi-tions in Chapter Eight).

Part Three

WOMEN'S CONDITIONS

& INNER MEDICINE

REMEDIES

Chapter Six

YOUR OWN ENERGY IS
YOUR BEST MEDICINE

The beauty of sadhana is that it affords you absolute
simplicity, the path that leads you to your inner harmony.

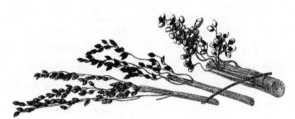

Figure 6.1 Coriander Plant

Our bodies are made of consciousness and spirit, and are connected to the greater continuum of energies through memory. In order to heal, we need to appease vital tissue memory and nourish and nurture the whole self. In essence, we need to reorder the same internal energy that goes into disorder that creates a disease, and bring it back into a state of harmony. In Inner Medicine healing, the main ingredient in any medicine is your own vital energy. Put simply—for you to be nourished and healed, your awareness along with the appropriate ingredients and proper timing must come together seamlessly in the preparation and imbibing of the remedies. In the Inner Medicine preparations that follow, you will be learning to use and enhance your internal forces—Shakti, buddhi, and elemental energies—which, in turn will strengthen your power to heal yourself.

Many women reject the idea of returning to nature's earthy ways. In the fast-paced, modern scheme of things, we tend to shy away from investing our own consciousness behind thoughts and activities we endeavor. In fact, the resistance you feel toward these sadhana measures bears a crucial clue to your disease. Had we maintained the harmonious ways of sadhana—using our highly-charged hands and feet to prepare our daily sustenance, plant the garden, reap the fruit, pound the whole grain into flour, grind the spice seeds with mortar and pestle, and thresh the fields—we would not be ill today. The same process of prana-generating life that we resist is the *identical* energy responsible for keeping us in good health and well-being! We have to want to reclaim these wholesome lifeways and vital energies if we are to heal ourselves.

The natural rhythmic practices gleaned from Mother Nature, which we call sadhana, will help you to accentuate your efforts in refining your energy and creating your perfect nourishment. Sadhana creates a life of balance. It is the natural way to heal and support the innate function of your vital tissue memory necessary for the healing process. Listen to your body, pay attention to the seasons. Your rhythms change with each season and therefore you must re-evaluate your conditions and needs at every seasonal juncture. Do not get into an endless cycle of taking medicines year after year. The more medicine you force into your body, the less effective *rasa's* operation becomes. Rasa, as you will see, is the Sanskrit name for the first vital tissue in your body.

After about three months of using the same remedy, rasa loses its effectiveness to project the medicinal essences into the tissue memory. Therefore, never take the same medicine for more than three months. Just a few weeks ago, I overheard a wonderful crone who is an accomplished medical practitioner tell a patient, "I am not just going to keep handing you bills and recommendations. You have to have the courage to get involved in your own healing." Ultimately, sadhana is about teaching the patient how not to be a patient. To get better, we need to dig deeply into our own understanding and start to embrace the practices that can strengthen our true nature.

Jennifer discovered this important lesson when she discontinued six different medicines she was taking over a two-year period for infertility. She came to this decision after spending one month at Wise Earth and engaging in the food and remedy sadhanas. One day she announced that she had a vision to go back to her birthplace of Ireland, where she lived until she was seven years old. When she returned from Ireland to the United States a few months later, she brought Finn, a 7-month old baby boy that she and her husband had adopted. Finn was born to a young mother out of wedlock in a small hamlet where Jennifer's ancestors originated. Now, Jennifer and her family are all enjoying a life devoid of medicines but filled with food sadhana practices that bring them joy.

Be conscious of your food choices and always try to eat in harmony with the organic provisions of each season. Eating the same foods season after season creates discontent in the vital tissue memory, and this brings uneasiness that is reflected in your mental, emotional, and physical activities. The practice of sadhana is not prescriptive; it is a natural tool for learning, teaching, and healing. Take your time with sadhana and put in a little bit of practice every day. After a short while, it will begin to call on you. Your confidence in the practice will grow as you start to see changes within you. The more you practice, the greater your self-confidence in this art of healing becomes, until finally, you are able to let go of the dependent way of existing that is merely a crutch.

The beauty of sadhana is that it affords you absolute simplicity, the path that leads you to your inner harmony. While practicing, evolutionary healing happens because you are increasing your personal awareness and sentience. As your memory evolves, you will begin to experience different dream states that reveal your unique karma. The more you recognize your karmas, the easier it will be to let go of those that have become appendages. When you have reconciled your karma, you will be free of disease; no negative energy will be left behind to create and reenact conflicts.

The cardinal rule of healing is to rid inner conflict. For this, we have to want to live a life of non-hurting, *ahimsa*. If you truly initiate a commitment to inner harmony, you will intuitively move away from and resolve anything that creates conflict and disturbs your peace. When you have become well-seated in your inner strength and harmony your energy will ward off and wash away conflicts. Indeed, within you there will be no conflict left for external energies to latch onto, pull on, or tangle with. Again and again, I will remind you that a life of ahimsa is about not hurting yourself, not hurting anyone else, not hurting your spirit and not hurting the spirit of any creature. Once you stop participating in the harmful activities of our present culture, you will find your breath, joy, and longevity. We do not have to kill the animals. We do not have to kill any part of nature to feed, nourish, or heal ourselves. In fact, in doing so, we irreparably hurt ourselves.

THE ART OF REMEDIES FOR INNER MEDICINE HEALING

Calling on the wisdom of the ancients, I've formulated many herbal essences and remedies for a vast range of women's disorders. The Inner Medicine remedies are natural and pure, prepared in such a way that they harmonize with the dynamic vibration that exists in the memory of each of the seven vital tissues, called *dhatus*. For this reason, they are proven extremely effective in correcting imbalances in your body. And when used at the appropriate cyclical junctures, you'll need only to take them in small measures for a short period of time.

But before we explore the wondrous art of making your homemade remedies, you'll need to know the nature of the six elemental tastes created by the seasons. These tastes play a crucial role in your everyday health, and knowing them will help you to understand the deeper levels of your unique metabolic constitution and the foods and herbs that support them.

THE SIX TASTES

Taste is part of the manifold function of rasa—the vast spectrum of aesthetics and emotions that influence your physical, mental, and spiritual preferences. According to Ayurveda, there are six tastes in nature. They are naturally produced by the revolving seasons as the earth makes its annual journey around the sun. In Ayurveda, there are six seasons—spring, summer, early fall, autumn, early winter, and late winter—each of which produces a specific taste: astringent, pungent, sour, salty, sweet, and bitter. Each dosha (Vata, Pitta, and Kapha) is primarily nourished by three tastes. For example, Kapha types are best nourished with pungent, bitter, and astringent tastes. I am not suggesting that the Kapha type cannot eat grains and fruits, which are mostly sweet, but that they must be mindful of the quality and quantity of sweets they eat. Pitta types do best with sweet, bitter, and astringent tastes, and Vata types thrive on sweet, salty, and sour tastes.

Keep in mind that all food consists of all six tastes, just as each one of us is composed of all five elements and all three doshas. The study of the doshas, which is based on the science of Ayurveda, teaches that the six tastes should be enjoyed proportionately. As a general rule, the sweet taste should be the most dominant taste in our daily nourishment. Pungent, salty, and sour tastes should be used moderately as secondary tastes, depending on the season. Bitter and astringent tastes are always used as minor or remedial tastes and should also be increased or decreased according to our condition and the particular seasons. Here are the descriptions of each of the six tastes and their qualities, listed according to their predominance in the universe.

Sweet is the dominant taste of all nourishment and sustenance, because almost all foods contain some degree of sweetness. Water and earth elements produce the sweet taste, which includes all carbohydrates, sugars, fats, and amino acids. The primary element of life, which is water, is considered sweet, as are milk and all sugars. Sweet increases bodily tissues, nurtures the body, and relieves hunger. Our diets should therefore be proportionately high in good quality "sweet" foods, including whole grains, root vegetables, and fruits. Herbs such as corn silk, cotton root, lily, and marshmallow are naturally sweet in taste.

Pungent is formed from the elements of air and fire and helps stimulate appetite and maintain metabolism and the balance of secretions in the body. This taste is most beneficial for the Kapha type and includes such foods as garlic, ginger, kale, mustard, tomatoes, and peppers. Examples of pungent herbs are cloves, eucalyptus, dill, horseradish, and lavender.

Salty is most beneficial for the Vata type, although it may be used in small quantities by all types as it helps to cleanse bodily tissues and activate digestion. The third most dominant taste, it is formed from the elements of water and fire and is found in all salts and seaweeds. Most watery vegetables, such as tomatoes, zucchinis, and cucumbers, are naturally high in saline. Few herbs boast the salty taste.

Remedies such as moss, kelp, seaweeds, and rock salt are predominantly salty.

Sour is formed from earth and fire elements and helps digestion and the elimination of wastes from the body. This taste may be used in small quantities by everyone, although it is most beneficial for the Vata type. Most fruits are considered somewhat sour with lemons, limes, and tamarind being the sourest. All organic acids and fermented foods, such as yogurt, soy sauce, and pickles, are also considered sour. The sour taste is also not predominantly used in medicines. This taste may be found in hawthorn and rosehips.

Bitter should be used by everyone in small quantities, and is especially good for the Pitta and Kapha types. Bitter detoxifies the blood, controls skin ailments, and tones the organs. This taste is formed from the elements of air and space and exists in all medicines, alkaloids, glycosides, and bitter foods such as aloe vera, arugula, radicchio, dandelion greens, and the spice turmeric. Examples of bitter herbs are blessed thistle, chaparral, chicory, and passion flower.

Astringent is formed from the elements of earth and air and intended to be used in medicinal measure by all types. The astringent principle helps to reduce bodily secretions and constrict bodily tissues. Examples of astringent foods are those high in tannins, such as dried legumes and bark teas. Herbs such as bistort, blackberry, cramp bark, hibiscus, raspberry, and uva ursi are highly astringent in quality.

THE SECRET OF RASA

Taste goes far beyond the preparation and consumption of food. Each one of us has an emotional, physical, psychic, and spiritual "taste" that influences all aspects of our daily lives. The choices we make are largely influenced by our individual sense of rasa: the emotions we express, clothing we prefer, the art we like, the careers we are attracted to, the people we cherish, the spouses we marry, etc. In Ayurveda, the vast spectrum of taste, rasa, begins long before we actually eat and taste food. Rasa says that "taste" begins with a complex chain of reactions that the body/mind experiences from its initial perception of that food by a sense organ to the stimulation of the brain cells that excite the appetite. Appetite is not simply the initial hunger for food, or yearning from a substance that will create balance in the mind/body. It is the principle of maternal emotions and natural aesthetics that upholds our nourishment and lives. By this means, rasa has gained its name as the first tissue layer of the body that is intrinsically linked to our creator, creation, and the sense of taste.

In Wise Earth Ayurveda, the sense of taste starts long before we actually taste a food. This sense operates through the water element of the body and is transported by the lymphatic system. Taste plays a prodigious role in the process of healing. When we do not taste the remedy, its essence arrives unannounced through the process of digestion into the vital tissue. Like an uninvited guest, the tissue is taken by surprise and does not have the necessary impetus (rasa desire) to project the essences into its memory. In the case of medicinal herbs and essences aimed at rebalancing tissue memory, the choices we make are even more relevant to the proper working of rasa in the body. The waters of rasa control the palate, the way in which an herb or food is absorbed into the body, and then projected as nourishment into the vital tissue. When the correct blend of unadulterated, natural ingredients is received on the tongue in a manner that promotes digestion, rasa responds positively. In this way, rasa works to transform the ingredients and send its medicine deep into the impaired tissue to prod its corrective memory. Rasa functions on the same vibrational level as that of the tissue memory. For this reason, its intrinsic vibrational structure can coalesce with the tissue memory.

Because it has an alien relationship to medicines that are chemically manufactured or produced in solidified forms such as in a pill, rasa is rendered inactive, or impotent in commuting the medicinal essences into the vital tissue. At best, these medicines operate at a superficial state addressing only the symptoms of disorders since they do not "speak the language" as the memory codes within the vital tissues. This is why diseases are not cured by taking conventional medicine.

More important than both the form and function of the medicines we imbibe is the state of awareness and consciousness we create when we prepare them. The more we know about the specific nature, quality, quantity of the herbs, powders, decoctions, and infusions that we use, the more efficient their effect will be in producing inner equilibrium. Rasa is the total intelligence of nourishment in the body acting in harmony with the external environment. As such, the power of rasa may be enormously enhanced when we use our inner dynamics to work with nature's nourishing materials.

For example, by using our hands to make or prepare our remedies, we call on the forces of the elements that course through our bodies. In my tradition, the hands and feet are called, "organs of action" because they can be transformed into the extension of healing energy from the five elements. As a Vedic custom, we eat with our hands because the mere touching of the food with the fingertips stimulates the five elements. Each finger is an extension of one of the five elements. Each element serves to aid in the transformation of food and herbs before they pass on to internal digestion to become nourishment. At this moment, if you rub them together for a few minutes, you will feel the tingling of elements coursing through the fingers, stimulating your hands. If you were to rest your energized right hand on the chest directly over your heart, you can actually feel the beat of the heart getting stronger while the breath becomes slower and deeper.

FOOD AS INNER MEDICINE

We are composed of energy, elements, rhythms, vibrations, and memory. The five elements continually transmute into each other creating atoms, molecules, minerals, foods, and life forms. Food is the keeper of the elements, and through its transformation the body of life is formed. Your relationship to food can unravel the vast mystery of your timeless karma. Food takes us through the complete cycle of evolution, from the original cosmic seed to the fragile sprout, to the flourishing plant and its fruits, our sustenance. The full cycle sustaining life begins with consciously sowing and harvesting the good earth, preparing its wholesome foods, and imbibing them with gratitude. To complete this cycle, we return the earth's food that has been transformed through the body's digestion and vital tissue operations as a gift back to the earth to uphold the unbroken continuum of the Mother Consciousness.

Food is memory. Eating is remembering. When we understand this cyclical wisdom onto which life is nourished, nurtured, and healed, we will be fully awakened to our intuition. Recognize every seed, herb, fruit, and bark used in your Inner Medicine course of healing to be food, the ever-sacred nourishment from the breast of the Mother.

The Wise Earth food sadhana includes the making of your own remedies. These practices are an inextricable part of a happy, fulfilled family life. Many cultures used these practices to bring family, friends, and community together. The children of Wise Earth practitioners who visit the monastery spend endless hours reveling in these breath-generating activities. They grind the herbs and spice seeds in mortar and pestles, called suribachis, pound the whole grain, beat on the drums, and chant to their hearts' desire. After taking to the practices at home with her mother, Erin, a 10-year old girl diagnosed with Attention Deficit Disorder (ADD) and put on the prescription drug Ritalin, is now fully recovered from ADD and no longer on the drug. Several children who attend ongoing yoga and sadhana classes at our MOM's charitable sites in New York have been weaned off a variety of medical drugs. Their parents have reported that as a result of Wise Earth Ayurveda's sadhana education, the children are calmer, sleep better, perform better with their schoolwork, have more focused energy and eagerly look forward to their time at MOM. Josephine, a young woman in her 30s who had breast cancer was so taken with crushing the herbs on the stone that she returned home and redesigned her kitchen, emulating the layout of sacred space in the Wise Earth kitchen. Instead of getting a mastectomy recommended by her doctor, she took her healing in her own hands and has been transforming her health by making the food sadhanas a central practice in her everyday life. Her latest medical examination shows a sizeable decrease of her breast tumor. Josephine is confident that with her newfound sadhana activities she can heal herself completely.

I have been doing these practices for more than a quarter of a century and have students who have been doing them for nearly two decades. Over these years, I have witnessed hundreds of women who have healed their cancers and reproductive disorders by simply putting these life-generating practices in the center of their lives. As you begin your conscious practices around food, breath, and sound, your health will improve, your happiness will increase, and you will become more awakened to your inner wisdom.

The blessing of the plants, fruits, leaves, herbs, seeds, grains and minerals, twigs, roots, and barks—called *annam* in Sanskrit—are intended to feed you and foster good health. Plant life is a special sacrifice decreed by the Supreme Goddess for the benefit of her children. She has never granted us permission to kill in order to feed and sustain ourselves. Remember, each herb is a goddess, every grain an icon, and every seed contains the power of Shakti. We need to recognize a remedy as being nourishing, nurturing, and life-sustaining food. To be healed, you must be fed, nourished, and nurtured. Drugs and medicines do not have the intrinsic authority to do this. The act of nourishment is a magical affair wherein every motion and moment is prayerful and meaningful. From the golden harvest to the green herb, buff-colored grain, and the multi-colored fruit, we are forever loved, served, and supported by Mother Nature. This is the support within we must continually enhance.

NATURAL TOOLS FOR PREPARING YOUR REMEDIES

In keeping with the principle of sadhana, you need to become comfortable with using your hands and limbs for all measuring. As you will see throughout these pages, learning to use your hands in the wise way of mudra practice allows you to invite in or dispel energy in accord with your needs at all times. Do not underestimate the powerful Inner Medicine Shakti of your hands! In Sanskrit, the term, *anjali* refers to the volume that can be held when two hands are cupped together. For example, you may measure rice, beans, or flour in the cup of your own hands. In determining appropriate quantities of food in each meal, you may use two of your own anjalis. According to the seers, this is the perfect quantity of food designed by nature to fit and fill your own stomach. *Angula* refers to the distance between the joints of each finger. This unit of measure is intended to gauge spices, herbs, such as cinnamon sticks, and the roots of turmeric and ginger. Here are some guidelines that might be helpful to memorize:

Anjali: Amount in your cupped hands, equivalent to 1 cup
Angula: Length of your finger joint, equivalent to 3/4 inch

Three finger pinch: Equivalent to 1/4 teaspoon
Five finger pinch: Equivalent to 1/2 teaspoon
Hollow of your palm: Equivalent to 1 tablespoon

It may be challenging at first to trust the accuracy of your own hands. But with time, you will become comfortable enough and begin to enjoy your body's most natural system of measurement. With constant application, this is a perfect tool to awaken intuition. Given the length of years you have spent using measuring cups and so on, I realize that many of you may find this ancient practice difficult to do since we have become infinitely dependant on a multitude of measuring tools. Easing into this naturally joyful way of life takes time and also a leap of faith. Using your limbs in the way of sadhana is a spiritual education that needs to be inculcated a bit at a time. As you grow into a life of balance with sadhana, so too will your intuition and the way you are drawn to move and flow through each day reflect this leap of faith. Look at dispensing with irrelevant tools in your kitchen as a metaphor for discarding the psychic co-dependency and personal attachments that do not serve your greater self.

That being said, you are advised to weave this healthful education slowly but surely into your life. As you develop more awareness you will glean more incentives to go the natural way and you will find yourself using less and less utensils to measure the quantities of your food. In the meantime, when you become more comfortable with preparing your own meals and exploring the exciting art of making your own homemade remedies, you will begin to make the vital connection to the Mother Consciousness through your sacred limbs by using your bare and beautiful hands to measure and gauge your foods, spices, herbs, etc. In this way, you will garner more personal security in and firm understanding of your True Self.

STONE SUPPORT FROM MOTHER EARTH

Stone supports the earth, lending her strength and security. We use stones to build dams, barriers, and bridges and the foundations of our homes—structures that give stability to our lives. The grinding stone and mortar and pestle are ancient symbols of the power of male and female energies. The mortar is *Parashakti*, primordial feminine power that brought forth manifestation. The pestle is *Parashiva*, the masculine force that represents all-pervasive Consciousness. When we grind our remedies by hand, we bring our feminine and masculine energies into a state of balance. Using the mortar and pestle to pound and grind your ingredients into powders and pastes helps to fortify your meditative state. All of these natural movements are meditations in motion.

Reclaim your hand tools for preparing your remedies. Since the invention of mechanical grinding tools, the vital connection of hand on stone or hand on clay has been lost. The rhythm of stone rubbing on stone renews our cosmic memory of our connection with the earth and enhances the energy of rasa. At once, your internal juices for appetite awaken as you experience the aroma, sound, and texture of the herb or seed. Each herb when crushed and grounded with your own hands may enliven a particular tissue memory and reunite your memory for healing with your ancestral pasts.

I have never met a woman or a child who did not instantly and immediately fall in love with the grinding stones and suribachi. Gayle and her 10-year old daughter, Andrea, attended a weekend herbal remedy workshop at the school. Gayle said that she had been suffering from insomnia for many years. Her physician had prescribed numerous medicines, none of which worked for her. In the herb preparation classes, all the women generally sit in a circle on a large hand-woven cotton quilt laid out on the floor as they passionately take to grinding, rubbing, pounding, and crushing the seeds and herbs, twigs and sticks with their hands on stone or on pestle. Gayle and Andrea gleefully joined in the ceremonious action. When Gayle first started to grind the herbs on the grinding stone in class, she reported a feeling of lightness in her head, almost as though she was going to faint. She would stop grinding for a little while and then rejoin the group activity. In one of the classes, Gayle fell soundly asleep and began to snore during the grinding session. Amused by the sound of her snoring, the women picked up rhythm and speed with their grinding, pounding, and chanting and created the most rambunctious atmosphere with music and fun. At the end of a two-hour session, they had produced more herbal powders than we had ever produced at any one sitting!

Through it all, Gayle slept deeply like a newborn baby, undisturbed by the sounds of the women and stones. In fact, somewhere along the way, the deep rhythm of the work had penetrated into her sleep state to silence her snoring. After completing the course, Gayle immediately gave up all medicines and took to gathering her own set of grinding stones with which she and Andrea grind their herbs and seeds to their hearts' content.

CREATING A KITCHEN SANCTUARY FIT FOR THE GODDESS

Because you are created from primordial space, recreating that space around yourself in your home is essential to reclaiming your personal rasa. In accordance with Vedic architecture, we leave the center of our living room wide open, cleared of heavy furniture and clutter. The center of our living spaces represents the heart of our physical and emotion being left open to receive the energies of the Mother

Goddess. You will be surprised at the joy and lightness you experience from clearing the center space of your home and ridding the excesses from your closets, cabinets, and hidden shelves. Lighten your load; give away the things you do not need like clothing, accessories, utensils, paraphernalia, and memorabilia. Healing begins from within, but the space you create around you can help to accelerate your healing. Space is essential to unearthing your joy.

Start with your kitchen and transform this space into a goddess sanctuary for the energized preparation of your natural remedies. This goddess is you. Do you envision yourself as a goddess? See the kitchen as a spiritual place for healing, complete with nature's utensils made from natural materials like stone, clay, straw, leaves, bamboo, and wood. Each utensil must be a means for extending your Shakti power into the creation of your Inner Medicine remedies. Choose a few good quality heavy stainless-steel and enamel pots and pans, as well as several cast-iron skillets. I recommend that you use utensils made from a variety of non-toxic materials, because they all lend different energies to the food. You will need some clay and wooden bowls; stainless-steel and wooden ladles; a ceramic hand-grater for your ginger, turmeric, and garlic; and most importantly, a grinding stone, suribachi, and mortar and pestle for your herbs, seeds, and remedies. Every sadhana kitchen must have a sharp knife or two.

The myriad aromas, sounds, tastes, and textures of nature's food enliven every one of our cells and memories. When looking around my own goddess sanctuary, I relish the delightful abundance of sensory stimuli around me: the smell and sound of roasted fennel seeds as I grind them with my mortar and pestle, and the rich aroma of golden ghee as it is boiled to perfection. My kitchen sanctuary displays nature's abundance; I hang fresh oregano, basil, mint, marjoram, and thyme from my kitchen rafters to dry. My shelves are open to view, lined with ceramic and glass jars filled with a variety of whole grains, beans, seeds, twigs, and barks. Each room of my sanctuary holds an altar for the gods and goddesses, and an earthen fire-pot and camphor cubes are set out on my kitchen altar. A small statue of Ganesha, the elephant-headed god, sits next to the fire-pot. Before every meal, I do a food offering to the deities. I place a small amount of food or remedy I have prepared into the pot, along with a tiny piece of camphor, light a fire, and say my prayers.

HOW TO USE INNER MEDICINE REMEDIES

The following chapters provide classical Ayurveda remedies presented in a simple and easy to follow way that will activate healing and transform your health. In Ayurveda, thousands of nature's herbs, minerals, resins, barks, roots, gels, and essences are used singly or compounded into powders, pastes, pills, gels, juices, infusions, and decoctions to bring reprieve and balance to the body, mind, and spirit. Dried or fresh herbs, barks, and roots are steeped, infused, or brought to a boil in water or milk to create simple tea remedies that can help us heal. Teas are aromatic and refreshing and are easy to make. They can bring a lasting sense of inner tranquility and wellness.

In the treatment of illness, Ayurveda targets the central dosha rather than the galaxy of symptoms that are produced as a result of that dosha's impairment. The easy to use homemade remedies and teas are a vital and natural means of keeping your doshas and internal rhythms in a state of balance. May you find your joy and enthusiasm in the practice and preparation of these simple Inner Medicine formulas.

Chapter Seven

HEALING PMS FOREVER

Rejoice plants, bearing abundant flowers and fruit
Triumphing together over disease like victorious horses,
Breaking free the earth, safe-guarding humans beyond disease.
                                        —*Rig Veda*

Health is more than the absence of disease; it is our individual undoing of disorder and continual unfolding of awareness as we strive to gain consciousness. In Wise Earth's Inner Medicine healing work, we educate you to cultivate and sustain excellent health of body, mind, and spirit by becoming aware of your own divine inner resources for healing. Through learning your own unique metabolic composition you may guide your menstrual health. Before we examine the nature of the menstrual cycle, let us explore the impact doshas have on your health and well-being. Understanding which foods, herbs, activities, goals, and desires better support or abate each dosha can help you to make appropriate choices that sustain your ongoing state of balance.

According to Ayurveda, each person has a unique metabolic type based on the principle of the three doshas—Vata, Pitta, and Kapha. Vata is formed from the air and space elements; Pitta from the fire and water elements; and Kapha from the water and earth elements. Indeed, your metabolic type is strongly influenced by your inherent genetics and is a blueprint of your entire physical, mental, and spiritual body. Since each dosha is formed from two elements, it bears the qualities of both. Vata types, for example, influenced by the reigning elements of air and space, tend to be somewhat ungrounded. Pitta types are generally fast, fluid, and fiery, patterned as they are after fire and water. And those in whom Kapha is dominant tend to be slow and methodical, since they are heavily affected by the characteristics of their main elements, water and earth. Every moment of every day, we are able to see the doshas in action through the elemental qualities we find in ourselves and the environment. (To discover your metabolic type, see Your Wise Earth Ayurveda Metabolic Type in Appendix One.)

THE MENSTRUAL CYCLE

Menstruation is the monthly cyclical means by which a woman's entire bodily organism is cleansed and rejuvenated. Through the menstrual process, the reproductive tissues and hormonal activities are revitalized while *ama*—accumulated matter that creates toxicity in the body that leads to disease—is involuntarily eliminated. This cycle is instrumental in the health, wellness, and happiness of women during their childbearing years. As you will see, your individual constitution sets up your disposition for certain intrinsic attributes—as well as specific conditions or disorders. And like all diseases, menstrual disorders manifest through the doshas—Vata, Pitta, and Kapha. However, just because you may have a Vata constitution does not mean that you will never have incident of a Pitta disorder.

Menstruation is intimately linked to the functions of the doshas. Apana vayu, one of the elemental air functions of the Vata dosha, is responsible for the downward flow of menstruation; Pitta dosha is responsible for cleaning and promoting blood quantity; and Kapha dosha adds the fluidity of tissue and mucus to the menstrual flow. Like all principles of energy, the doshas are not implacable in nature. Formed from the greater energies, they are heavily influenced by the lunar wheel of time, the solar cycle of the seasons, and the interplay of external and internal conditions. For example, the quality of Vata, Pitta or Kapha changes under specific conditions.

For example, having a fever is considered to be a Pitta condition. To successfully treat this condition, we would need to know not only your internal energetic conditions, but also the external environment and how you as a whole person are responding to your condition and to your potential treatment. Both your metabolic type as well as the dosha of your disorder play a primary role in your condition and would impact how we create the appropriate sadhana recommendations for you.

Time, place, and seasonal considerations are also important factors in your healing. For instance, to dispel fever in spring we would provide a different set of recommendations than we would give in the autumn. Moreover, your program will need to be adjusted to harmonize with the climatic conditions—temperate, tropical, and so on. In the spring, as in the colder climates, we would need to consider the role Kapha plays in your fever condition since coldness and spring are both largely pervaded by Kapha energy. Likewise, in autumn, we would also take into consideration Vata, which is most prevalent in this season; or Pitta, which is the dominant dosha of the tropics. Ultimately, to successfully help you heal your condition we want to closely examine the whole person—your physical, mental, and emotional disposition, and gauge your response to all the above mentioned factors in order to take complete charge of your disorder.

The same dynamic interplay of the doshas holds true in external nature. A red pepper, for example, is considered Pitta because it is hot in nature and grows during the Pitta predominant season of summer when solar energy is also plentiful. However, the nature of the same pepper will change if grown under different conditions, for instance, in a greenhouse during the full moon. It will still be Pitta in nature but grown in the safeguarded environment affected by the cooling energy of the moon, it will bear different color tones and not be as hot or have the same energy as the pepper grown in the outdoor conditions of a garden.

As we now know, all reproductive disorders relate to Shakti energy. When this energy is out of balance with the lunar cycles it influences the doshas, which in turn impacts the menstrual cycle. When the menstrual flow is out of tune with the new moon phase of the lunar wheel, it is an invitation for trouble and reproductive disorders like PMS, and the appallingly increasing number of diseases relating to our reproductive health and well-being such as, leucorrhea, genital herpes, sexually transmitted diseases, Candida, yeast infections, and so on. And remember that in addition to menstrual disorders, which represent a large fraction of a woman's reproductive problems, there are also the more severe conditions such as breast, ovarian, and uterine cancers; endometriosis; osteoporosis; hormonal imbalance; and infertility, which we'll address in the upcoming chapters.

REGAINING THE GRACE OF MOTHER CONSCIOUSNESS

Disruption of the natural menstrual cycle speaks to the symptoms of a larger, more insidious development. We are in disfavor with Mother Nature and in disharmony with her whole cosmic cycle. When women stopped convening in the privacy of their bleeding sanctuary to gather Shakti's wisdom and to commune with Mother Earth, we lost a part of ourselves and halted the innate joy and intuition of acting as emissaries of the Divine Mother. With modern civilization came the loss of women's memory of her precious feminine energies and her role as the keeper of nurturance.

Besides being out of touch with the lunar calendar, many other factors can contribute to disrupting the menstrual flow such as: poor nourishment, stress, exhaustion, excess physical exercise, inactivity, overwork, and genetic disposition. Recent studies indicate that more than 80 percent of women in America experience irregular cycles, or have their cycle begin at the opposite end of the lunar cycle, the full moon rather than the new moon. Interventions such as contraceptive devises, birth control pills, and hormone replacement therapy have intervened so that a female's menstrual cycle often happens at the exact opposite time in the lunar calendar that it should. As a direct result, she is losing touch with her primordial inner rhythms, which not only control her menstrual cycles, but also her physical, mental, emotional, and intuitive well-being. This reality serves to increase her dependency on the medical caregiver and a barrage of medicines. Despite the current situation, however, we can regain the grace of the Mother Consciousness.

To permanently rid yourself of menstrual ailments, you will need to bring your menstrual cycle in alignment with the new moon phase. The Uttara Vasti home therapy set out in Chapter Five will help you to accomplish this wonderful feat and bring you reproductive health.

ANATOMY OF MENSTRUATION: THREE METABOLIC TYPES

Ayurveda's entire approach to health is to uncover and treat the root cause of the disease. Recognizing that manifold conditions and symptoms can appear from one central cause, it focuses on a person's metabolic constitution and traces its connection to how they respond to both their internal and external environment.

Vata types have a short, irregular, and variable cycle usually punctuated by spotting either before or after the period. The menstrual flow tends to be sparse, brownish-red in color, darkish and may contain clots. Cramping and pain in the lower back may also occur. Premenstrual mood swings, accompanied by anxiety, fear, nervous tension and insomnia are common. Constipation or abdominal distension may also occur. Symptoms are worse during pre-dawn and pre-dusk, the heights of Vata time.

Pitta types generally experience regular cycles with excess bleeding which can last for several days. The blood is usually warm and red in color with a purple or bluish hue and occasional clotting. Burning sensations, sweating, fever, migraine headaches, skin rashes, or inflammations, and acne may occur. Premenstrual irritability, outbursts of anger, and food cravings are common occurrences. Symptoms are at their worst during midnight and noon, the heights of Pitta time.

Kapha types experience a regular, slow, and steady cycle, which tends to be late. Menstrual flow is thick and whitish in color with mucus or clots. Kapha tends to generate dull pain, or cramps, water retention, nausea, swollen breasts, edema, stiffness in joints, and sluggishness. Emotionally overwrought, tearful, and sentimental, Kapha types have great need for love, attention, care, and companionship during this time. Symptoms are worse during the early morning and early evening, the Kapha times of day.

PMS

Premenstrual syndrome is one of the most common ailments for women, affecting more than one third of the female population between the ages of 18 and 52. Katharina Dalton, M.D., a British physician who has conducted extensive research on treating women with PMS, documented that the probability of women injuring themselves, having accidents, using alcohol, attempting suicide, and committing crimes is far greater during this period. This means that millions of women around the world spend more than half their time feeling sick, depressed, or miserable!

Until recently, women with PMS were ambivalently treated with tranquilizers, mood suppressants, sleeping pills, and were sent to receive psychiatric help. Evidenced by the popularity of thousands of self-help books, along with wholesome nutritional guidelines now being introduced into many clinical health facilities and hospitals across the country, the perception and response of the medical community is beginning to change. But it is neither knowledgeable enough or soon enough. Another reason for the change is an increase in research: in 1991, a research study reported in the *Annals of Medicine* stated that women with PMS showed no more sign of psychiatric or personality disorders than women without PMS. As this idea catches on, the medical community has no choice but to take note.

EASING BODY & MIND DURING MENSTRUAL FLOW: FIRST STEPS

Menstrual disorders are caused by an imbalance of energy and matter within the body. For a growing number of women and young girls, menstruation is a difficult time of emotional hurt, pain, discomfort, and fatigue. At the physical level, metabolic activity during the menstrual cycle naturally increases ama, metabolic toxicity, which may manifest as menstrual cramps, physical pain, diarrhea, nausea, nervous tension, and emotional distress. For this reason, most women experience a feeling of incredible lightness after the cycle is over. To minimize pain, fatigue, and discomfort and ease challenges during the period, we need to make certain crucial changes in our living environment. Here are some simple Ayurvedic recommendations that will help you maintain your reproductive health in a state of balance:

- **Focus on proper nutrition.** Eat fresh, organic, nutritious meals that are light, soft, and warm. Imbibe in small portions and keep a regular schedule of meals. Avoid eating junk foods, frozen and refined foods, animal flesh, cold drinks, carbonated beverages, and dairy products.
- **Keep a regular schedule of daily routines and lighten your daily activities.** Take a few days off from work or maintain a moderate schedule. Retreat inward; this is a time to replenish your Shakti energy within by paying attention to your thoughts and dreams and by being mindful of your miraculous life-generating process.
- **Create a stress-free environment at home and at work.** Avoid potentially volatile situations, giving or receiving bodywork, and sexual activity.
- **Perform light exercise.** Take some time every day if possible for mild yoga

stretches, gentle tai chi, or short daily walks. Keep a regular sleeping schedule and avoid sleeping during the day.

WISE EARTH REMEDIES FOR PMS

In Ayurveda, we consider both the individual constitution and condition. Therefore I have set out the remedies for PMS in accord with each type, Vata, Pitta, and Kapha. Each formula has a two-pronged approach: it provides you with the remedy for a deep or serious condition, as well as a mild or temporary condition. Mild conditions are those that tend to occur occasionally and go away quickly: headaches, indigestion, bodily aches and pains, nausea, fatigue, and so on.

Deep conditions are serious ones, which tend to be long-term and grow incrementally into deep and sometimes life threatening diseases. For example, if you are experiencing a Vata type PMS with severe cramping and pain or relentless anxiety and fear, you will use the Vata formula for a deep PMS condition. On the other hand, if you are having a mild symptom, such as the sweating or irritability that can occur with Pitta type PMS, you would want to use the Pitta formula for a mild PMS condition.

WISE EARTH REMEDIES FOR VATA TYPE PMS

Let us quickly review the menstruation disorders as they associate with the Vata type person:

Vata Type Menstruation
- Most vulnerable time: pre-dawn and pre-dusk
- Irregular, variable with spotting
- Brownish red, dried with clots
- Scanty flow with painful cramps
- PMS discomfort comes at the beginning of the cycle
- Lower back and abdominal pain
- Constipation prior to menstruation
- Insomnia, dizziness, nervous tension, vertigo
- Premenstrual mood swings
- Forgetfulness, anxiety, fearfulness
- Cravings for salty and savory foods

Inner Medicine Guidelines for Vata Type PMS
- Never take medicine every day.

- Do not use more than three herbs at any given time.
- Always take your remedies after a meal.
- Drink half a glass of water after taking a soft pill or paste.
- Do not take more than two of your homemade pills at any given time.

Ayurvedic Herbal Powders for Vata Type PMS

The most effective Ayurvedic herbs for Vata PMS are sweet and stimulating and include: triphala, gokshura, ashwagandha, vidari, jatamansi, and shatavari. Other common herbs which can also help relieve Vata PMS are nutmeg, cinnamon, valerian, turmeric, dill, fennel, and wild yam. The *anupana* (medium used to create soft pills and pastes from powders explained on the pages following) specific to Vata, are ghee, honey, aloe vera gel, Sucanat, and milk.

Note: As you become more familiar with your needs and the energy of each of these herbs, you may follow the steps below and use any one to three herbs in equal portion to prepare the paste or soft pill of your choice as you need them.

Cyclical Timing for Vata

Challenging Time: 2:00-6:00 (morning and afternoon)
Challenging Seasons: Early fall (rainy season) and autumn
Challenging Moon Phase: Last phase of waning cycle

The PMS remedies that follow are to be taken for five to seven days starting one week prior to the day you anticipate the commencement of your menstrual cycle. If your cycle is not in alignment with the new moon, you may start the remedy on the day of the new moon and take it for three days total. Then resume taking the remedy for five days prior to the commencement of your cycle. You may use the remedies for a maximum period of three months. Avoid taking the remedy during your cycle. The times of day most suitable to take the remedy are indicated in each formula.

For Deep Vata PMS Condition

- Ashwagandha & Vidari Paste
- Shatavari & Aloe Soft Pill

ASHWAGANDHA & VIDARI PASTE | SERVES ONE

1/2 teaspoon ashwagandha powder
1/4 teaspoon vidari powder (ancient relative of wild yam)
1/4 teaspoon licorice powder
1 1/2 teaspoons honey

Combine the three powders in a small bowl and add honey. Mix into a paste and take it twice daily, once after breakfast and then again after lunch for a period of seven to eight days. Chase with half a glass of warm water.

SHATAVARI & ALOE SOFT PILL | SERVES ONE

1/2 teaspoon shatavari powder
1/4 teaspoon turmeric powder
1/4 teaspoon valerian powder
1 teaspoon ghee or aloe vera gel

(The recipe for making ghee is provided on page 122)

Combine the three powders in a small bowl and add aloe vera gel. Mix into a paste and place in the palm of your left hand. Rub the palms together to roll the paste into a soft pill. The size of the pill that fits in the space between your palms is designed to flow effortlessly down your trachea as you swallow it. Take once after breakfast and then again after lunch for a period of seven to eight days. Chase with half a glass of warm water.

For Mild Vata PMS Condition
• Jatamansi & Nutmeg Milk

JATAMANSI & NUTMEG MILK | SERVES ONE

1 cup organic cow's milk or almond milk
1/2 teaspoon jatamansi powder
1/4 teaspoon nutmeg powder
1/4 teaspoon valerian powder
1/4 teaspoon Sucanat

Bring the milk to a boil. Remove from heat. Stir in the powders and add the Sucanat. Drink about an hour before bed. Take for a period of five to seven days.

Ayurvedic Herbal Teas for Vata Type PMS
Some of the most effective herbal teas for Vata PMS are basil, cardamom, cinnamon, cloves, comfrey, chamomile, ginger, hyssop, lavender, lemon balm, lemon verbena, licorice, marshmallow, orange peel, peppermint, rose flower, orange peel, peppermint, rosehips, saffron, and spearmint. You may drink as many as three cups of tea per day prior to and during your menstrual cycle.

Note: Using the steps on the next page, prepare teas of your choice as needed.

BREWING TEA INFUSIONS & DECOCTIONS

There are two classical ways to brew a tea remedy: infusion and decoction. For infusion, add one part of the herb to eight parts of hot water, cover and steep for 10 to 15 minutes. To make a decoction, add one part herb to 16 parts water or milk and bring to a boil on low heat for one hour or so. Depending on the desired strength of the tea, you may reduce the liquid content and boiling time accordingly. Follow the directions set out for making a tea infusion or decoction with any of the herbs mentioned on the previous page.

PEPPERMINT & ROSEHIPS TEA INFUSION | SERVES TWO

4 cups of water
1 tablespoon dried peppermint leaves
1 tablespoon dried orange peel
1 tablespoon rosehips
1 tablespoon honey

In a heavy stainless-steel saucepan, bring four cups of water to a boil. Put the herbs and orange peel in the boiling water and remove from heat. Cover and let simmer for 15 minutes. Strain and add honey directly before drinking.

CINNAMON, CLOVES & CARDAMOM TEA DECOCTION | SERVES TWO

2 cups of water
2 cups of organic cow's milk or almond milk
1 tablespoon cloves
1 teaspoon cinnamon powder
1 teaspoon cardamom powder
1/2 teaspoon ginger powder
1 pinch of saffron

In a heavy stainless-steel saucepan, bring the water and milk to a boil. Put the cloves and spice powders in the boiling decoction and leave to simmer on medium heat for 30 minutes. Remove from heat, add the saffron, cover and let stand for a few minutes. Strain and drink while still warm.

TRIPHALA INFUSION | SERVES ONE

This remedy may be taken on an ongoing basis. It helps to remove internal toxicity, reactivate digestion and bodily elimination, strengthen tissue function, and aid sleep.

1/2 teaspoon triphala powder
1 cup water

In a heavy stainless-steel saucepan, bring one cup of water to a boil. Put the triphala powder in the boiling water and remove from heat. Cover and let simmer for five minutes. Strain and drink an hour or so after dinner.

Nourishing Foods for Vata Type PMS

To buffer the cold, dry, and cranky qualities of Vata, eat easy to digest, warm, and nourishing foods during your menstrual cycle. Use fresh, organic, or local, family farm-grown foods; unhydrogenated oils; unrefined brown sugar; Sucanat; rock salt and sea salt; organic milk, butter, cheese, and yogurt; and organic almond milk.

The following food recommendations are the most appropriate for long-term use by the Vata type. They are also the most effective foods to relieve Vata type menstrual disorders, including PMS.

Vegetables (Use Seasonally):
Sweet potatoes, yams, pumpkins, winter squashes (acorn, butternut, buttercup), summer squashes (yellow, crookneck, zucchini, patty pan), watercress, bok choy, asparagus, carrots, daikon, green beans, leeks (cooked), onions (cooked), broccoli, cauliflower, and leafy greens (occasionally).

Fruits (Use Seasonally):
Avocados, bananas, berries, cherries, coconuts, grapefruit, oranges, kiwi, lemons, limes, tangerines, mangos, melons, papayas, peaches, pineapples, plums, rhubarb, tamarind, dates, figs, raisins, grapes, and strawberries. (Dried fruits are to be cooked before using.)

Grains (Whole, Cracked, and Cereal):
Brown rice (short, medium, and long), Basmati white and brown rice, Arborio Rice, sushi rice, wild rice, oats, cracked wheat, spelt, and kamut; whole wheat, spelt, or kamut berries; barley, quinoa, and amaranth.
Use Occasionally: soft cooked millet.

Legumes (Use Occasionally):
Aduki, mung (whole and split), tofu (cooked), kidney, lima, lentils, and black beans.

Foods that Exacerbate PMS Symptoms (To Be Avoided):

Caffeine, alcohol, saturated fats, excess salt, and most dairy products; highly processed junk foods, meats, and refined foods; frozen, canned, stale, commercially grown, bioengineered, transgenic foods, and irradiated spices; refined salts, sugars, flours and oils.

WISE EARTH REMEDIES FOR PITTA TYPE PMS

Pitta Type Menstruation
- Most vulnerable time: noon and midnight
- Excess bleeding
- Bright red with clots
- Lasts for a long time
- Fetid smell and sweating
- Burning sensations in bladder and down leg or bottom of feet
- Fever, migraine headaches, skin rashes, diarrhea
- Irritability, anger, fatigue
- Increased appetite
- Cravings for sweets and spicy foods

Inner Medicine Guidelines for Pitta Type PMS
- Never take medicine every day.
- Do not use more than three herbs at any given time.
- Always take your remedies after a meal.
- Drink half a glass of water after taking a soft pill or paste.
- Do not take more than two of your homemade pills at any given time.

Ayurvedic Herbal Powders for Pitta Type PMS
The most effective Ayurvedic herbs for Pitta PMS are bitter, sweet, and calming, as follows: shatavari, manjishta, bhringaraja, kutuki, gotu kola, brahmi, and triphala. Common herbs which can also help relieve Pitta PMS are fennel, coriander, black cohosh, gentian, motherwort, yarrow, skullcap, and echinacea. The anupana specific to Pitta used to create soft pills and pastes from the powders are ghee, aloe vera gel, Sucanat, maple syrup, and milk.

Note: You may follow the steps below and use any one to three herbs in equal portion to prepare the paste or soft pill of your choice as you need them.

Cyclical Timing for Pitta
Challenging Time: 10:00-2:00 (morning and evening)
Challenging Seasons: Spring and summer
Challenging Moon Phase: Mid-phase of waning cycle

The PMS remedies that follow are to be taken for five to seven days starting one week prior to the anticipated commencement of your menstrual cycle. If your cycle is not in alignment with the new moon, you may start the remedy on the day of the new moon and take it for three days. Then resume taking it for five days prior to the commencement of your cycle. You may use the remedies for a maximum period of three months. You should avoid taking the remedy during your menstrual cycle. The times of day most suitable to take the remedy are indicated in each formula.

For Deep Pitta PMS Condition
- Shatavari & Turmeric Paste
- Gotu Kola & Bhringaraja Soft Pill

SHATAVARI & TURMERIC PASTE | SERVES ONE

1/2 teaspoon shatavari powder
1/4 teaspoon turmeric powder
1/4 teaspoon licorice powder
1 1/2 teaspoons ghee or aloe vera gel

Combine the shatavari, turmeric, and licorice powders in a small bowl and add the ghee or aloe vera gel (whichever you prefer). Mix into a paste and take it twice daily, once after breakfast and then again after lunch for a period of seven to eight days. Chase with half a glass of warm water.

GOTU KOLA & BHRINGARAJA SOFT PILL | SERVES ONE

1/2 teaspoon gotu kola powder
1/4 teaspoon bhringaraja powder
1/4 teaspoon fennel powder
1 teaspoon aloe vera gel or ghee

Combine the gotu kola, bhringaraja, and fennel powders in a small bowl and add the aloe vera gel or ghee. Mix into a paste and place in the palm of your left hand. Rub the palms together to roll the paste into a soft pill. As noted earlier, the size of the pill that fits in the space between your palms is designed to flow effortlessly down your trachea as you swallow it. Take once after breakfast and then again after lunch for a period of seven to eight days. Chase with half a glass of warm water.

For Mild Pitta PMS Condition
- Manjishta, Saffron & Fennel Milk

MANJISHTA, SAFFRON & FENNEL MILK | SERVES ONE

1 cup organic cow's milk or soya milk
1/2 teaspoon manjishta powder
10 strands saffron thistles
1/4 teaspoon fennel powder
1/2 teaspoon Sucanat

Bring the milk to a boil. Remove from heat. Stir in the manjishta and fennel powders, saffron thistles, and Sucanat. Drink an hour or so before bed. Take for a period of five to seven days.

Ayurvedic Herbal Teas for Pitta Type PMS

Some of the most effective herbal teas for Pitta PMS are birch bark, blackberry leaves, catnip, chamomile, chrysanthemum, comfrey, dandelion leaves, elder flowers, hops, jasmine, lavender, lemon balm, licorice, lotus, marshmallow, passion flower, peppermint, raspberry leaves, red rose flower, saffron, spearmint, violet, and wild cherry bark. You may drink as many as three cups of tea per day prior to and during your menstrual cycle.

Note: Using the steps below, you may use any one to three herbs in equal portion and prepare teas of your choice as you need them.

RASPBERRY & ROSE FLOWER TEA INFUSION | SERVES TWO

4 cups of water
1 tablespoon dried raspberry leaves
1 tablespoon dried rose petals (organic)
1 teaspoon Sucanat (optional)

In a heavy stainless-steel saucepan, bring four cups of water to a boil. Put the herbs in the boiling water and remove from heat. Cover and let simmer for 15 minutes. Strain and add Sucanat directly before drinking.

LAVENDER, FENNEL & GINGER TEA DECOCTION | SERVES TWO

1 cup of water
1 cup of organic cow's milk or soya milk
1 teaspoon roasted fennel seeds
1 tablespoon lavender petals
1 tablespoon hops

1/2 teaspoon ginger powder
1 pinch of saffron

In a heavy stainless-steel saucepan, bring water and milk to a boil. In a small cast-iron skillet, dry roast the fennel seeds for a few minutes until you smell an aroma. Be careful to not over roast them. Add the seeds, lavender petals, hops, ginger powder, and saffron to the boiling decoction and leave to simmer on medium heat for 15 minutes. Then remove from the heat, add one pinch of saffron, and cover and let stand for three to five minutes. Strain and drink while still warm.

Nourishing Foods for Pitta Type PMS

To reduce the hot, penetrating, and volatile qualities of Pitta, eat plenty of fresh, warm, and nourishing foods during your menstrual cycle. The following food recommendations are the most appropriate for Pitta type menstrual disorders and for long-term use by the Pitta type. Use fresh, organic, or local, family farm-grown foods when available; unhydrogenated oils, unrefined brown sugar, Sucanat, rock salt and sea salt; organic milk, butter, and yogurt, and organic soya milk.

Vegetables (Use Seasonally):
Greens (kales, collards, bok choy, mustard, landcress, watercress), bitter greens (arugula, radicchio, dandelion, lettuces, endives), asparagus, green beans, artichokes, broccoli, cauliflower, brussel sprouts, cabbage, cucumber, jicama, Jerusalem artichokes, karela, okra, parsnips, peas, potatoes, sprouts, sweet potatoes, yams, pumpkins, winter squashes (acorn, butternut, buttercup), and summer squashes (yellow, crookneck, zucchini, and patty pan).

Fruits (Use Seasonally):
Apples, apricots, berries, cherries, coconuts, dates, fresh figs, grapes, oranges, pears, pomegranates, sweet tangerines, mangos, melons, pineapples, plums, raisins, cherries, watermelon, and sweet strawberries.

Grains (Whole, Cracked, and Cereal):
Barley oats, cracked wheat, spelt, and kamut; whole wheat, spelt, or kamut berries; and barley.
Use Occasionally: long grain brown rice, sweet brown rice, Basmati white and brown rice, Arborio rice, and sushi rice.
Use Rarely: Quinoa, amaranth, and millet.

Legumes:
Aduki, mung (whole and split), soya, kidney, lima, lentils, navy, black, pinto, split peas, and tofu.

Foods that Exacerbate PMS Symptoms (To Be Avoided):
Caffeine, alcohol, saturated fats, excess salt, oily and spicy foods, and most dairy products; highly processed junk foods, meats, and refined foods that are packed with additives, and refined sugars; frozen, canned, stale, commercially grown, bio-engineered, transgenic foods, and irradiated spices; refined salts, sugars, flours, and oils.

WISE EARTH REMEDIES FOR KAPHA TYPE PMS

Kapha Type Menstruation
- Most vulnerable time: early morning and early evening
- Deep, dull ache resonating in back of belly
- Pain comes at end of cycle
- Flow is thick and whitish with mucus or clots
- Discharge before or after cycle
- Bloating, cramping, and water retention
- Nausea, tender and swollen breasts
- Teary-eyed and sentimental
- Craving sweets and attention
- Lethargic, drowsiness
- Depression and day sleeping

Inner Medicine Guidelines for Kapha Type PMS
- Never take medicine every day.
- Do not use more than three herbs at any given time.
- Always take your remedies after a meal.
- Drink half a glass of water after taking a soft pill or paste.
- Do not take more than two of your homemade pills at any given time.

Ayurvedic Herbal Powders for Kapha Type PMS
The most effective Ayurvedic herbs for Kapha PMS are bitter, pungent, and astringent in quality with a highly stimulating effect such as: gokshura, kutki, manjishta, trikatu, punarnava, vacha, and vidanga. Common herbs and spices that are also excellent for reducing Kapha PMS are black pepper, barberry, uva ursi, black cohosh, cloves, cardamom, cinnamon, turmeric, ginger, and goldenseal. The anupana, medium, specific to Kapha, used to create soft pills and pastes from the powders are aloe vera gel, and honey.

Note: As you become more familiar with your personal needs and the energy of each of these herbs, you may follow the steps on the following page and use any one to three herbs in equal portion to prepare the paste or soft pill of your choice as you need them.

Cyclical Timing for Kapha
Challenging Time: 6:00-10:00 (morning and evening)
Challenging Seasons: Early winter and late winter
Challenging Moon Phase: Early phase of waning cycle

The PMS remedies that follow are to be taken for five to seven days starting one week prior to your anticipated menstrual cycle. If your cycle is not in alignment with the new moon, you may start the remedy on the first day of the new moon and take it for three days. Then again, you may resume taking it for five days or so, prior to the commencement of your cycle. You may use the remedies for a maximum period of three months. Avoid taking the remedy during your cycle unless you have forgotten to take it earlier.

For Deep Kapha PMS Condition
• Gokshura & Vacha Paste
• Trikatu Soft Pill

GOKSHURA & VACHA PASTE | SERVES ONE

1/2 teaspoon gokshura powder
1/4 teaspoon vacha powder
1/4 teaspoon ginger powder
1 teaspoon honey

Combine the three powders in a small bowl and add the honey. Mix into a paste and take it twice daily, once after breakfast and then again after lunch for a period of seven to eight days. Chase with half a glass of warm water.

TRIKATU SOFT PILL | SERVES ONE

1 teaspoon trikatu powder
3/4 teaspoon aloe vera gel

Combine powder and aloe vera gel. Mix into a paste and place in the palm of your left hand. Rub the palms together to roll the paste into a soft pill. As noted earlier, the size of the pill that fits in the space between your palms is designed to flow effortlessly down your trachea as you swallow it. Take once after breakfast and then again after lunch for a period of seven to eight days. Chase with half a glass of warm water.

For Mild Kapha PMS Condition
- Manjishta, Clove & Cinnamon Milk

MANJISHTA, CLOVE & CINNAMON MILK | SERVES ONE

1 cup soya milk
1/2 cup water
1/2 teaspoon manjishta powder
1/2 teaspoon clove powder
1/4 teaspoon cinnamon powder

Combine the milk and water and bring to a boil. Remove from heat. Stir in the powders. Drink an hour or so before bed. Take for a period of five to seven days.

Ayurvedic Herbal Teas for Kapha Type PMS
Some of the most effective herbal teas for Kapha PMS are alfalfa, basil, chamomile, chicory, chrysanthemum, dandelion, elder flower, eucalyptus, hawthorn berries, hibiscus, jasmine, lavender, lemon balm, nettle, orange peel, pennyroyal, sage, sassafras, spearmint, violet, and fresh and dried ginger. You may drink as many as three cups of tea per day prior to and during your menstrual cycle.

Note: Using the steps below, you may use any one to three herbs in equal portion and prepare teas of your choice as you need them.

HAWTHORN BERRIES & ROSEHIPS TEA INFUSION | SERVES TWO

4 cups of water
2 tablespoons dried hawthorn berries
1 tablespoon dried rosehips
1 tablespoon dried orange peel
1 tablespoon ginger powder

In a heavy stainless-steel saucepan, bring four cups of water to a boil. Put the herbs in the boiling water and remove from heat. Cover and let simmer for 25 minutes. Strain and drink while still warm.

LEMON BALM & HIBISCUS TEA DECOCTION | SERVES ONE

3 cups of water
1 tablespoons lemon balm
1 tablespoon dried hibiscus leaves

1 tablespoon dried nettle
1/2 teaspoon fresh lemon juice
1 teaspoon honey

In a heavy stainless-steel saucepan, bring the water to a boil. Add herbs to the boiling water and leave to simmer on medium heat for 15 minutes. Remove from heat, add the lemon juice, cover and let stand for a few minutes. Strain and drink while still warm.

TRIKATU INFUSION | SERVES ONE

Trikatu is a classical Ayurvedic formula consisting of pippali, black pepper, and ginger. It is a powerful digestive aid, a highly stimulating spice combination Kapha types may use frequently. It may also be used occasionally to reduce Vata and Pitta disorders.

1/2 teaspoon trikatu powder
1/2 cup water

In a heavy stainless-steel saucepan, bring one cup of water to a boil. Put the trikatu powder in the boiling water and remove from heat. Cover and let simmer for three minutes. Strain and drink an hour or so after breakfast.

Nourishing Foods for Kapha Type PMS

To ward off the cold and sluggish qualities of Kapha, warm, stimulating, and nourishing foods should be taken during your menstrual cycle. Use fresh, organic, or local, family farm-grown foods; unhydrogenated oils, unrefined brown sugar, Sucanat, rock salt and sea salt; and soya milk—dairy products are regressive for Kapha types. The following food recommendations are the most appropriate for long-term use by the Kapha type, and the most effective foods to relieve Kapha type menstrual disorders, including PMS.

Vegetables (Use Seasonally):
Greens (kales, collards, bok choy, mustard, landcress, watercress, turnip greens), bitter greens (arugula, radicchio, dandelion, lettuces, endives), asparagus, green beans, artichokes, broccoli, bell peppers, peppers, carrots, carrot tops, celery, corn, eggplant, karela, jicama, leeks, cauliflower, brussel sprouts, cabbage, okra, parsnips, peas, summer squashes (yellow, crookneck, zucchini, patty pan), spinach, sprouts, and turnips.

Fruits (Use Seasonally):
Apples, apricots, berries, cherries, peaches, pears, persimmons, pomegranates, and quince.

Use Occasionally: grapes, tangerines, mangos, oranges, limes, lemons, raisins, and strawberries.

Grains (Whole, Cracked, and Cereal):
Barley, buckwheat, millet, rye, and corn.
Use Occasionally: long grain brown rice, Basmati white and brown rice, quinoa, and amaranth.
Use Rarely: Cracked wheat, spelt, and kamut.

Legumes:
Aduki, mung (whole and split), soya, kidney, lima, red lentils, black beans, navy, pinto, split peas, and Tofu

Foods that Exacerbate PMS Symptoms (To Be Avoided):
Caffeine, refined sweets, alcohol, saturated fats, excess salty, oily and spicy foods, and most dairy products; highly processed junk foods, meats, and refined foods packed with additives; frozen, canned, stale, commercially grown, bioengineered, transgenic foods, and irradiated spices; refined salts, sugars, flours and oils.

GHEE: GOLDEN ELIXIR OF HEALING

Ayurveda considers milk to be the first and most complete food on earth. Ghee, made from milk, is thought of as the golden elixir of health, a pristine food source for cultivating ojas and the Mother Consciousness. This gentle food comes from the cow's ability to churn grass into milk, a phenomenal ability that is intrinsic to the cosmic memory of the cow. Milk was traditionally collected well after the delivery of the cow's calf, so that it could be properly digested by the human system. From this salubrious food comes buttermilk, butter, yogurt, and ghee. But milk is *sattvic*, peaceful, only when its quality remains pure and unadulterated.

Milk has been used widely but not wisely throughout the ages. Because of the corruption prevalent in today's animal husbandry, we are in danger of losing this sacred food. The cruel treatment of animals as well as the arsenal of poisons, chemicals, and hormones used in cows' feed contribute to the misery of this beneficent animal and the impairment of its life-sustaining milk. When butter, yogurt, and ghee are made from organic milk they are our most nourishing and healing foods. Ghee is regarded as an intelligence building principle that fosters the body's strength and virility when used internally. The Ayurveda sage Charaka praises its ability to promote memory and immunity. Like honey, ghee is able to penetrate deep within the tissues, making it a potent anupana for conveying herbal powders, essences, and medicines into the vital tissues.

Ghee is made by boiling sweet butter, which rids it of enzymes that encourage bacteria. The ghee quality stems from the quality of the butter, and how it is made and stored. Medicinal quality ghee is made in an earthen pot and is stored under strict conditions. It requires no refrigeration, as the elements that cause butter to spoil have been removed. It does need to be kept covered, away from direct sunlight or heat, and free from water or any other contaminants. Used in small quantities in cooking, ghee is a powerful rejuvenator. It blends with food nutrients without losing its medicinal quality, so that it soothes and nourishes bodily constituents.

From the perspective of sadhana, ghee is associated with *sneha*, the vital tissue element of love. By following this sadhana practice of making ghee, we may strengthen ojas and bring our "love tissue" into a state of balance. Making ghee is one of the simplest, most rewarding forms of meditation I know. Ghee is good for all doshas and is specifically recommended for Pitta and Vata types.

To maintain excellent perennial health and well-being all year long, try the following sadhana practices of making ghee and Inner Medicine spice masalas. Observing the meditative, aromatic, and vibratory practices that follow will help you to refine the Mother Consciousness within and alleviate all disorders relating to your sacred reproductive anatomy.

THE PRACTICE: MAKING GHEE

1 pound organic sweet butter
heavy stainless-steel saucepan
stainless-steel spoon

Sterilize the saucepan, spoon, and storage jar in advance by immersing them in boiling water. Melt the butter in the saucepan over a very low flame. Continue to heat the butter until it boils gently and buff-colored foam rises to the surface. It's important not stir the melted butter or remove any of the foam. Allow the ghee to cook gently until the foam thickens and settles to the bottom of the pan as sediment. When the ghee turns a golden color and begins to boil silently, with only a trace of air bubbles on the surface, it is done. (At this point it will have a wonderful aroma!) Once it is cool, pour the liquid into a clean glass jar, making sure that the sediment remains on the bottom of the pan and does not go into the jar. The sediment may be eaten as a luxurious snack.

HERBAL MASALAS:
HEALING IN HARMONY WITH THE SEASONS

Masalas are significant everyday Inner Medicine to bolster immunity and heighten your rhythmic dance with nature. To maintain good health all year long, you can learn to prepare and enjoy your masalas with the rhythms of each season. As you continually make masalas, you will find that your reproductive health and self-love will blossom. Soon you will want to create your own masala combinations from a variety of herbs and spice seeds available to you that you find especially appealing. These wonderful masalas can also be used to wisely add flavor to your meals and heighten their remedial value. By this means, you are using the rasa, essences of the herbs and spices, to safeguard your health and prevent ailments, while also adding variety and energy to your meals.

Learning to use your grinding stones and suribachi, mortar and pestle, to prepare your herbal masala remedies will also stimulate your Shakti energy and bring you great joy. The postures you assume and sounds and aromas you produce while you grind your spices will make this delightful practice a musical and healing one as well. Making your own masala is a great way to personalize the remedies you may need on a daily and seasonal basis. In this way, you may keep in gentle touch with your physical and emotional needs from day to day by tuning into your own body's cues as to what's appealing to you. As you progress in your mastery of masalas, you may be interested in using the spices of your own ancestry, which will be especially potent in reordering your ancestral memories. Here are a few general guidelines for masalas:

- When using the spice seeds, begin by roasting them. The heat helps renew the energy and memory of the seeds. Using a cast iron skillet, roast one type of seed at a time for a few minutes over moderate flame until they begin to crackle or pop. Be careful not to burn the seeds.
- Next sit on the clean kitchen floor, preferably in the squatting or diamond posture, if you can comfortably do so, and place a mortar and pestle on the ground. Grind the seeds one kind at a time, in a clockwise motion.
- Allow yourself to become immersed in the circular movement of your hands. Be mindful of the blissful aroma and blissful resonance of each herb or spice as it is ground. Be mindful, as well, of the inner tranquility you feel as you grind away the cares and fears of the day. Be aware of the rasa essences and rich taste this sadhana gives to your food remedy.

Use a grinding stone (sil and batta) for ingredients such as cinnamon sticks, cloves, fresh ginger, garlic or turmeric root, fresh or dried chilies, dried leaves, and dried tamarind. Generally, we use the grinding stones to prepare a wet or moist paste or masala. When using the grinding stone to crush fresh roots or dried fruits, use a quarter palmful of water to help blend the ingredients. Wet masala must be used at once and cannot be stored. The quantities provided in each recipe will last a family of two people about one week. Use these healing masalas with your vegetable stir-fries, bean dishes, and grains to prepare wholesome meals for yourself and family.

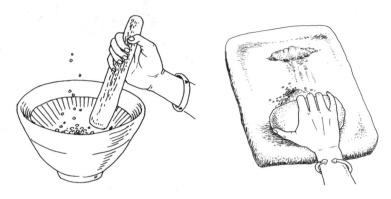

Figure 7.1 & 7.2   A Hand Grinding Spice Seeds in a Suribachi and on a Sil Batta

THE PRACTICE: MAKING SEASONAL MASALAS

SPRING MASALA:

1 teaspoon cumin seeds
2 tablespoons coriander seeds
1 tablespoon yellow mustard seeds
1 teaspoon black peppercorns
1 teaspoon cardamom seeds

SUMMER MASALA:

2 tablespoons coriander seeds
1 tablespoon fennel seeds
1 tablespoon poppy seeds
1 teaspoon cardamom seeds
10 saffron thistles

Grind the saffron thistles along with the fennel seeds. Do not roast them.

EARLY FALL MASALA:

2 tablespoons celery seeds
1 tablespoon black mustard seeds
1 tablespoon white peppercorns
1 teaspoon ginger powder
1/2 teaspoon grated nutmeg

Roast and grind the spice seeds before adding the ginger powder and grated nutmeg.

AUTUMN MASALA:

1/2 cup sesame seeds

I teaspoon freshly ground cayenne powder

I teaspoon rock salt

Roast and grind the sesame seeds before adding the cayenne and salt.

EARLY WINTER MASALA:

2 tablespoons cumin seeds

2 tablespoons caraway seeds

I teaspoon yellow mustard seeds

I teaspoon turmeric powder

I teaspoon garlic powder

Roast and grind the seeds before adding the spice powders.

LATE WINTER MASALA (WET):

2 cloves garlic

2" piece of fresh ginger root

3 dried red chilies

2 tablespoons coriander seeds

I teaspoon turmeric

Peel the garlic and ginger, roast the coriander seeds, and grind all the ingredients together on a grinding stone. Use half of a palmful of water to meld the ground ingredients. Add turmeric powder toward the end of grinding.

Begin by taking the organic approach to this new (ancient) education by incrementally deepening your sadhana practices in your daily life at your own pace. The more practice you do, the more incentive you'll glean from breathing and flowing in this harmonious river of sadhana. By using your hands to measure your food quantities, you'll find your intuition blossoming—not only in the way you intuitively "measure" your herbs, grains, legumes, seeds, and spices, but in the way you appraise your dreams, goals, and choices in life. In the meantime, I am accommodating your transition by presenting to you the measurements with which you are familiar. However, I strongly recommend that you begin to use your naked hands and fingers to convert these measurements into your own unique angula and anjali so that you may strengthen the pranic energy of your limbs to cultivate the hands of sadhana—the hands whose touch have the power to heal everything they encounter: the good earth, your food, children, friends, and community.

As you will discover, through your act of daily sadhana everything that appears to be external—herbs, foods, remedies, thoughts, and actions—is melded into the fine weave of your personal Inner Medicine resource. No medicine, however powerful, can replace your own. Life is simple. We've made it complex by adding massive amounts of material appendages to it, living in over-stress and contributing to the fallacy that more is better! It is not. Healing is simple. It is a subtle thing—your relationship to the earth, sun, moon, sky, water, forest, animals, and children—is an ongoing initiation. Your love and regard for these things transfer them within your heart, thereby transforming the external to the internal. What you love becomes part of your vital tissues, your ojas, and your destiny.

You'll find the remedies offered in this book simple to prepare and easy to digest. (And no need to worry—you'll develop a taste for the various powders. Women who had first complained about the taste of these herbs now share a tome of compliments about how much they have grown to love their tastes.) These remedies are an extension of your own being—they will work for you immediately—especially when you invest your own energy of sadhana. You'll feel instant tranquility as you start to prepare them. In this way, healing begins long before you imbibe the actual remedy. You'll begin to look forward to your time in your kitchen apothecary, grinding herbal pastes, rolling soft pills, scrubbing grains in your bare hands, feeling the energy in your fingertips as you sprinkle powders and seeds. The more of you that you apply to the preparation of your foods and remedies, the more health, joy, and abundance you and your family will gain. Indeed, your being will become transformed into the very act of darshana—all life that surrounds you will begin to glow from the healing light emitting in and from your presence. Everything you touch will nourish, nurture, and heal. This is my profound desire for you.

Chapter Eight

HEALING DIFFICULT
MENSTRUAL DISORDERS

Through dedication to the Wise Earth Ayurveda healing practices,
you can finally regain your inner calm and strength.

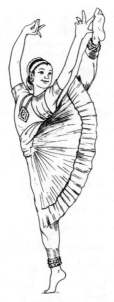

Figure 8.1 Dance of Light

The beauty of Ayurveda is that rather than lump all women together, it addresses the different doshas—Vata, Pitta, and Kapha. As we have learned, the doshas work together to produce the menstrual flow, and when they are out of balance, the menstrual cycle becomes irregular. Some of these common reproductive system disorders include menorrhagia, heavy menstrual bleeding; dysmenorrhea, difficult menstruation with cramps; amenorrhea, delayed or absent menstruation; and leucorrhoea, abnormal vaginal discharge. Luckily, some simple Ayurvedic cures can help alleviate and often cure these discomforts. When experienced by women of different metabolic types, each one of the disorders I'll discuss will reflect particular symptoms allied with each dosha. The longer a disorder lasts the more chronic it becomes and, invariably, it adapts a more Vata-like nature, which is characterized by symptoms such as mental vagueness, loss of appetite, sleeplessness, and a persistent feeling of weariness.

Since we take into consideration both the individual constitution and its condition for each disorder, I will set out the food and remedies for each type—Vata, Pitta, and Kapha. The Uttara Vasti home therapy presented in Chapter Five when applied in the new moon cycle with the Triphala-Aloe Decoction is one of the most effective measures for all of these disorders.

HEALING MENORRHAGIA: HEAVY MENSTRUAL BLEEDING

Lindsey, a 40-year old Pitta type woman who attends our classes regularly told me that her heavy menstrual flow each month felt like "letting the rage out of my body." For years before she had summed up the courage to leave her abusive, alcoholic husband, Lindsey kept her torment and anger bottled up inside of her. After her divorce, she said that she bled almost nonstop for more than six months. Finally, she has given herself permission to release her rage. Through her dedication to Wise Earth Ayurveda's healing practices, she has finally been able to regain her inner calm and strength. Her menstrual flow is now back to normal in consonance with the new moon cycle.

Menorrhagia is characterized by heavy bleeding with prolonged menstrual cycles punctuated by spotting between periods. Pitta is predominant in menorrhagia, since it relates to the blood tissue; Pitta controls the fire element of the body and relates also to the emotion of anger and excess. According to Ayurveda, the condition of menorrhagia arises from the *rakta dhatu*, blood tissue, and is caused by an excess Pitta condition in the blood. Other contributing factors may be endometriosis, adenomyosis, fibroids, tumors, and polyps. (A common cause of painful, heavy bleeding, adenomyosis is a condition in which the glands that normally grow in the endometrium pierce deeply into the walls of the uterus.) Menorrhagia may also be caused by incomplete miscarriages, abortions, cervical erosions, IUD contraceptives, and birth control pills.

Emotional sources at the root of this condition may be unresolved anger, resentment, and hostility. Menorrhagia may be aggravated by poor lifestyle habits such as binging on spicy, hot, oily, sour, and poor quality foods; irregular sleeping habits; drinking alcohol; and excessive work. This condition is related to stress and is generally experienced by the Pitta type who is driven by career, work, creativity, and financial and material power. Menorrhagia is both a condition of excess and deficiency, since heavy bleeding can ultimately lead to malnourishment and anemia (low red blood-count caused by insufficiency of iron and minerals necessary to keep the blood tissue happy).

Menorrhagia is such an extreme Pitta condition that all constitutional types need to observe a strong Pitta-reducing course of food, herbs, and cosseting therapies to heal the condition. In Sanskrit, internal bleeding is called *rakta-pitta*, meaning heat in the blood. However, in Ayurveda we must consider the individual constitution. Therefore I have set out the remedies for menorrhagia in accordance with each of the three types. All constitutional types may follow the Pitta type food recommendations. The Uttara Vasti Therapy presented in Chapter Five when used with the Triphala-Aloe Decoction and applied in the new moon cycle is one of the most powerful remedial measures for menorrhagia.

Symptoms of Menorrhagia
- Heavy menstrual bleeding
- Chronic menstrual bleeding
- Sharp pain during periods
- Fatigue and stress
- Anger, hostility
- Anemia, with low red blood-count
- Spotting in between periods
- Diarrhea, fever
- Cravings for spicy, hot, salty, and sour foods, and intoxicants

WISE EARTH REMEDY FOR VATA TYPE MENORRHAGIA

As noted earlier, menorrhagia is a Pitta condition characterized by excess menstrual bleeding and may be experienced by all three constitutional types. Vata type bleeding is generally caused by dryness of the mucus membranes and is dark red, dry, and frothy in quality. Immediate treatment to lessen bleeding requires the same herbs and roots that are astringent: Arjuna, manjishta, ashoka, fresh turmeric root, alum powder, and triphala. Long-term treatment to bring Vata into a state of harmony requires rejuvenating herbs such as: ashwagandha, shatavari, licorice, and bala. The most effective common herbs for Vata type menorrhagia are tannins from barks such as white oak and wild cherry, along with blessed thistle, yarrow, plantain, turmeric, and licorice. Aloe vera gel and ghee act as a terrific anupana to carry the herbal essences deeply into the blood tissue. A simple remedy consists of half a teaspoon of any of these herbal powders infused in half a cup of warm water and taken as tea. You may use these remedies as needed.

Ideally, choose one of the two remedies presented and take it for a period of seven days each month for three consecutive months, starting on the first day of the new moon. However, if the condition persists during your menstrual cycle, take the remedy once daily after breakfast for the duration of your cycle, starting two days prior to the commencement of your menstrual cycle. Be especially alert with your nutrition and activities during the crucial periods, noted below, when Vata tends to go out of balance.

Symptoms of Vata Type Menorrhagia
- Excess menstrual bleeding
- Dryness of mucus membrane
- Thin, dryish, dark red blood
- Blood in the stool
- Intermittent constipation and diarrhea
- Dry cough
- Anxiety, fearfulness
- Cravings for spicy, salty, and sweet foods

Cyclical Timing for Vata
Challenging Time: 2:00-6:00 (morning and afternoon)
Challenging Seasons: Early fall (rainy season) and autumn
Challenging Moon Phase: Last phase of waning cycle

SHATAVARI & ALUM PASTE | SERVES ONE

1/2 teaspoon shatavari powder
1/4 teaspoon alum powder
1/4 teaspoon licorice powder
1 1/2 teaspoons aloe vera gel

Combine powders in a small bowl and add the gel. Mix into a paste and take it once daily after breakfast for the rest of your cycle, starting two days prior to the start of your cycle. If the condition persists, take it after dinner for a period of seven days each month for three months, starting on the new moon. Chase with half a glass of warm water.

WILD CHERRY & RASPBERRY TEA | SERVES ONE

2 cups water
1 tablespoon wild cherry bark
1 tablespoon raspberry leaves
1 tablespoon aloe vera gel

Bring the water to a boil on medium heat in a stainless-steel saucepan. Add the wild cherry bark and raspberry leaves and remove from heat. Cover and let simmer for 15 minutes. Strain and stir in the gel before drinking. Take once after breakfast and then again after lunch during your menstrual cycle.

WISE EARTH REMEDY FOR PITTA TYPE MENORRHAGIA

For the Pitta constitution, the effects of heavy and prolonged menstrual bleeding can be devastating. The best treatments to immediately stop the bleeding are astringent, haemostatic, cooling, and soothing herbs such as: Arjuna, ashoka, amalaki, bhringaraja, manjishta, and shatavari. The most effective common herbs for assuaging Pitta are rose flower, raspberry leaves, wild cherry bark, white oak bark, coriander, and saffron. Alum powder, aloe vera gel, and ghee act as terrific anupanas to carry the herbs deeply into the blood tissue. A simple remedy consists of half a teaspoon of any of these herbal powders in half a cup of warm water, taken as tea. Use these remedies as needed. Follow the same timeline for Vata type menorrhagia as a preventative measure or if the condition persists.

Because you are treating a condition of excess, you can use the remedies below on a longer-term basis than usual. Choose one of the two remedies presented below and take it for a period of seven days each month for three consecutive months, starting on the first day of the new moon. However, if the condition persists during your menstrual cycle, take the remedy once daily after breakfast for the duration of your cycle, starting two days prior to your menstrual cycle. Be especially alert with your nutrition and activities during the crucial periods, noted below.

Symptoms of Pitta Type Menorrhagia
- Heavy menstrual bleeding
- Chronic menstrual bleeding
- Sharp pain during periods
- Fatigue and stress
- Anger, hostility
- Anemia, with low red blood-count
- Spotting in between periods
- Diarrhea, fever
- Cravings for spicy, hot, salty, sour foods, and intoxicants

Cyclical Timing for Pitta
Challenging Time: 10:00-2:00 (morning and evening)
Challenging Seasons: Spring and summer
Challenging Moon Phase: Mid-phase of waning cycle

MANJISHTA & SHATAVARI PASTE | SERVES ONE

1/2 teaspoon manjishta powder
1/4 teaspoon shatavari powder

1/4 teaspoon alum powder
1 1/2 teaspoons aloe vera gel

Combine the three powders in a small bowl and add the aloe vera gel. Mix into a paste and take it twice daily—once after breakfast and then again after lunch for a period of seven days, starting three days prior to your menstrual cycle. Chase with half a glass of warm water.

YARROW & MUGWORT TEA | SERVES ONE

2 cups water
1/2 teaspoon yarrow powder
1/2 teaspoon mugwort powder
1/4 teaspoon alum powder
1 teaspoon aloe vera gel

Bring the water to a boil on medium heat in a stainless-steel saucepan. Add the powders and remove from heat. Cover and let simmer for 15 minutes. Drain with a cotton strainer and stir in the aloe vera gel before drinking. Take once after breakfast and then again after lunch for the duration of your menstrual cycle.

WISE EARTH REMEDY FOR KAPHA TYPE MENORRHAGIA

Kapha type bleeding is largely due to blockage of the blood vessels by phlegm, which can cause the blood to be rerouted through the wrong channels. Herbs that act as a haemostatic along with mildly astringent and stimulating herbs are required to treat Kapha type menorrhagia. The most effective Ayurvedic herbs are some of the same used for Pitta type: Arjuna, ashoka, manjishta, and shatavari, with the addition of more stimulating herbs such as triphala and trikatu. Common herbs that may be used are agrimony, nettle, blessed thistle, yarrow, mullein, and cattail for assuaging Kapha bleeding. Alum powder, aloe vera gel, and ghee act as a terrific anupana to carry the herbal essences deeply into the blood tissue. A simple remedy consists of half a teaspoon of any of these herbal powders infused in half a cup of warm water and taken as tea. You may use these remedies as needed.

In all types, menorrhagia is an exhaustive condition of excess. The ideal course for all types is to choose one of the remedies presented on the following page and take it for a period of seven days each month, once after breakfast, for three consecutive months, starting on the first day of the new moon. However, if the condition persists during your menstrual cycle, you may take one of the remedies once daily after breakfast for seven days starting three days prior to the commencement of your cycle. In particular, Kapha types need to be especially alert with their nutrition, sleeping habits, and activities during the crucial periods, noted below, when Kapha tends to go out of balance. The times of day most suitable to take the remedy are indicated in each formula.

Symptoms of Kapha Type Menorrhagia
- Heavy menstrual bleeding
- Blood is thick, pale, and slimy
- Dull pain during periods
- Resentment and attachment
- Increase of mucus discharge
- Sluggishness
- Anemia, low red blood-count

Cyclical Timing for Kapha
Challenging Time: 6:00-10:00 (morning and evening)
Challenging Seasons: Early winter and late winter
Challenging Moon Phase: Early phase of waning cycle

MANJISHTA & TRIKATU PASTE | SERVES ONE

1/2 teaspoon manjishta powder
1/4 teaspoon trikatu powder
1 teaspoon aloe vera gel

Combine the powders in a small bowl and add the aloe vera gel. Mix into a paste and take it twice daily—once after breakfast for a period of seven days beginning three days prior to the start of your menstrual cycle. Chase with half a glass of warm water.

AGRIMONY & NETTLE TEA | SERVES ONE

2 cups water
1/2 teaspoon agrimony powder
1/2 teaspoon nettle powder

Bring the water to a boil on medium heat in a stainless-steel saucepan. Add the agrimony and nettle powders and remove from heat. Cover and let simmer for approximately 15 minutes. Drain with a cotton strainer, stir, and drink while still warm. Take twice daily, once after breakfast and then again after lunch for the duration of your menstrual cycle.

HEALING DYSMENORRHEA: DIFFICULT MENSTRUATION WITH CRAMPS

Pamela, a tall, willowy 32-year old Vata type woman attended the satsanga I held at Integral Yoga Center in Greenwich Village to offer nourishment to the ancestors and the departing souls a week after the September 11th disaster. The event was packed; the raw pain and horrific shock was palpable in everyone's demeanor. At the end of the satsanga, I stayed back to give darshana to each and every person. When Pamela arrived at the head of the line to see me, she was bent over with pain. Apparently she was in her monthly cycle.

Pamela lived only 20 blocks away from the World Trade Towers, and unfortunately, from her southern exposed windows she saw the flying debris plummeting out of the exploding towers. Witnessing the massive onslaught firsthand had spurred on her menstrual cycle two weeks earlier than it was due. Her cycle came on the last quarter of the full moon—twelve days earlier than the optimum time with the new moon. I asked two of my female instructor aides to help her to a private room where they did Abhyanga—a vigorous Ayurvedic body rub down, concentrating on her lower back. Within 30 minutes her pain was relieved. After the event, she told me that when she first started her cycle at the age of 14 she was plagued by dysmenorrhea and haunting nightmares with visions of ghosts in flight. In her own words Pamela shared how she spent her last 18 years: "I hid from everyone, felt invisible like I was living out of my body." This haunting continued until she turned 20. Now all of a sudden, her experience of September 11th had brought back the awful cramps and frightening visions.

What most people did not realize was that September 11th occurred at the very midst of *Pitri Paksha*, an auspicious time when Vedic people honor ancestors. The ceremonies we performed that evening were also to remember and nourish the ancestors whom we'd forgotten. As you may not know, our ancestors play an imperative role in our daily lives, in our deaths, and especially in the Hereafter. I encouraged Pamela to continue reciting the Vedic prayers she had learned at the satsanga to appease her ancestors, and to begin studying with the two local Wise Earth Ayurveda instructors who had so caringly massaged her. As a result of her dedicated practice, her nightmares were transformed into visions of peaceful forebears. Not surprisingly, she was quickly able to restore her good health. Within two months she had brought her menstrual cycle back to the new moon phase and the cramps and pain were gone.

Dysmenorrhea, menstrual cramping, often starts during the teenage years and can be a young woman's introduction to pain and discomfort surrounding the menstrual cycle. According to Ayurveda, this difficult menstruation is primarily due to an imbalance in the Vata dosha. This imbalance registers in the uterus as dryness caused by insufficiency of chemical secretions naturally produced by the uterus; it may also be the result of spasms occurring in the uterus's smooth muscles. In accordance with Ayurveda, scientific research shows that dysmenorrhea is an imbalance of chemicals called prostaglandins produced in the uterus. Although dysmenorrhea is mostly common in those with Vata type constitutions, it may also be experienced by Pitta and Kapha types. In the Pitta type, symptoms include burning sensations and diarrhea, whereas the Kapha type may experience congestion, edema, and mucus. Both doshas may also combine to produce a congestive disorder caused by the obstruction of torpid blood.

Dysmenorrhea is characterized by physical and psychic fragility with an overwhelming feeling of disconnect from our physical bodies. It is a condition that is rooted in the ungroundedness of Vata's emotional experience. It expresses isolation, lack of trust of our caretakers, and self-doubt. According to Wise Earth Ayurveda, Vata types are highly spiritually charged, and equipped with a sensitive psyche. Because of their ethereal prowess, their physical stability is often challenged. Dysmenorrhea is also linked to strong physical and emotional experiences with the forebears, and in particular, with the mothers. Inability to interact with warmth, sweetness, or love is symptomatic of the dysmenorrheal experience, which may be linked to the occurrence of coldness and dehydration during pregnancy. This frigid memory is transferred to the child. These conditions may result in nervous system imbalance and a message of distrust in the menstrual memory. Genetic disposition to fear, anxiety, and nervousness can also factor into this condition. For Vata types, dysmenorrhea can be a dominant condition in the developmental years of the female. According to the *Journal of Obstetrics and Gynecology* as many as 60 percent of the world's menstruating teenage population suffers from difficult cramps.

Dysmenorrhea is divided into two types. Primary dysmenorrhea is caused by a spasm of the uterine muscles, with pain occurring in the lower back, lower abdomen, and thighs. It is often associated with bloating, gas, and constipation and may also be accompanied by nausea and vomiting. Secondary dysmenorrhea occurs mostly in women who are over 30, with cramps caused by pelvic disorders such as pelvic inflammatory infections, fibroid tumors, and endometriosis.

Symptoms of Dysmenorrhea
- Difficult menstruation with painful cramps
- Dryness of uterus
- Spasms in smooth muscles of uterus
- Bloating, gas, constipation
- Congestive disorder (relating to Pitta and Kapha)
- Blockage of stagnant blood
- Burning sensation, diarrhea (relating to Pitta)
- Edema, congestion of phlegm
- Pelvic disorders (relating to secondary dysmenorrhea)

WISE EARTH REMEDY FOR VATA TYPE DYSMENORRHEA

Herbs that are antispasmodic, muscle relaxing, and pain reducing make the best remedies for Vata type dysmenorrhea. The most effective common herbs for assuaging Vata type menstrual cramps and pain are turmeric, nutmeg, valerian, asafetida, ginger and licorice. A simple remedy consists of half a teaspoon of any of these herbal powders infused in half a cup of warm water and taken as tea. You may use these remedies as needed. Be especially alert with your nutrition and activities during the crucial periods, noted below.

Symptoms of Vata Type Dysmenorrhea
- Severe colicky pain and cramps
- Constipation
- Abdominal distention and flatulence
- Headaches
- Anxiety, fearfulness
- Palpitations

Cyclical Timing for Vata
Challenging Time: 2:00-6:00 (morning and afternoon)
Challenging Seasons: Early fall (rainy season) and autumn
Challenging Moon Phase: Last phase of waning cycle

SHATAVARI & LICORICE PASTE | SERVES ONE

1/2 teaspoon shatavari powder
1/4 teaspoon licorice powder
1/4 teaspoon jatamansi powder
1 1/2 teaspoons aloe vera gel

Combine the three powders in a small bowl and add the aloe vera gel. Mix into a paste and take it twice daily—once after breakfast and then again after lunch for a period of seven to eight days. Chase with half a glass of warm water.

TURMERIC & NUTMEG SOFT PILL | SERVES ONE

1/2 teaspoon turmeric powder
1/2 teaspoon nutmeg powder
1/4 teaspoon valerian powder
1 teaspoon honey

Combine the powders and honey. Mix into a paste and place in the palm of your left hand. Rub the palms together to roll the paste into a soft pill. The size of the pill that fits in the space between your palms is designed to flow effortlessly down your trachea as you swallow it and creates an ideal dosage. Take once after breakfast and then again after lunch for a period of seven to eight days. Chase with half a glass of warm water.

WISE EARTH REMEDY FOR PITTA TYPE DYSMENORRHEA

Herbs that are cooling and soothing, such as manjishta, shatavari, and gotu kola, make the best remedies for Pitta type dysmenorrhea. The most effective common herbs for assuaging Pitta type menstrual cramps and pain are rose flower, licorice, passion flower, raspberry leaves, skullcap, hops, coriander, fennel, and saffron. A simple remedy consists of half a teaspoon of any of these herbal powders prepared as an infusion in half a cup of warm water to be taken as tea. You may use any of the following remedies as needed. Be especially alert with your nutrition and activities during the crucial periods, noted below, when Pitta tends to go out of balance. The times of day most suitable to take the remedy are indicated in each formula.

Symptoms of Pitta Type Dysmenorrhea
- Severe piercing pain and cramps
- Abdominal distention
- Blockage of stagnant blood
- Burning sensation, diarrhea
- Pelvic disorders (relating to secondary dysmenorrhea)
- Congestive disorder (relating to Pitta and Kapha)

Cyclical Timing for Pitta
Challenging Time: 10:00-2:00 (morning and evening)
Challenging Seasons: Spring and summer
Challenging Moon Phase: Mid-phase of waning cycle

GOTU KOLA & LICORICE PASTE | SERVES ONE

1/2 teaspoon gotu kola powder
1/4 teaspoon licorice powder
1/4 teaspoon fennel powder
1 1/2 teaspoons aloe vera gel

Combine the three powders in a small bowl and add the aloe vera gel. Mix into a paste and take it twice daily—once after breakfast and then again after lunch for a period of seven to eight days. Chase with half a glass of warm water.

SAFFRON & SHATAVARI SOFT PILL | SERVES ONE

1/2 teaspoon shatavari powder
1/4 teaspoon coriander powder
10 saffron thistles (ground into powder)
1 teaspoon aloe vera gel

Combine the powders and ground thistles into the aloe vera gel. Mix into a paste and place in the palm of your left hand. Rub the palms together to roll the paste into a soft pill. Take once after breakfast and then again after lunch for a period of seven to eight days. Chase with half a glass of warm water.

WISE EARTH REMEDY FOR KAPHA TYPE DYSMENORRHEA

Herbs that are stimulating and antispasmodic such as vacha, guggulu, and pippali serve as the best remedies for Kapha type dysmenorrhea. The most effective common herbs for restoring balance to Kapha type menstrual cramps and pain are ginger, cinnamon, nutmeg, cardamom, calamus, turmeric, rosemary, myrrh, rosemary, and pennyroyal. A simple remedy consists of half a teaspoon of any of these herbal powders infused in half a cup of warm water and taken as tea. You may use these remedies as needed. Be especially alert with your nutrition and activities during the crucial periods, noted below, when Kapha tends to go out of balance.

Symptoms of Kapha Type Dysmenorrhea
- Dull pain and cramps
- Increase of mucus discharge
- Edema, swelling of the breasts
- Susceptibility to colds or flu
- Abdominal distention
- Blockage of stagnant blood
- Sluggishness
- Congestive disorder (relating to Pitta and Kapha)

Cyclical Timing for Kapha
Challenging Time: 6:00-10:00 (morning and evening)

Challenging Seasons: Early winter and late winter
Challenging Moon Phase: Early phase of waning cycle

VACHA & GINGER PASTE | SERVES ONE

1/2 teaspoon vacha powder (or calamus powder)
1/2 teaspoon ginger powder
1 1/2 teaspoons aloe vera gel

Combine the three powders in a small bowl and add the aloe vera gel. Mix into a paste and take it twice daily—once after breakfast and then again after lunch for a period of seven to eight days. Chase with half a glass of warm water.

CINNAMON & CARDAMOM SOFT PILL | SERVES ONE

1/2 teaspoon cinnamon powder
1/2 teaspoon cardamom powder
1/4 teaspoon turmeric powder
1 teaspoon aloe vera gel

Combine the powders in the aloe vera gel. Mix into a paste and place in the palm of your left hand. Rub the palms together to roll the paste into a soft pill. Take once after breakfast and then again after lunch for a period of seven to eight days. Chase with half a glass of warm water.

HEALING AMENORRHEA: DELAYED OR ABSENT MENSTRUATION

Vrinda was a frightened young woman who had just migrated from New Delhi, India to South Carolina when I met her a few years ago. She came to me for advice because she hadn't menstruated in two years. She was definitely not pregnant, and at 28 years old, she was much too young for menopause. Besides her lack of a period, Vrinda also felt lethargic, complained of indigestion and insomnia, and would often sleep during the day. In reading her facial diagnosis, I could see that she was on the verge of anemia and that her hormonal levels were unbalanced.

My first question, as always, was, "What's going on in your life right now?" She told me that she was upset because she couldn't find a job and she was unhappy living with her aunt. She also said she missed her family, but didn't want to talk to them because it was too painful, making their distance from one another feel more profound.

She said that her father was an alcoholic who badly mistreated her mother. Although she was glad to be away from her unhappy home, she felt guilty about leaving her mother—now divorced from the abusive husband—alone in India. The reason for her missed periods was obvious to me, and it had nothing to do with the stress of not finding a job. She was obviously in conflict with herself, as well as malnourished, depressed, and feeling isolated from her mother and friends. In her despair, her Shakti prana had become stagnant, and as a result, her lethargy had rapidly increased. Apparently, she had been sleeping until noon on most days and had disrupted her body's rhythms, which are meant to be synchronized with the rhythms of nature.

My first advice was that she return to a more normal schedule by waking at six or seven in the morning and going for a walk. I also provided her with information on where to find inexpensive calling cards to India so she could speak more frequently to her mother, and suggested she visited the local agencies that help find the right jobs for her computer skills. I also counseled her to help her aunt with the chores, to visit the local health food stores and organic farmers' market, and to cook wholesome foods, which I knew would not be a hardship since she loved to cook. To regulate her digestive fire and to get stagnated energy moving again, I told her that a week before and after the new moon, she should take twice-daily doses of trikatu, a combination of pippali (a type of pepper), black pepper, and ginger, which are meant to give fire to the body. Finally, I "prescribed" the Uttara Vasti therapy, which she was instructed to do in accord with the new moon cycle.

Vrinda began menstruating again within three months—on the new moon. When I last spoke to her, six months later, she still hadn't found work, but she was having regular periods at the new moon, and was conversing with her mother regularly. By taking interest in cooking and the general care of the home, she was feeling more nourished and cared for, and at the same time she was cementing a more loving relationship with her aunt. Vrinda was on the menstrual mend.

Amenorrhea tells a deeply emotional story of feeling unworthy as a woman. It is a condition that expresses a lack of self-love, self-esteem, and nourishment. According to Wise Earth Ayurveda, amenorrhea is a deep condition that can start in the embryo and take form in the developmental years of the female. It is linked to strong physiological and emotional experiences of the mother such as violence, trauma, poor nutrition, anemia, emaciation, and dehydration, the memory of which has been transferred to the child. These conditions may result in the displacement of the uterus at birth, hormonal imbalance, and a message of fear in the menstrual memory. Excessive exposure to cold may also contribute to this disease, especially if the mother was cold during the child's birth or her pregnancy. Genetic disposition to diabetes and low blood pressure can also factor in to this complex condition.

Amenorrhea is considered a deficiency disease largely attributed to Vata dosha. As it goes on, it may develop a strong presence in the Kapha bodily humor, tracing its condition all the way back to the maternal building block of the body. For this reason, rasa—the greater sense of appetite and taste—is also impaired. As a result, food-related disorders such as binging, overeating, anorexia, and bulimia are common habitual behaviors in the amenorrhea experience. In all conditions of amenorrhea, the body's deeply principled immunity, ojas, is seriously diminished. I have guided numerous women with amenorrhea who exhibit the same deep emotions, including maternal distrust, low self-esteem, and a conditioned sense of repulsion to any form of nurturance. Despite the range of ages, what I have noticed is that each of the women was subconsciously trying to hold back the biological clock of coming into their womanhood and maternal nature.

WISE EARTH REMEDY FOR VATA TYPE AMENORRHEA

Stimulating and warming herbs that help promote menstrual flow, and rejuvenating tonics that can recreate reproductive health, are the best remedies for Vata type amenorrhea. The Ayurvedic herbs for healing Vata type amenorrhea are ashwagandha, kapikacchu, shatavari, trikatu, and hingu. The most effective common herbs are turmeric, ginger, black pepper, cinnamon, cardamom, cloves, tansy, rue, motherwort, and pennyroyal. Myrrh tincture is also an excellent palliative for amenorrhea in Vata types. Simply add four or five drops of myrrh tincture to half a cup of warm water and take after meals. You may use any of the above mentioned herbal powders to make a tea remedy by using half a teaspoon of any powder and infusing it in half a cup of warm water. These teas can also be brewed from the dried leaves, bark, or seeds of the herbs by using one tablespoon of the herbs and infusing them in a cup of hot water. Any of these teas may be taken when desired. Be especially alert with your nutrition and activities during the crucial periods, noted on the following page, when Vata tends to go out of balance.

Because you are treating a condition of deficiency or insufficiency, you may use these remedies on a longer-term basis than usual. Choose one of the two remedies presented and take it for a period of seven days, once after breakfast each month for three to five months, starting on the first day of the new moon. The times of day most suitable to take the remedy are indicated in each formula.

Symptoms of Amenorrhea
- Associated with Vata dosha
- Poor nutrition, emaciation
- Emotional trauma
- Displacement of uterus from birth

- Hormonal imbalance early in life
- Dehydration
- Feelings of maternal lack, low self-love
- Fearful of becoming a woman
- Long term exposure to cold
- Impairment of ojas (relating to Kapha)

Cyclical Timing for Vata
Challenging Time: 2:00-6:00 (morning and afternoon)
Challenging Seasons: Early fall (rainy season) and autumn
Challenging Moon Phase: Last phase of waning cycle

ASHWAGANDHA & TRIKATU PASTE | SERVES ONE

1/2 teaspoon ashwagandha powder
1/4 teaspoon trikatu powder
1 teaspoon honey

Combine the powders in a small bowl and add the honey. Mix into a paste and take it twice daily, once after breakfast and then again after lunch. Chase with half a glass of warm water. Take for a period of seven days each month, once after breakfast for three to five months, starting on the first day of the new moon.

CARDAMOM, CLOVE & CINNAMON SOFT PILL | SERVES ONE

1/2 teaspoon cardamom powder
1/2 teaspoon clove powder
1/4 teaspoon cinnamon powder
1 teaspoon ghee

Combine powders with the ghee. Mix into a paste and place in the palm of your left hand. Rub the palms together to roll the paste into a soft pill. Take once after breakfast, for a period of seven days each month, for three to five months, starting on the first day of the new moon. Chase with half a glass of warm water.

WISE EARTH REMEDY FOR PITTA TYPE AMENORRHEA

Pitta type amenorrhea is usually mild in nature and can be treated with gentle yet stimulating remedies such as saffron, rose flower, raspberry leaves, licorice, hops, fennel, coriander, and dandelion leaves. A simple remedy would consist of half a teaspoon of any of these herbal powders infused in half a cup of warm water and taken as tea. These teas may be taken regularly as needed. Be especially alert with your nutrition and activities during the crucial periods, noted below, when Pitta tends to go out of balance.

Because you are treating a condition of deficiency or insufficiency, you may use the remedies on a longer-term basis than usual. Choose one of the two remedies presented below and take it for a period of seven days each month for three consecutive months, starting on the first day of the new moon. The times of day most suitable to take the remedy are indicated in each formula.

Cyclical Timing for Pitta
Challenging Time: 10:00-2:00 (morning and evening)
Challenging Seasons: Spring and summer
Challenging Moon Phase: Mid-phase of waning cycle

WARM MILK & SAFFRON BREW | SERVES ONE

1 cup organic cow's milk (or soya milk)
12 saffron thistles
A pinch of ginger
1/2 teaspoon Sucanat

In a medium size stainless-steel saucepan, bring one cup of organic cow's milk or soya milk to a boil and remove from heat. Stir in the saffron thistles, ginger powder, and Sucanat, then cover and let stand for a three to five minutes. Drink the brew after eating breakfast. Take for seven days each month for three consecutive months, starting on the first day of the new moon.

SAFFRON & SHATAVARI SOFT PILL | SERVES ONE

1/2 teaspoon shatavari powder
10 saffron thistles (ground into powder)
1/4 teaspoon coriander powder
1 teaspoon aloe vera gel

Combine shatavari and coriander powders and ground saffron thistles into the aloe vera gel. Mix into a paste and place in the palm of your left hand. Rub the palms of your hands together to roll the paste into a soft pill. Chase with half a glass of warm water. Take for seven days each month for three consecutive months, starting on the first day of the new moon.

WISE EARTH REMEDY FOR KAPHA TYPE AMENORRHEA

Kapha type amenorrhea is caused by sluggishness and congestion in the body. Herbs that have a warm and stimulating effect generally move Kapha into a state of balance. The most effective common herbs for restoring balance to Kapha type are trikatu, guggulu, ginger, cinnamon, cardamom, calamus, turmeric, rosemary, myrrh, and pennyroyal. A simple remedy consists of half a teaspoon of any of these herbal powders infused in half a cup of warm water and taken as tea. These teas may be taken regularly, when desired. Be especially alert with your nutrition and activities during the crucial periods noted below, when Kapha tends to go out of balance. The times of day most suitable to take the remedy are indicated in each formula.

Cyclical Timing for Kapha
Challenging Time: 6:00-10:00 (morning and evening)
Challenging Seasons: Early winter and late winter
Challenging Moon Phase: Early phase of waning cycle

CAYENNE & GINGER BREW | SERVES ONE

2 cups water
1/2 teaspoon cayenne powder
1/2 teaspoon ginger powder
1/4 teaspoon black pepper powder
1 teaspoon honey

In a medium size stainless-steel saucepan, bring the water to a boil and remove from heat. Stir in the cayenne, ginger, and black pepper powders, cover and let stand for a few minutes. Add the honey, and drink the brew after breakfast. Take for seven days each month for three consecutive months, starting on the first day of the new moon.

TRIKATU & ALOE VERA GEL SOFT PILL | SERVES ONE

1/2 teaspoon trikatu powder
1/2 teaspoon aloe vera gel

Mix the trikatu powder in the aloe vera gel and create a paste. Place the paste in the palm of your left hand. Rub the palms together to roll the paste into a soft pill. Chase with half a glass of warm water. Take for seven days each month for three consecutive months, starting on the first day of the new moon.

HEALING LEUCORRHOEA:
ABNORMAL VAGINAL DISCHARGE

When Sandra swaggered into the classroom to attend the Women's Health Program, the floorboards shook. Goddess-like with her voluptuous body, jet black wavy hair, and moonlit complexion—she was obviously a Kapha type. She was a professional dancer who had performed in several Broadway musicals and appeared vibrant. But after classes, she shared that for the last three months she had been having a severe case of leucorrhoea, malodorous vaginal discharge. She was on the road traveling with her dance troupe and had been eating poorly with lots of fast foods and sodas. Moreover, she began an affair with one of her dancing partners whom she suspected had many ongoing affairs at the same time. I recommended that she stop her sexual relationship for a while and start on a strict regimen of Kapha nourishing foods, along with doing the Uttara Vasti therapy as recommended in earlier pages. Six months later, on her 30th birthday, she wrote me a letter:

> I've been doing UV and Kapha nourishing food for four months. I can't believe the beauty and ease I feel in my body, no more awful discharges or smells, thank God. I don't know if it's your energy which I feel so close to me, or if it's UV, but I came back from Wise Earth feeling no attraction to Rick and have ended my affair with him. I have faith that the right partner will come when I'm ready. Right now, I'm enjoying every minute of caring for myself as a woman and feeling so whole again.

Leucorrhoea is an abnormal discharge from the vaginal passage linked to excess mucous common to the Kapha dosha, but it can also be caused by the other humors. It occurs when the natural stasis within the vaginal canal goes out of kilter. The vagina has a natural acerbic environment that safeguards it from adverse pathogens. When the acidic balance is off, various bacteria and fungi can exist and thrive. Other contributing factors are lack of personal hygiene, use of antibiotics, sexual indulgence and sexually transmitted diseases, infections, and poor quality foods.

Although this disorder is mainly Kapha produced, it may be experienced by all constitutional types. Vata type discharge is dry, brownish, and sticky, with severe pains in the lower body. Pitta type discharge is yellowish, odious, and sometimes mixed with blood followed by burning sensations. Kapha type discharge is thick and whitish with mucous, with feelings of sluggishness and dullness.

Whatever your constitution, the Kapha humor must be restored to its natural state within the body. The most effective herbs used to heal the condition of leucorrhea are trikatu, vacha, ashwagandha, and shatavari. Common herbs that may be used are barberry, ginger, calamus, prickly ash, tansy, rue, alum root, goldenseal, gentian, and echinacea. The Kapha nurturing foods mentioned in Appendix Two are also essential to alleviate this condition. A simple remedy consists of half a teaspoon of any of these herbal powders in an infusion of half a cup of warm water and taken as tea. You may use these remedies as needed. Ideally, as a preventative measure, you would prepare the remedy Licorice & Ashwagandha Paste below and take it for a period of five days each month, once after breakfast for three consecutive months, starting on the first day of the new moon. You may also use the remedy during the period of the abnormal discharge.

Many of the herbs used to heal leucorrhea are also highly remedial for tricamosis, the yellow-smelling discharge that is produced as a result of a sexually transmitted disease. These herbs may also be prepared and used by men for similar discharges. Ashwagandha, calamus, prickly ash, white oak bark, pine bark, and saw palmetto are some of the most effective herbs used for abnormal reproductive discharges in men.

The most potent therapy practice for leucorrhoea is Uttara Vasti to be applied with the Triphala-Aloe Decoction in harmony with the new moon cycle. Details on Uttara Vasti are presented in Chapter Five.

WISE EARTH REMEDY FOR VATA TYPE LEUCORRHEA

LICORICE & ASHWAGANDHA PASTE | SERVES ONE

1/2 teaspoon licorice powder
1/4 teaspoon ashwagandha powder
1/4 teaspoon shatavari powder
1/2 teaspoon ghee

Combine the three powders in a small bowl and add the ghee. Mix into a paste and take it twice daily—once after breakfast and then again after lunch for a period of five days during the period of the discharge. Chase the remedy with half a glass of warm water.

WISE EARTH REMEDY FOR PITTA TYPE LEUCORRHEA

SHATAVARI & GOLDENSEAL PASTE | SERVES ONE

1/2 teaspoon shatavari powder
1/2 teaspoon goldenseal powder
1/2 teaspoon alum powder
1 tablespoon aloe vera gel

Combine the three powders in a small bowl and add the aloe vera gel. Mix into a paste and take it twice daily—once after breakfast and then again after lunch for a period of five days during the period of the discharge. Chase the remedy with half a glass of warm water.

WISE EARTH REMEDY FOR KAPHA TYPE LEUCORRHEA

TRIKATU & HONEY PASTE | SERVES ONE

1/2 teaspoon trikatu powder
1/2 teaspoon honey

Combine the powder and honey and mix into a paste. Chase the remedy with half a glass of warm water. Take it twice daily—once after breakfast and then again after lunch for a period of five days during the period of the discharge.

STRONG HERBAL TEA FOR LEUCORRHEA (FOR ALL TYPES) | SERVES TWO

3 cups water
1/2 teaspoon tansy powder
1/2 teaspoon rue powder
1/2 teaspoon goldenseal
1 teaspoon honey

Bring the water to a boil on medium heat in a stainless-steel saucepan. Add the powders and remove from heat. Cover and let simmer for 15 minutes. Drain with a cotton strainer, stir, and drink warm. Take it twice daily, once after breakfast and then again after lunch for the duration of the discharge.

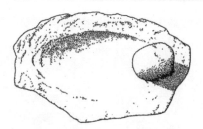

Figure 8.2 Primitive Grinding Stone

Part Four

CARE OF THE WOMB WOMEN'S BEAUTY, FERTILITY & SEXUALITY

Chapter Nine

CARING FOR
THE SACRED YONI

*Caring for the physical sanctum, replenishing the womb in
its inner sanctuary, reconnecting with lunar rhythms, and
performing the rites and ceremonies that safeguard sacred yoni
are necessary if you are to remember your Shakti power.*

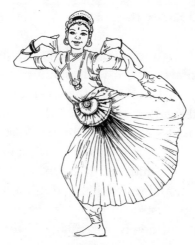

Figure 9.1 Dance of Shakti

As women, sexuality makes us powerful. This largess comes directly from the primeval energy of the Goddess Shakti and her power of creation and regeneration.
Women's sexuality is tied to the yoni, the cosmic gateway through which primordial feminine energy enters and replenishes the heart and womb, and by which it
leaves to nourish and heal the entire world. Yoni in Sanskrit means "womb, vulva,
source, origin, abode, nest, and family." In essence, it is the channel through which
each and every human life must enter the world. Regarded by the Vedic tradition
as sacred, Shakti's cosmic yoni is the source of life, joy, and pleasure. Shakti Yoni
is the primordial cradle from which all creation emerged.

Western cultures refer to the vulva as *vagina*, a word derived from Latin, meaning "sheath for a sword," the sword a metaphor for the penis which is intended to
be sheltered in the safe space of the vagina. By extreme contrast, in Sanskrit the
vulva is described as *bhaga*, the one who contains the overriding power, wealth,
fame, and beauty. In other words, the yoni is a woman's opening or awakening to

consciousness. The yoni behaves like a lotus flower—naturally opening its petals to allow the flow of the menstrual cycle during the new moon phase and closing them slightly after the menses is over. At the end of each day, the yoni performs an almost imperceptible closure of its petals. Understanding the cosmic nature of your yoni will help you reclaim your feminine authority, heal old scars and karmas of the heart and womb, and transform your relationship with your own cosmic body into a thing of wisdom and beauty.

Endowed with creative and sexual divinity, the yoni has been worshipped for thousands of years in India. In South India, an exquisitely carved wooden rendition of the yoni (19th century C.E.) is stained red with the sacred *sindhur* powder worshippers have daubed onto it since it was made. Hundreds of yoni images appear in other parts of the world, many of them from the European Paleolithic period. Today in the United States, the horseshoe, a yoni-shaped symbol, is still rubbed for good luck.

The yoni is directly connected to sexual activity. To protect it, you must first become mindful of your sexual practices, understanding that your yoni is also the gateway to spiritual ascension. The yoni is the most ancient image from which the female's moon-faced vulva and moon-crested womb took its shape. Likewise, the male's sexual organ took its shape from the pestle shaped lingam of Shiva. Unfortunately, under patriarchal rule in Europe, during the destructive course of events that occurred between the 10th and 16th centuries, the goddess power fell into grave demise in the West and took with it all things of the feminine sacred. Witch hunts and inquisitions destroyed the rites of women's divine sensuality. These actions have brutally cut down the female power and its inherent force of nourishment, creativity, and sexuality, leaving a legacy of irretrievable damage to women's relationships, especially the one they have with themselves. As a result, women's rites of passage and vital exchanges with nature have been severely fractured. Moreover, with the continued rise of poverty in the rural areas of India comes societal and familial angst and ignorance resulting in horrendous acts of violence and brutality against women; each year thousands of young girls undergo female genital mutilation. The psychic implications of these far reaching acts of sexual violence against women the world over pervade the collective female buddhi. We must change these detrimental concepts that contribute to the physic pain of women all over the world.

At present, we are still nursing these wounds, paying the price as we strive to regain a wholesome sense of our physical and spiritual anatomy and a nourishing relationship with the Mother Consciousness. As you will see in the wholesome practices set out in this chapter, you can reclaim your voice hidden in the primordial recesses of the Mother's vulva. You can allow your tears to naturally flow in the form of menstruation and urination without medical imposition and scientific intervention. In fact, you must completely lose the latter to reclaim your natural voice and tears and ojas. You can reclaim your ojas, ovulation of pearl-translucent joy, all of which will flow like nectar from the greater maw of wisdom, when you remember who you really are. Ultimately, your yoni represents the continuum of creation and the fulfillment of desire.

The energies of the yoni guide our health, sexuality, creativity, and our intrinsic interdependence on nature. The impairment of the yoni reflects the breakdown of human nourishment, the demise of nature's wholesome foods, the loss of collective memory, the disintegration of family and community, the erosion of sensuality, and the disharmony between the genders—in other words, the fracturing of the Mother Consciousness. Little wonder the scourge of diseases relating to female reproduction and human sexuality continues to grow unabated. At the deepest level of our physiological constituent is *shukra* (sperm), and *artava* (ovum), in that order, the male and female reproductive tissue that is the culmination of the body's nourishment chain, where ojas is built and fortified for the purpose of safeguarding and promoting the procreation of new life. Through a lack of knowledge of our sacred yoni, we have neglected to care for it physically, emotionally, or spiritually.

THE LESSON OF THE YONI

The lesson of the yoni is about unearthing your feminine prowess through healing your feminine fragility. For this you need to employ deep self-care. Knowing the yoni to be the gateway of the inner temple within, you must endeavor to safeguard it at all levels of your being. Caring for the physical sanctum, replenishing the womb in its inner sanctuary, reconnecting with lunar rhythms, and performing the rites and ceremonies that safeguard sacred yoni are necessary if you are to remember your Shakti power.

Participating in indiscriminate sexual liaisons and activities has produced an entire subculture that is inadvertently propagating violence against women and children, and increasing the number of sexually transmitted diseases. The proliferation of venereal diseases is an endemic symptom of the popular culture we live in. It speaks to the erosion of ojas, the yoni's natural cervical mucosa that safeguards it against viral and pathogenic invasions. According to medical science, more than 80 percent of the body's immune cells are located in the mucosal membranes, such as the vulva, vagina, cervix, and urethra. These regions of the female body are greatly affected by stress hormones, and are therefore vulnerable to the manifold layers of real and/or perceived physical threats and physic disturbances put upon them every day.

Claudia's painful story of genital herpes reminds us of the threat that women are exposed to when they exploit the rule of the yoni. Soon after her 32nd birthday,

Claudia discovered that she had genital herpes. Being a Pitta type, her outbreak was devastating. After returning from a late night tryst with one of her boyfriends, she woke up the next day with a high fever and a painful outbreak of red, swollen genital ulcers that persisted for several days. A few months after her initial outbreak, Claudia attended the Wise Earth Ayurveda Women's Program I was teaching in New York. After the workshop, she approached me and asked if I had an Ayurvedic solution to her condition. She confided that she had been "sexually involved" with three men and was so mortified by her condition that she has had stopped seeing all of them.

I told her that although celibacy is a compelling way to heal the symptoms of her problem, she first needed to dig deep and find the reasons behind her sexual habits. Quickly, she was able to trace some of her behavior to the anger she felt toward her mother who had been the one to initiate a divorce from her father who was having an affair with his secretary. As Claudia began to explore her past, she discovered that she had underscored her fragility by exposing her yoni to untoward experiences and circumstances. She was eager to learn the lesson of the yoni and followed the recommendations that I gave her: a year of celibacy practice, the Ayurvedic food sadhana practices, and the Pitta herbal recommendations for herpes (see pages 160-161). At first it was difficult for Claudia to embrace the sacred practice of sexual restraint, but as she cogitated on the true nature of her yoni and stayed with the Wise Earth Ayurvedic healing regimen, she was able to become deeply reflective of her feminine health and her life purpose.

Within three months of her dedicated practice, she had restored health to her yoni and was free of all symptoms. Three years later, she got married to a wonderful young man with whom she shares a spiritual life. She has never had a recurrence. Claudia wrote me these special words:

> My husband, Tim, is awed by the reality that I take such care of my sacred yoni. I teach him what you have made me understand about myself, that my yoni is the passage through which our child will first come through to see the world. He is eager to meet Mother and learn more about his own reproductive sanctity as a man.

WELCOMING SHAKTI PRANA WITH YONI MUDRA

Women are the gatekeepers to life. We hold within our bodies and minds the breath of the goddess called, Shakti prana, the central prana in a woman's body that safeguards her primordial feminine energies. In the body, Shakti prana congregates in the lower chakras located around the perineum and sacrum. Shakti prana is the body's inherent reproductive life force; when in a state of balance, it protects the health of the reproductive organs, genitals, womb, belly, and breasts. Working in tandem with apana vayu, it gives tremendous power to bring forth life as in the birthing process, and helps the uterine lining extract from the body at its appropriate time in the lunar cycle. Strengthening Shakti prana is imperative if we are to protect the hallowed gateway to life, along with the vagina, cervix, and urinary tract. In Tantric Sri Vidya tradition, the goddess is invoked through 10 hand gestures. The most powerful mudra to draw Shakti's power within a woman is called the Yoni Mudra ("womb seal"). You can reclaim the remarkable power of the womb by practicing Yoni Mudra, which strengthens Shakti prana and redirects the menstrual blood back in accordance with the new moon. Use this powerful practice to balance hormonal activity in the body even if you are no longer menstruating or sexually active.

In this practice, we gather Shakti's energy within our womb or belly, strengthening and enhancing her prana within us. The Yoni Mudra is especially sacred to women. Among other benefits, it acts as a *bandha* in yoga, locking the aperture to the womb, thereby intensifying the circulation of Shakti prana in this region. As you continue to practice this meditation, you will feel the subtle movement of this breath in the root chakra area. You may experience the breath as a light, serpentine movement along the spine or as a pulsating pressure in the womb region.

Practice Yoni Mudra for three days directly before the new moon and the full moon phases, or at any time you want to revitalize Shakti prana, except during your menstrual cycle, pregnancy, or when bleeding from the lower pathways. Circle these important dates in your moon calendar as a reminder to do this practice every month.

THE PRACTICE: YONI MUDRA

- Sit in a meditative posture and cup your hands together, palms facing up.
- Intertwine the little fingers and fully extend the middle fingers, which meet at the tips to form a pyramid shape.
- Cross the ring fingers behind the extended middle fingers and hold them down with the index fingers.
- Tuck in your thumbs to touch the base of the middle fingers.
- Hold the hand gesture for five minutes.
- Allow your breath to flow freely by taking quiet inhalations and exhalations while holding the mudra pose.
- Visualize your breath flowing freely throughout your body, keeping your mind centered on mudra.
- This mudra will help to bring your mind into a deep state of calmness.

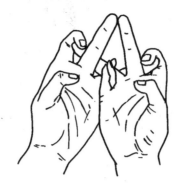

Figure 9.2 Yoni Mudra

WATER CARE OF THE YONI

Millions of Hindus go to the sacred Mother River of India to pray, offer oblations, chant, and take reprieve in the cool flowing arms of Ganga, the River Goddess. These sacred waters are said to have emerged from the head of God Shiva. On my frequent visits to Sri Swami Dayananda's ashram in Rishikesh, India, I never miss the chance to take *snanam*, a bath in the holy river, Ganges. Mother River penetrates to the core, surrounding me with her cool, rushing embrace as I continually rediscover my ancient karma.

At the Sringeri Shrine, a small village in the mountains of Karnataka, the present day avatar, Sri Sankaracharya, continues the unbroken tradition of identifying with and serving Shakti, Mother of the Universe. There at the Goddess Sarada Temple, Hindus bathe in the cool, crystal waters of the Tunga River before entering the stone sanctuary where the breathtaking stone image of the goddess resides. Several priests preside over the sacraments of flowers, incenses, fruits, rice, milk and water, thereby offering their obeisance to the goddess. They use special mudras for each elemental offering. In flawless spiritual choreography and syncopated Vedic rhythms, they chant the Devi Mantras in Sanskrit and toll the bells and ripple the *damaru*—a small double-headed hourglass shaped hand drum. With a flaming camphor brass lamp they offer *aarti* to the goddess employing circular motion from her from head to her toe. In the end, they transport the goddess's light and blessings to the pilgrims by pouring sacred water on their heads.

Millions of pilgrims visit the various sacred rivers around the world to pay homage and take the blessings of Mother Water. In fact, water is the most powerful element in the universe. Like all elements, water is composed primarily of energy. By this means, it has the ability to cleanse, nurture, purify, comfort, and heal. "Crossing the ocean of samsara," is an expression used by Hindus as a metaphor for enduring the lengthy rebirth process of human evolution, finally to merge into the Pure Consciousness.

AMAZING WISE EARTH HERBAL HIP BATHS

There is a holy river within each one of us that has the power to cleanse and revive the mind and body. In the Hindu tradition, the sacred Ganges is seen pouring out from the head of God Shiva carrying the Goddess Ganga in its flow. In ways both big and small, you too may take the blessings of the goddess every time you touch water. This goddess element shapes and supports the biological foundation of life within and without. In a deeper way, it manifests as embryonic fluid within the womb. Transcend the meaning of your bath into that of a snanam, a sacred dip that can help to revitalize your yoni energy, and heal its ailments. Let the bath water buffer you and transport your healing experience into that of being afloat in the cosmic embryonic fluid of the Mother. For numerous conditions of the vulva, vagina, cervix, urethra, and bladder, prepare the Herbal Hip Bath with warm water and soothing herbs—a combination of aloe, gentian, and lemongrass—to gently wash the negative karmas and pathogens, sores and lesions, stagnant energies, and toxicities. These baths are an excellent measure to nourish the mucosa surfaces of the womb and repair hurtful conditions of the yoni. (There is more on sacred rejuvenative baths in Chapter Fourteen.)

Preparing Herbal Decoctions for Your Bath
The herbal hip baths that follow may be used to heal a number of conditions relating to your female reproductive and vaginal health and wellness.
Lunar Timing: New moon phase is the most effective timing for all conditions relating to the health of the reproductive organs, vagina, vulva, cervix, and lower urinary tract. You may also perform the herbal bath practice at any time of the moon phase that you may be experiencing vaginal symptoms or an outbreak.
Time of Day: Evening

THE PRACTICE: HERBAL HIP BATHS

LEMONGRASS & ALOE BATH DECOCTION
Conditions: Genital herpes, venereal warts

1 gallon water
1/4 cup dried lemongrass
2 tablespoons gentian powder
2 cups aloe vera gel

Bring the water to a boil over medium heat in a stainless-steel pot. Place the dried herbs and powder into the water and bring to a boil. Lower the heat and simmer for five minutes. While the decoction is boiling, prepare your bath by filling the tub about a quarter full with warm water. Remove herbs and powder from heat and use a colander to strain the decoction. Add the aloe vera gel into the warm decoction and pour into bath.

Sit in the bath for 15 minutes, preferably while squatting. Use the bath decoction to wash the vaginal lesions. After drying your body, apply a dab of comfrey-goldenseal ointment or salve on the lesions. (You may purchase the ointment from health food stores. Most carry an excellent range of locally made ointments.)

TRIPHALA, GOLDENSEAL & GENTIAN BATH DECOCTION

Conditions: Candida, vaginitis, yeast infection, vaginal sores or itching, vulvar pain

1 gallon water
2 tablespoons triphala powder
2 tablespoons goldenseal powder
2 tablespoons gentian powder
1/4 cup aloe vera gel

Bring the water to a boil over medium heat in a stainless-steel pot. Add the herbal powders to the water and bring to a boil. Lower the heat and simmer for five minutes. While the decoction is boiling, prepare your bath by filling the tub about a quarter full with warm water. Remove from heat and use a colander to strain the decoction. Add the aloe vera gel into the warm decoction and pour into bath.

Sit in the bath for 15 minutes, preferably while squatting. As with the Uttara Vasti Bath, contract the vaginal muscles to allow some of the bath decoction to enter the uterus. Hold the decoction for a few minutes before releasing the vaginal muscles. Repeat this practice once or twice. After drying your body, daub a bit of comfrey-goldenseal ointment in the vaginal passage. (You may purchase the ointment from health food stores. Most carry an excellent range of locally made ointments.)

SARSAPARILLA, TRIPHALA & SAFFLOWER BATH DECOCTION

Conditions: Syphilis, gonorrhea, HIV, AIDS, venereal warts, candida, yeast infections

1 gallon water
2 tablespoons sarsaparilla powder
2 tablespoons triphala powder
2 tablespoons safflower threads
1/4 cup aloe vera gel

Bring the water to a boil over medium heat in a stainless-steel pot. Add the herbal powders and threads to the water and bring to a boil. Lower the heat and simmer for five minutes. While the decoction is boiling, prepare your bath by filling the tub about a quarter full with warm water. Remove from heat and use a colander to strain the decoction. Add the aloe vera gel into the warm decoction and pour into bath.

ALOE VERA GEL & TURMERIC BATH INFUSION
Conditions: Miscarriage, abortion, sexual abuse, rape

For Miscarriage and Abortion: Take the following bath for three days. This warm and mildly stimulating bath will help to remove the stagnant blood from the uterus and comfort it with special herbs such as aloe vera gel, myrrh, and turmeric. You may also follow the herbal recommendations, set out below.

For Sexual Abuse and Rape Victims: Take the bath for ten consecutive days. You may also follow the herbal recommendations, set out below.

1 gallon water
1/4 cup aloe vera gel
2 tablespoons turmeric powder

Bring the water to a boil over medium heat in a stainless-steel pot. Add the aloe vera gel and the turmeric powder. Remove from heat and let stand for five minutes. In the meantime, prepare your bath by filling the tub about a quarter full with warm water. Pour the infusion into the bath. Enter the bath with care and support yourself by bracing on the rim of the tub while slowly sitting in the bath.

GENITAL HERPES

Genital herpes is a tenacious viral infection that is contracted through sexual activity. Once infected, the virus remains stored in the DNA of the contaminated tissue or spinal nerve and can remain inactive for years. When activated, the virus causes characteristic lesions on the genital organs. A highly Pitta condition, the initial outbreak of herpes may include fevers, swollen and painful genital lesions, swollen lymph nodes in the groin, urinary infections, angst, and anxiety.

From the standpoint of Ayurveda, herpes produces excess heat in the liver that is then transported along the liver meridian into the urinogenital area of the body. This heat can contaminate the blood with bile. Although herpes disorder is largely Pitta in nature, it can involve the other two humors particularly when there is toxicity in the system. Vata type herpes is less painful and exhibits mildly inflamed wart-like lesions that are hard and dryish, and may be accompanied by insomnia, dry skin, constipation, and general fearfulness. Kapha type herpes involves oozing lesions with little pain or redness, and mucus-like vaginal discharge along with excess phlegm and lethargy in the body.

In all cases, food and herbs with antiviral blood cleansing qualities are needed like coriander, gotu kola, sarsaparilla, aloe vera gel, barberry, gentian, and licorice. Rejuvenating tonics are also important to maintain mental and emotional calmness and clarity. Using the Herbal Hip Bath on pages 157-158 to gently wash the sores and lesions is an excellent measure to assuage this condition. Ayurveda recommends avoiding hot, sour, and spicy foods, junk foods, refined carbohydrates, alcohol, excess sugar and salt. In addition, use the food recommendations set out in Appendix Two for both the Pitta type and your individual body type.

WISE EARTH REMEDY FOR VATA TYPE GENITAL HERPES

Note: Venereal diseases such as syphilis, gonorrhea, and venereal warts may also be treated with the Gotu Kola & Sarsaparilla remedy as directed below.

GOTU KOLA & SARSAPARILLA TEA | SERVES ONE

1 cup cow's milk (organic)
1/2 teaspoon gotu kola powder
1/4 teaspoon sarsaparilla powder
1 teaspoon ghee

Bring the milk to a boil on medium heat in a stainless-steel saucepan. Add the powders and remove from heat. Cover and let simmer for a few minutes. Drain with a cotton strainer, and stir in the ghee while the infusion is still warm. Take once after breakfast and then again after lunch for the duration of the outbreak.

Note: If you prefer, this remedy may also be prepared as a soft pill by omitting the milk and using one and a half teaspoons of ghee instead. Take with one cup of warm water.

WISE EARTH REMEDY FOR PITTA TYPE GENITAL HERPES

SHATAVARI & GOKSHURA TEA | SERVES ONE

1 1/2 cups water
3/4 teaspoon shatavari powder

1/2 teaspoon gokshura powder
1/2 teaspoon lemongrass powder
1 tablespoon aloe vera gel

Bring the water to a boil on medium heat in a stainless-steel saucepan. Add the powders and remove from heat. Cover and let simmer for a few minutes. Drain with a cotton strainer, and stir in the gel while the infusion is still warm. Take once after breakfast and then again after lunch for the duration of the outbreak.

Note: If you prefer, this remedy may also be prepared as a soft pill by omitting the water. Take with one cup of warm water.

WISE EARTH REMEDY FOR KAPHA TYPE GENITAL HERPES

SARSAPARILLA & TRIKATU TEA | SERVES ONE

1 1/2 cups water
1/2 teaspoon trikatu powder
1/2 teaspoon sarsaparilla powder
1/4 teaspoon clove powder
1 tablespoon aloe vera gel

Bring the water to a boil on medium heat in a stainless-steel saucepan. Add the trikatu, sarsaparilla, and clove powders, and remove from heat. Cover and let simmer for a few minutes. Drain with a cotton strainer, and stir in the aloe vera gel while the infusion is still warm. Take twice daily, once after breakfast and then again after lunch for the duration of the outbreak.

Note: If you prefer, this remedy may also be prepared as a soft pill by omitting the water. Take with one cup of warm water.

BALA TEA FOR GENITAL HERPES (FOR ALL TYPES) | SERVES TWO

3 cups water
1/2 teaspoon bala powder
1/2 teaspoon lemongrass powder
1/2 teaspoon sarsaparilla powder
1/2 teaspoon licorice powder
1 teaspoon aloe vera gel

Bring the water to a boil on medium heat in a stainless-steel saucepan. Add the powders and remove from heat. Cover and let simmer for 15 minutes. Drain with a cotton strainer, stir in the aloe vera gel and drink warm. Take once after breakfast and then again after lunch for the duration of the outbreak.

CANDIDA ALBICANS

The more ravaged the world's food sources become, the more prevalent the diseases relating to our food quality and their negative impact on the digestive system become. In the past year, I have seen more than 100 women who suffered from debilitating Candida, an invasion of the Candida albicans yeast. Yeast infections and Candida are usually caused by a weakened or low digestive fire, which in turn produces ama, the accumulation of undigested food in the intestines. These conditions begin in the gastrointestinal tract. Most people take long courses of antibiotics and strong herbs to alleviate the pathogens. Antibiotics and antifungal herbs can quickly compromise the immune system, especially in Vata types.

According to Ayurveda, Candida can occur in all constitutional types but is most common in Kapha and Vata types. Vata type symptoms include insomnia, fatigue with erratic energy, weight loss, nervousness, lower back pain, chronic flatulence, abdominal distention, and constipation. Pitta type symptoms are fevers, hyperacidity, burning sensations, thirst, frequent infections, irritability, and diarrhea. And Kapha type symptoms include chronic colds and flus, congestion, mucus, swollen glands, edema, lethargy, and excessive sleeping.

Effective treatment of this condition involves strengthening the digestive fire, as well as nourishing the immune system while ridding the yeast pathogens from the body. Healthful nutrition serves a very important role in getting rid of pathogens from the body. Stimulating spices such as black pepper, cayenne, basil, bay leaves, asafetida, cardamom, and garlic help to promote healthy digestion and assist the body in releasing toxins that promote Candida.

Foods to be avoided are yeast producing wheat, and mucus forming foods, sweets, dairy products (except for ghee and yogurt), sweet fruit juices, dried fruits, cold drinks, raw foods, peanuts, and alcohol. Follow the herbal recommendations below and on the following page for alleviating vaginal yeast infections, in addition to the food recommendations set out in Appendix Two for each body type.

WISE EARTH REMEDY FOR VATA TYPE CANDIDA

Note: Vaginitis and yeast infections may also be treated with the remedy that follows. The same timing and schedules for taking the remedy should be observed.

VIDANGA & VACHA PASTE | SERVES ONE

1/2 teaspoon vidanga powder
1/2 teaspoon vacha powder (calamus powder)
1/4 teaspoon cardamom powder
1 1/2 teaspoons ghee

Combine the three powders in a small bowl and add the ghee. Mix into a paste and take it twice daily, once after breakfast and then again after lunch for a period of five days during the period of the discharge. Chase the remedy with half a glass of warm water.

WISE EARTH REMEDY FOR PITTA TYPE CANDIDA

KATUKI & GOLDENSEAL PASTE | SERVES ONE

1/2 teaspoon katuki powder
1/2 teaspoon goldenseal powder
1/2 teaspoon barberry powder
1 tablespoon aloe vera gel

Combine the three powders in a small bowl and add the gel. Mix into a paste and take it twice daily, once after breakfast, and then again after lunch for a period of five days during the period of the discharge. Chase the remedy with one half a glass of warm water.

Note: The Ayurvedic remedy Mahasudharshan may be taken for fevers. Mix half a teaspoon of powder with half a glass of warm water to be taken after breakfast and again after lunch until fever desists.

WISE EARTH REMEDY FOR KAPHA TYPE CANDIDA

TRIKATU & CLOVE PASTE | SERVES ONE

1/2 teaspoon trikatu powder
1/2 teaspoon clove powder
1 teaspoon aloe vera gel

Combine the powder and gel and mix into a paste. Chase the remedy with half a glass of warm water. Take it twice daily, once after breakfast and then again after lunch for a period of five days during the period of the discharge.

YEAST INFECTIONS

When the natural balance of the acid environment (pH levels) in the vaginal canal is disturbed, it attracts unhealthy pathogens that deplete the friendly bacteria that control the yeast. For each constitutional type, follow the same food and herbal recommendations stated for Candida. Other herbs that are curative for yeast infections are echinacea, lady's mantle, gentian powder, barberry, basil, goldenseal, and neem. Acidophilus (Lactobacillus bifidus), the friendly bacteria which helps to restore a healthy bacterial environment in the digestive system, may also be used as a supplement. The most potent therapy practice to alleviate yeast infection is Uttara Vasti to be applied with the Triphala-Aloe Decoction in harmony with the new moon cycle. Details on Uttara Vasti are presented in Chapter Five.

HIV/AIDS

According to Wise Earth Ayurveda, HIV and AIDS result from a compromised autoimmune system wherein the body's ojas is significantly depleted. Ojas is the essence of Kapha, the building block of the body. When it is impaired, the other humors will also be impacted. As noted earlier, there are many factors that compromise ojas such as excessive sexual activity, poor nutrition, erratic and stressful schedules, use of drugs, and lack of sleep.

The treatment for both HIV and AIDS evolves around creating a nourishing physical, emotional, and spiritual regimen beginning with food and activity. Observing celibacy is an imperative measure for the healing of HIV/AIDS. When sexual activities are excessive or perverted, they quickly diminish ojas. Any activity that over exerts apana vayu—downward-flowing air of the body—tends to negatively impact ojas, which in turn decreases vital autoimmunity. Lack of sexual activity not only bolsters the sufficiency of ojas in the body but also gives the health challenged person the opportunity to examine, reflect, and change their understanding and attitude toward their spiritual and sexual lives.

Peaceful, conflict-free, and harmonious life supporting sadhana activities tend to be ojas producing. All of the sadhana practices—chanting, yoga, meditation, mudra, mantra, and handmade food practices, to name a few—presented in this work cater to the development of consciousness through the restoration of ojas. Many people who have tested positive for HIV have been able to heal themselves completely by adhering to Wise Earth's healing work.

At the MOM sites, we see more and more women in inner cities and Third World countries that are experiencing the challenges of living with this debilitating virus. To add to their distress, their own family members often ostracize them. Last year, we visited with a family in a very poor village in Guyana where a woman with three young children had been infected with the virus by her husband, an abusive alcoholic. When the woman's mother discovered that her daughter had the dreaded disease, she shot and killed her son-in-law. In these less informed communities like New York's inner cities and rural areas of Guyana, the common person's response to HIV/AIDS is often times more lethal to the person infected than the condition itself. These populations live with manifold layers of pathologies, with the root cause of disease and disorder often deeply hidden in their ancestral memories. These are some of the most challenging areas in which we work. For the last seven years, MOM's instructors have made great strides reaching and opening the hearts of poor people with Wise Earth's Inner Medicine healing programs. As in the case of all profound diseases, the root cause of HIV/AIDS is often deeply hidden and it takes a sadhaka, an informed educator who is aligned with her own strong sense of intuition, to unearth the disorder and bring it to light so the individual person and the greater family may embrace healing.

The treatment for HIV/AIDS combines Vata and Pitta protocols. Naturally sweet, salty, and pungent tastes help to support the immune system. Foods such as sesame seeds, almonds, chickpeas, milk, yogurt, ghee, and coconut and sesame oils are ojas promoting and rebuild prana. Recent scientific studies have shown that coconut oil naturally retards the growth of HIV/AIDS. Herbs that are sweet and gentle in nature like gokshura, guggulu, myrrh, triphala, guduchi, ashwagandha, shatavari, sandalwood, and coriander are excellent for cleansing toxicity from the deep tissues that can cause fevers. They also help to replenish ojas and rebuild immunity in the body. Taken in combination with natural diuretics, they work well to cleanse the genitourinary tract.

Following are the Wise Earth Ayurvedic remedies that may be used by all constitutional types for assuaging and healing HIV/AIDS. You may also follow lifestyle sadhana practices set out in my book, *The Path of Practice*, as well as both the Vata and Pitta food recommendations set out in Appendix Two for each body type.

WISE EARTH REMEDY FOR HIV & AIDS

Note: You are also advised to seek the help and guidance of a qualified Ayurvedic physician.

Symptoms Include:
Chronic fevers, frequent flus and colds, pneumonia, insomnia, fatigue with erratic

energy, weight loss, anxiety, nervousness, irritability, lower back pain, chronic flatulence, diarrhea or constipation, emaciation, intermittent loss of memory, palpitations, and vertigo.

GOTU KOLA, GOKSHURA & GUGGULU PASTE | SERVES THREE

1/2 teaspoon gotu kola powder
1/2 teaspoon gokshura powder
1/2 teaspoon guggulu powder
1/2 teaspoon triphala powder
1/2 teaspoon ashwagandha powder
2 tablespoons coconut oil

Combine the powders in a small bowl and add the coconut oil. If the guggulu is available only in resin or pill form, ground it to a powder with a mortar and pestle. Mix into a paste and take it three times daily, once after breakfast, once after lunch, and then once again after dinner. Chase the remedy with half a glass of warm water. Take for a period of three to six months with the supervision of an Ayurvedic practitioner.

- In the event of flus and colds, add 1/2 teaspoon of ginger powder to the existing remedy.
- In the event of fevers, add 1/2 teaspoon of guduchi powder to the existing remedy.
- In the event of insomnia, add 1/2 teaspoon of nutmeg to the existing remedy.

MISCARRIAGES

Growing up in the Corentyne Village in Guyana, I often watched the women working and plying the fields. One day I witnessed a woman giving birth right in the rice fields while other women came to her aid. After giving birth on the straws under a shade of a tree, she stayed there to rest with her newborn child in her arms while the other women continued with their work. It was a common sight to see women sitting in the shade on their verandas in the still serene afternoons and nursing not only their own baby, but also those of other women who were working in the fields. This was life in a community where people worked arduously and lived in harmony with Mother Nature. Although not a single one of the village women knew how to read or write, the wisdom they had of their bodies and their maternal beauty and functions went far beyond any formal education.

Through hard work in the fields and their continual touching upon the spirit of Mother Nature, they were able to keep their Shakti power in exquisite form. It would have seemed incongruous to these women to think of running to the doctor or hospital to do what they perceived to be such a natural part of their womanhood: giving birth to their newborns. They made no association between the act of birthing babies and medical or scientific institutions. There were two mid-wives in my village, Auntie Mitchell and Aunt Sarah, the latter of whom helped my mother to bring me into the world. These beautiful African Guyanese women with skilled hands and profound intuition brought most of the village children, whether poor or affluent, into the world. There would have been no reason why my mother would have wanted to go to a doctor to give birth to her child unless she was experiencing a major problem with her pregnancy or the birthing process. Even so, going to the doctor was a last resort for these women.

Recently, I asked my mother about the rate of miscarriages in the villages as she was growing up. She told me that in her time miscarriages were infrequent, and that when they did occur they were mainly caused by excessive physical exertion on the part of the pregnant women. Among the women who did miscarry, she said, they all seemed to share the fact that they lived in a conflicted environment with their mothers-in-law and received very little emotional support from their husbands. The infrequent miscarriages of the Corentyne Village women are in stark contrast to the present day scenario where one in six pregnancies ends in miscarriages.

I believe that these miscarriages can be due to both physical and emotional causes. For example, endocrinological imbalances induced by emotional stress may lead to miscarriage; stressful emotions have also been known to affect the immune system as well as cause long-term hormonal imbalances, which in turn can have devastating effects on pregnancy. Fears around motherhood; fear of pain or of giving birth; maternal anger hoarded for generations; and psychological imprints of the memory of sexual abuse or incest can all compromise pregnancy. Physical irregularity of the womb, what is called an "incompetent cervix," an abnormally narrow vaginal passage, vitiated apana vayu, and poor lifestyle habits such as smoking and excess caffeine can also negatively impact pregnancy.

There is no doubt in my mind that the bombardment of troubled energies afflicting the maternal psyche in our present culture plays a pivotal role in women's reproductive challenges in general, and specifically in infertility and miscarriage. As we mislay our maternal memory and the Mother Consciousness of the world slackens, women appear to be literally losing the cervical grip and proper rhythmic dilation imperative to maintain the fetus in their wombs. Besides, the more Mother Consciousness women lose, the lesser the ability for communion between themselves and their fetus. The communion to the great Goddess Mother enhances our ability to "speak" to our unborn child as we carry and sustain them within the inner sanctum of the womb for nine or ten months.

Our emotions play a crucial role in the carrying, safeguarding, and birthing of life. When the internal maternal energies are impaired, our emotions are negatively affected. Medical research shows that women who frequently miscarry demonstrate endocrinological imbalances as a result of high levels of emotional stress. Miscarriages speak to a more inured problem than that of the physical competence of the cervix. Women who experience frequent miscarriages may be hoarding conflicts and fears around motherhood and the process of birthing a child. In the *Psychosomatic Medicine Journal*, researcher R. L. VandenBergh, wrote an article on the emotional illness referring to what are unfortunately called "habitual aborters" in the medical arena. He demonstrates that women who miscarry their fetuses have a challenging time fulfilling their own expectations. In other words, in trying to please the needs of others, they suffocate their own desires and as a result hoard hostility and anger in their bodies. Miscarrying the child helps to relieve the tension and stress in their bodies. VandenBergh reported that when many of these women later sought psychotherapy and learned how to directly cope with their anger and release pent up hostility, 80 percent went on to have successful pregnancies.

I believe that psychotherapy is not the ideal path to healing. The Inner Medicine way of thinking is a more profound way to heal anger, hostility, pain, and hurt. To reclaim the brilliant health of the womb, we must ignite the feminine wisdom, power, and security within us. We must take back the authority to serve our reproductive glory, and in so doing, we may serve our family to restore health and energy to the larger community that surrounds us.

According to Wise Earth Ayurveda, miscarriages have numerous causes, all of which are hinged on the vitiation of Pitta dosha and its fiery tendency, which may exacerbate the movement of downward-flowing air and cause excessive pressure to the fetus. For this reason, a Pitta type is more susceptible to miscarriages. A Kapha type is generally very fertile and may experience a false pregnancy—with many of the signs of pregnancy like nausea, swollen breasts, and lack of menstrual cycle appear—when they are not pregnant. Vata type is more likely to have challenges with fertility and conceiving. Therefore, Ayurveda recommends a strong Pitta nourishing and recuperative regimen to restore a state of mental and physiological balance within the body. Ample rest and avoidance of emotionally-conflicting situations are advised before and during the pregnancy. Exposure to heat and sunlight should be limited. A healthy food regime includes foods that are nourishing and good for Pitta types. Avoid stale, frozen, commercial foods, especially those that are oily or spicy. Animal flesh should also be avoided.

Ayurveda herbal therapy includes assuaging and calming the mind, body, and spirit of the mother. To remove torpid blood and heal the uterus after a miscarriage, you may use the Aloe Vera & Turmeric Bath as recommended on page 159. You may also observe the following healing practices:

- Pitta food recommendations set out in Appendix Two.
- Uttara Vasti procedure with Triphala-Aloe Decoction. Apply during the new moon cycle—at least two to three weeks *after* the miscarriage.

Ayurvedic herbs such as manjishta, shatavari, ashwagandha, turmeric, aloe vera gel, and gotu kola act as an excellent emmenagogue to help heal the womb and restore emotional tranquility. Following are the Wise Earth Ayurvedic remedies that may be prepared and used by all constitutional types for restoring strength to the uterus and/or repairing its health after a miscarriage.

WISE EARTH REMEDY FOR MISCARRIAGES

Note: You are also advised to seek the help and guidance of a qualified Ayurvedic physician.

MANJISHTA, SHATAVARI & ASHWAGANDHA PASTE | SERVES THREE

1/2 teaspoon manjishta powder
1/2 teaspoon shatavari powder
1/2 teaspoon ashwagandha powder
1/2 teaspoon triphala powder
2 tablespoons aloe vera gel

Combine the powders in a small bowl and add the gel. Mix into a paste and take it three times daily, once after breakfast, once after lunch, and then once again after dinner. Chase the remedy with one half a glass of warm water. Take for a period of one month following the miscarriage.

ABORTION

My tradition sees abortion as an act of violence against life, creating a difficult karma for both the mother and the unborn. However, it does not judge a person for their actions. Obviously, no girl or woman cherishes the thought of enduring the physical and emotional hurt that comes from having an abortion. This is a profound problem that all of society must come to terms with. For women to find themselves on this divisive plane, having to struggle with the hurt and hurtfulness of it all, not to mention the ethical and spiritual issues involved, points us directly to the underlying virus of it all: the willful erosion of the Mother Consciousness. Still, this is not an issue for political intervention. It is deeply personal and a social concern for and about women. For this reason, women must take responsibility for their sexual, emotional, and physical roles in this dark pall. We have to reckon with the fact that abortion is one of the most egregious issues relating to the well-being of women. Let us examine a woman's human gift of free will and what should amount to her unfettered ability to make her own choices.

Equipped with the unique and phenomenal human birthright of free will, we are allowed to make our own choices, even those which may not serve our karma or dharma well. It is essential to keep within our wisdom the idea that our actions, whatever they may be, all bear consequences in this life or in the hereafter. When we make choices that come from inner conflict, we must know that they will attract other challenging karmas that we will need to face, negotiate, and resolve at some point in the future. This is the story of life. Any form of *himsa*, hurt and harm, whether performed by our sacred mind and hands or by another, contributes to the difficult karma accruement of our sanchitakarma account, mentioned earlier. In the present culture, who would dare stand up and tell a woman that she does not have the right to control her own fertility? We do have a right to "control" our fertility. Likewise, we also have the right to own the karmas we may create from our actions. No other human force should usurp this right. But is our Shakti power entirely under our own control? If so, why do we need the energy medicines— mantra, mudra, yoga, rituals, rites, moon rites, sun rites, love, food, nourishment, and nurturance? If we each had complete control of our body, mind, intuition, and consciousness, we would be in no need of prayer. We do not own the body. Indeed, we are simply the keepers of the entire world.

The *Lalita Sahasranama*, a Vedic invocation that honors the Divine Mother through a thousand names, deftly describes our relationship to her. In the following excerpt we are told that we are the privileged *Ksetrapala*, keeper of the body, and not its owners.

Om Ksetra-svarupayai Namah
Om Ksetr'esyai Namah
Om Ksetra-ksetrajna-palinyai Namah
Om Ksetra-pala-samarcitayai Namah.

Reverence to the Supreme Goddess who is the body of all beings
Reverence to Her who is the ruler of all bodies
Reverence to Her who protects both the soul and the body
Reverence to Her who is worshipped by the Ksetrapala
—the individual who is the keeper of the body.

We all have the power of the Goddess Mother within us, and when we are awakened to her consciousness we may begin to understand our complete and infinite nature. Each one of us has a greater power that lives within us; the Goddess's Shakti that does not judge, condemn, or decry our actions no matter how much hurt we may create. When we have a disease or suffer from despair, she assumes this disorder. But unlike the human, she does not die. She is eternal. She is unconditionally there for you in each and every birth. The lesson here is that we have inherited from the goddess the supreme power to make choices as long as we recognize that each and every choice we make, both positive and negative, comes with its own set of karma.

At MOM, we see countless young women who come to us for counseling and blessings when they are faced with the dilemma of whether or not to have an abortion. Most of these women are at extremely difficult crossroads. At these heart wrenching meetings, we listen to women tell the stories of their deeply conflicted lives. We spend as much time as it takes to help these women gain a better understanding of the nature of Shakti and help them find the most supportive environments for nourishing themselves and giving birth to their babies. Some of these women have actually managed to give birth and keep their babies by rallying the support of their extended families; many have chosen to carry their babies to term and put them up for adoption; and an equal number have gone ahead to abort their fetuses. In all cases, regardless of the outcome, MOM's instructors have helped these women come to terms with their decisions. In my journey as a Spiritual Mother, I pray for each and every woman that comes to these extremely difficult crossroads, and I die a little every day for each soul that hurts.

You will find the healing remedies and recommended practices for abortions below. Although the genetic factors and personal psyche behind miscarriages are quite different from that of abortion, there is a certain commonality of treatment that addresses the healing of both conditions. To remove stagnant blood and heal the uterus after an abortion, you may use the Aloe Vera & Turmeric Bath as recommended on page 159. You may also observe the following healing practices:

- Pitta food recommendations set out in Appendix Two.
- Uttara Vasti procedure with Triphala-Aloe Decoction. Apply during the new moon cycle—at least two to three weeks after the abortion.

Moreover, certain specific ceremonies and invocations need to be performed by women who have had a miscarriage or an abortion. The energies of the spirit must be ceremoniously sent back to the higher ethers. If they are not cleared or freed from their thwarted arrival onto the earthly plane, they can remain fixated or stuck around the aggrieved person, often causing unimaginable unhappiness. Following are the ritual practices for freeing the spirit of the unborn child and healing the reproductive energy of the woman.

RITUAL FOR WOMEN RECOVERING FROM MISCARRIAGE, ABORTION & SEXUAL ABUSE

Moon Timing: Starting on the morning following the new moon, you may perform this ritual for the 15 days during the waxing phase of the moon.

Ritual Utensils: A small 8" clay pot, a piece of organic camphor resin, a handful of dried white sage, matches, and a stone or tile base on which to rest the fire pot. These utensils should be used exclusively for your rituals and need to be kept in a serene, dedicated space within your home.

THE PRACTICE: RECOVERING FROM MISCARRIAGE, ABORTION & SEXUAL ABUSE

- Facing east in the early morning light, prepare a ritual space in the privacy of your meditation/altar room, or in a clean and serene room in your home.
- Take a warm bath with drops of lavender and sandalwood essential oils. Soak you body from head to toe for about 15 minutes.
- Wear a very large and spacious white cotton frock, with no undergarments.
- Facing east again, sit and recite the following mantra for 10 minutes to invoke the Divine Mother's grace. Ask the Mother to help you heal the womb space and to restore the innocence of your sexual energies. Recite:

   Om Srim Hrim Klim Ambikayai Namah

- After you recite the mantra, light a piece of organic camphor resin in a clay pot on the floor. After the fire burns down, add the dried white sage, which will smoke.
- Be careful to ensure that the pot is not hot and that the fire is out (with only smoke remaining) before the next step.
- Still facing east, assume the squatting position and carefully lift your frock over the smoking sage.
- Let the smoke envelop your belly and genital area under the garment while you mentally ask for the womb to be cleansed.
- In the event of miscarriage or abortion, ask the Mother to allow the spirit of the thwarted life to be gently released from your body. Ask for your womb to be restored to good health and to be able to own your motherhood and be able to carry your child to fruition when the time is right.
- In the event of an abortion, ask for the Mother to show you the way to forgive yourself and to bring you the wisdom to realize the sanctity of your limbs, body, mind, and spirit.
- In the event of sexual abuse, ask for the womb space to be cleaned and for the negative, toxic energy of the perpetrator to be released. You may also ask Mother to help shift the demented mind space of the attacker to one of awareness so that he may recognize the brutality of his actions.
- Afterwards, clean your utensils and neatly put them away. Change your garment and wash it and put it away. It may be used as a meditation frock and for other rituals.

Chapter Ten

ANATOMY OF
WOMEN'S FERTILITY

Every woman must arrive at the pivotal juncture in life when the choices she makes about procreation are entirely conscious.

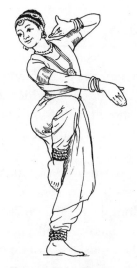

Figure 10.1 Dance of Fertility

Fertility depends on nature's rasa of fruitfulness, sweetness, wetness, and happiness. When these rasas are depleted, sterility, dryness, loneliness, and isolation are bound to set in. The rishis predicted that the increase of fear in modern culture would result in the decline of the earth's fertility.

Referred to as *vandhyatva* in Ayurveda, infertility is generally associated with the Vata condition, although it may involve all three doshas. At the mundane level, a woman's infertility may stem from a variety of physiological and psychological factors such as age, lack of proper development in the reproductive organs, unwholesome lifestyle, depression, stress, fear, anxiety, nervousness, and sexual immorality. However, before we examine the physical causes and remedial measures for infertility, let's shift our understanding to the cosmic energies that support women's strength and fertility.

In the greater vision, a woman's fertility is fashioned by the immortal heart rather than the act of reproduction. Across cultures and entrenched in the infinite span of time, the persona of the Mother Goddess has represented a multiplicity of paradoxes that have shaped the feminine identity of every woman.

The complex nature from which a woman's fertility is derived may be traced to the multi-dimensional role of the goddess in the Hindu pantheon. She is the Mother Goddess as well as the non-physiological mother. At once, she is a virgin and a mother; a consort and yet pure; a fierce warrior and also the embodiment of harmony and compassion. The ancient psyche of the Mother transcends cultural and geographical diversities as well as matrilineal and patrilineal principles, irretrievably linked to the conception of fertility. With the notable absence of masculine antecedents throughout history, she has been identified with nature, earth, fertility, reproduction, food and nurturance.

SEXUALITY, LIFE & DEATH

A woman's fertility is the nexus for the growth and sustenance of offspring, food, agriculture, consciousness, and life—all of which are connected to her power of sexuality. This primeval urge should not be underestimated.

According to Hindu mythology, even the gods and sages themselves are said to have experienced moments when they were unable to control their sexual urges. Human sexuality arises from the psyche of attachment. Tracing the genesis of human attachment would necessitate going back to the beginning of creation. The *Bhagavata Purana*, whose wisdom wields the greatest influence on modern Hindu life, metaphorically states: "Man has only half a body, woman being the other half. Since the body of a person is their most treasured possession, it is only natural that they would feel strongly drawn to the opposite gender to complete their body."

The coming together of two people is an act that makes each person complete within the human psyche of who they are; in other words, they are emulating the cosmic union of Shiva-Shakti. This may be one explanation why the primeval attraction forged between the sexes is such an irresistible force. When sexual relationships are not managed properly, they can produce great confusion and unhappiness and most of all, an insurmountable sense of attachment.

At the profound extreme, the act of completing oneself within the other is symbolic of nature's way of reconciling the experience of life and death. The only experience we have of life is an embodied one. We exist corporally and therefore create a tenacious attachment to the physical body because it is our most fundamental and cherished possession. By this means, we are provided with the natural desire to live. Through it we also forge all other attachments that find their place into the heart. We identify the body with the precious life force and naturally try to protect and sustain it against even the most painful circumstances. Unfortunately, we tend to forget that everything we are attached to is perishable, including the physical body. But death dispossesses the body, the physical entity to which we are firmly attached. As Subhash Anand, Professor of Hindu philosophy and religion, puts it, "It is precisely because death is certain that man feels his sexual urge, his faculty of life, so strongly. Sex is the embodiment of man's refusal to die." In this sense, sexual attachment becomes a primary source of fear.

FEAR DEPLETES FERTILITY

When this potent sexual power is not understood or managed, sexual activity can adversely affect your fertility. Through inappropriate sexual liaisons, we tend to collect and engorge the emotion of fear. In turn, fear adversely impacts your ojas, the essence of virility and vitality.

To renegotiate our fears and to reclaim our Shakti power of fertility, we must re-examine the binding relationship we have with our own bodies. The sages say that absolute freedom from fear can only be achieved once we are able to detach the greater self of consciousness from the binding sense of identification with the physical body. This is not to say that we should not mindfully care for the physical body, but rather find a gentle balance that frees the mind and spirit from the unnatural relationship of possessiveness of the body. Bit by bit the physical body dies. Staying present with every moment of life as it dies is a powerful tool by which you may cultivate joy, freedom, fertility, and complete immunity. Unless we are able to simultaneously care for and let go of this prized physical possession, we will find ourselves continually struggling against fear, unhappiness, and aging. We are cautioned to be mindful of the certain, impending return of the physical body to the subtle elements at the end of each life's journey. The *Lalita Sahasranama* tells us that we are, "Ksetrapala—the individual who is the keeper of the body."

Every woman must arrive at the pivotal juncture in life when the choices she makes about procreation are entirely conscious. A woman's fertility and her pro-creative Shakti ability have become complex since we live in a culture that has completely reversed our sacred feminine priorities. Because the woman's psyche is filled with fear, she is losing control of her procreative rights and power. She is almost compelled to play the divisive game of choosing between pro-life and pro-choice. From a sacred viewpoint, your fertility should never have filtered down to this end game. Conceiving and bringing forth new life must be an act of conscious contemplation. Difficult as it may seem, there is a solution.

TAKING SEXUAL PAUSE

To begin with, consider taking a sexual pause for six months to a year and observing a loving environment of celibacy with your spouse. This is not as hard as it may seem. In India, many couples who take to a spiritual life observe celibacy for years while maintaining a loving bond and companionship with each other. In fact, abstinence has enabled them to foster a deeper, more caring relationship. Look at this pause as a journey to the internal woods within you—*vanaprastha ashrama,* or retreating into the forest—which is recommended in my tradition for those of us in our mid years.

The story of Anne, a beautiful young woman in her early 30s, shows how this pause can replenish and refresh. Anne, an executive in a large public relations firm in New York, came to me out of desperation. She and her husband Todd had been trying to get pregnant for three years without success. Her physician had just informed her that her fertility count was so low that she could probably never conceive. To "solve" the problem, he recommended artificial insemination. Anne was amenable to this drastic technological approach, but Todd was adamantly opposed to the idea. By the time she arrived at Wise Earth, she was dejected and depressed. I recommended she put aside her concerns for a day or two and stay present in the meditation classes.

I arranged for a meeting with her and Todd, who joined us during the meditation class. My eyes caught hers during the first class after Todd had arrived and she broke down in tears. Todd rushed to embrace his wife and rocked her in his arms. They stayed close to each other throughout the sessions. It was evident that they cared deeply for each other. The day before the course ended, I invited them to join me in meditation. My intention was to find a harmonious path to bring their child into the world. I advised them to keep their intention to naturally conceive clearly in their hearts. I saw that Anne was not barren and that her inability to become pregnant was linked to her difficult relationship with her mother and stress at work. At the end of the meditation, both of them were at ease. Anne said, "It's as though a big load has been lifted from my heart." Todd nodded his head in agreement, their faces softly lit by the northern light peering in from the window. "Can you maintain the inner peace you feel now in my presence?" I asked, and they both nodded to the affirmative. "What did you discover about your fertility during your time at Wise Earth?" I asked Anne. After a moment's thought, she replied. "I'm capable of conceiving without being inseminated!"

Before they left, they asked for a spiritual practice that they could do together. I suggested they spend two hours every day in a loving and intimate way with each other in any activity of their choosing, except cohabitation. They gasped for a moment, looked at each other and broke out in laughter like children do. "Mother!" exclaimed Anne, "how am I supposed to get pregnant without sex?" In response, I asked them how many times they'd had sex. Looking at Todd with a puzzling grin, she sheepishly replied, "about 100 times." They understood my point without my having to say it. I advised them to consider observing six months of celibacy to ease their minds and hearts of the stressful demand "to get pregnant."

I strongly recommended to Anne that she prioritize her time to de-stress and spend more time doing things that made her happy. I assured them that the chances of becoming pregnant following sexual abstinence are far greater than they were at the present time.

I knew that they would take my advice on faith. Three months later, I received a letter from Anne detailing their progress with abstinence. Anne said she was actually cultivating a gentler relationship with her mother and she and Todd had continued their meditation practice. She reported they were both experiencing a serenity within that they had not felt before. They practiced the fine sadhana of celibacy for nine months, and it was no surprise when they soon after announced the conception of their baby. Todd said that Elijah, their son, came out of his mother's womb smiling.

ANATOMY OF CONCEPTION

Statistics show that one out of every two couples may be infertile. The gradually diminishing egg and sperm count has more to do with the mental and emotional condition of the human heart than with increasingly toxic lifestyles, contamination of food sources, and the polluted environment. Although these factors do adversely affect our health and fertility, the greater impact is from the underlying subtle effects operating within our psyche as a response to the gradual deterioration of the Mother Consciousness.

The anatomy of conception goes directly to the cosmic heart of human matter and energy. The journey of birth begins with each one of us carrying the imprint of all previous lives in our cosmic memory, embedded in the buddhi. While we are nestled in the mother's womb, we transcend those memories of our collective past in preparation for our arrival into the physical elements of the Planet Earth. To help prepare the mind of the newborn for its new set of karmas and experiences, the child is held and nourished in the mother's womb for about nine months as it slowly completes its passage into birth. More so than other species, the human child is in an entirely dependent and underdeveloped state so that it can be nurtured and weaned with the milk of the mother, which is packed with cosmic memory-rich nutrients. The unique care of the human child is intended to allow ample space, time, and nurturance for the reformatting of its memory so that the newborn may meet the challenges of a new life. In the present state of motherhood, we have denigrated this wondrous process of procreation to such a point that all we appear to be left with are the endless fears around fertility drugs, reproductive diseases, hormonal therapies, medical bills, birth controls, abortions, and miscarriages. Have you wondered about the spiritual magic and mystery that surrounds the energetic continuum of conception, birth, life, death, and rebirth?

It is imperative that women who are intending to bring forth new life make the connection between fertility and the nurturance of the child within your belly. We must reconnect to the continuum energy of life. Take a proactive position in being present in the awesome process of giving life to life.

THE BEAUTY OF THE EMBRYO

In the Hindu tradition, the mother is revered and treated with rites, prayers, mantras, medicinal remedies, along with sacred amulets, and talismans that relate to her pregnancy, childbirth, and post-partum care.

From the inception of the universe, the Vedic ancients have recorded the physiological and pyschospiritual development of the fetus long before modern science discovered the reality of chromosomes and hormones. They recognized that the human seed is more than the DNA of the human body that bears the characteristics of the parents. They knew that it contained the imprints of cosmic memory and that in its magical replication into life it reveals the entire universe within itself.

During the time of coalescence of the male and female seeds in the uterus, the soul enters the embryo, *garbha*, along with the eightfold material for creation. These are mind, intellect (buddhi), ego, and the five pure elements of space, air, fire, water, and earth. These elements are transformed into developmental forces that are intended to safeguard the embryo; air helps in the continual segmentation process of the embryo's growth while fire creates the digestive process. The water force provides moisture to the embryo while supplying and maintaining the balance of the embryonic fluid. The earth principle gives stability and strength to the embryo, while the space element gives the appropriate freedom for the necessary development of the embryo.

The awesome beauty of the living process of the embryo as it is safeguarded in the soft internal light of the womb's embryonic fluid reveals the magical power of the Mother Shakti. The mouth of the fetus is closed by a thin membrane, the throat is closed by natural mucus, and all the passages for air within the body are closed. There is no wind, excreta, or urination by the fetus since it has no access to the colon or bladder. In essence, the fetus does not breathe or cry in the mother's womb. Its respiration, movement, and sleep pattern are crucially linked to the mother's physical and emotional functions.

THE EMBRYONIC STAGES

Ayurveda sages gave remarkable insights and information into the awesome development of the embryo as it grows in the mother's womb. In the first month, the embryo is a soft mass, *kalala*. In the second month, the five elements meld and express themselves in the form of the three humors—Vata, Pitta, and Kapha. By this means, the soft mass assumes a ball-like shape when the embryo is a male and the shape of an egg if it's a female. Incredibly, the gender of the fetus is not formed or fixed until the third month. According to Ayurveda, the mother has the power to influence the gender of her fetus even into its second month by taking special herbs and performing ceremonial mantras and prayers. In the pivotal third month of pregnancy, a definitive structure of the embryo is formed, along with budding protrusions for the head and limbs. The eleven organs of the body are also introduced in the third month, which continue to develop in the fourth month, as the heart assumes full performance of its vital functions. As a result, the fetus begins to exhibit certain desires that replicate themselves as cravings or longings by the pregnant mother, such as wanting savory foods, ice cream, chocolates, or pickles. The embryo's desires are largely patterned after the mother's physical and psychic aspirations. Fulfilling these cravings helps to safeguard the health and strength of the embryo.

In the fifth month, the physical structure of the brain takes shape. The mind begins to register subtle imprints. In the sixth month, the fetus begins to display emotions. At this time a discerning mother can read feelings like pain or pleasure coming from the child. By the end of the seventh month, the physical structure of the fetus is distinctly formed along with the progressive growth of the primary and secondary organs of the body. In the crucial eighth month, ojas begins to propagate and promote stability in the entire organism of the child. For this reason, if premature delivery occurs it is at very high risk because the autoimmunity of ojas is yet to be fully formed in the body.

The optimum time for the birth of the child is somewhere between the beginning of the ninth month to the end of the tenth month. In the Hindu tradition, the birth of a newborn child is celebrated with stupendous ceremonies. Special sacraments are performed at specific astrological and numerological junctures of time in accord with the child's birth. These powerful samskaras (sacraments) are intended to impress upon the psyche of the child its infinite nature and purpose for spiritual advancement.

My reason for exploring these traditional sacraments is not to convert you to Hinduism, but to share the importance of cultivating and maintaining magical rites of passage for safeguarding your fertility and consciousness. Modern culture has reversed these priorities for us, and therefore we will need to make every effort to re-establish them. In so doing, we regain our awareness and joy of the cosmic heart. The Vedic tradition is unique; its vast and ancient wisdom is universal, intended for the benefit of every human being and all life on earth. You may imbibe its wellspring of knowledge in the same way you may take a yoga or meditation class while still preserving the identity of your own ancestral tradition.

SACRAMENTS THAT PRESERVE
MATERNAL LIFE FORCE

The Vedic ancients established a system of 16 primary sacraments, samskaras, intended to safeguard the entire continuum of revolving life from birth to rebirth. In other words, each person's life is marked by 16 rites of passage. These rites coincide with the significant transitions relating to the 16 lunar Shaktis of Tripurasundari, as described in Chapter Sixteen. They are performed to ensure the safe and conscious passage of the individual from the onset of its new birth through the challenges of life. The rites following mid-life are intended to prepare us for life's ultimate experience in life—detachment from the physical body and evolution into death. According to Vedic thought, we have the power to transcend the physical body even as we live within it. This detachment prepares us for the incredible event of death and the transcendent journey that follows.

Through the practice of these significant sacraments, which most Hindus faithfully observe, the human person may safeguard mind, body, and spirit while expending personal karma and promoting the collective awareness. Even amid the massive identity and spiritual crisis that the world is experiencing, practicing Hindus still adhere to these crucial rites of passages. But, as we know, the impact of modernity has had a devastating effect on our consciousness. Evidenced by the gradual erosion of nature and distortion of native traditional sacraments across the world, we are in desperate need of reordering the wisdom we need to reclaim these vital Inner Medicine rites necessary for maintaining fertility.

Let us briefly examine this truth. Every day Mother Nature endows the world with more than 50 trillion dollars' worth of her bounty and nourishment in the form of forests, trees, plants, herbs, fruits, air, water, sun, moon, stars, and sky. In response, we have introduced fertilizers, pesticides, chemicals, poisons, and bio-engineering to the good Earth, altogether individually and collectively perpetuating disease and destruction on what has been handed down to us for free. According to a recent British Broadcasting Corporation news report, we have accomplished the near impossible—the "slow death" of the ocean and the destruction of almost two-thirds of the world's natural resources. This means that, at present, more than 80 percent of the world's food source is contaminated. Nature is the bedrock of life that sustains the earth's fertility, and when it is compromised, as it is at present, it has a significant impact on human fertility. According to the Vedic way of thinking, infertility is connected to our individual karma from the actions of our past lives. In the last century, however, this karma has more to do with what has been created for us in the present; technological, scientific, and medical advances—which have polluted the environment, poisoned our natural food sources, and denigrated the feminine principle of life—have collectively deteriorated the Mother Consciousness.

VEDIC FERTILITY RITES—CONCEPTION

According to the Vedic fertility rites, *garbhadhana*, the rite of conception, is keenly observed. From conception throughout the crucial stages of pregnancy and birth, sacred ceremonies are performed by the couple with the guidance of elders and the family priest. First, their physical union is consecrated with prayer, mantra, and invocation, with the intention of invoking an enlightened soul into its physical birth. To accomplish this feat, the couple sets out to cultivate a state of inner peace and tranquility before cohabitation, when the husband places his seed into the wife's womb. In the Vedic calendar, there are certain auspicious days for cohabitation that align with the ascendance of specific lunar mansions such as *Asvini, Utthiradam, Satayam, Uttaram, Hastham, Chitthirai,* and *Svati.*

The impending father plays a pivotal role in the support of the soon-to-be new mother. He demonstrates his affection for his pregnant wife and pledges his support to her by giving her gifts and offering a prayer for her well-being. During pregnancy, three critical phases are observed by the couple. First, the husband blesses his consort by presiding in a ceremony marking the third month of her pregnancy and offers special prayers for the protection and safe development of both the child and mother. During the mother's fourth month of pregnancy, the hair-parting sacrament is endeavored wherein the husband demonstrates his affection for her by combing his wife's hair, parting it in the center, and uttering gentle words of praise to her beauty. (A woman's hair is vitality connected to her sensuality.) Traditionally, this is an elaborate ceremony filled with many magical symbolisms. In the presence of the ceremonial fire, the wife places her hand on her husband's as he parts her hair using the quill of a porcupine that has three spots on it. The quill is to ward off negative energies and spirits, the three spots representing the three major Vedas, as well as the three worlds: earth, mid-region, and sky. A necklace of small, unripe udumbara fruits are tucked within three strands of sacred grass and worn by the mother-to-be. The fruitful, milky, udumbara fruits symbolize a woman's fertility whose protection is prayed for by the husband during this ceremony.

These magical themes are held as sacred by the couple and are carried throughout their married life. They begin life as a unified force with the ritual of seven steps, *Saptapadi*, taken by bride and groom during the marriage ceremony. The bridegroom leads the bride in the northern direction around the ceremonial fire while they keep their intention in mind: "We take the first step for food; second step for strength; third step for prosperity; fourth step for happiness; fifth step for progeny; sixth step for the welfare of the seasons, and the last step for friendship between us." In Christianity, three is also a symbolic number representing the Father, Son, and Holy Ghost. Among the Aztecs, a variation of the Saptapadi Ritual appears in their tradition.

SACRED LIFE TAKES BIRTH

In the third phase of the ceremony, the couple heralds the newborn child into the world by reciting gentle mantras to invoke the grace of the Divine toward its well-being. Afterwards, the father introduces a mixture of honey and ghee, which has been rubbed onto a piece of gold, to the lips of the child, and feeds the child while reciting the appropriate mantras. By this means the child's first experience in the world is one of sweetness of food, breath, and sound. The Vedas inform, "The hearts of all beings are interwoven in nature's songs and nourishments that are firmly fixed like spokes in a wheel." In the Brahmin home, a thin leaf of gold is placed on a piece of vacha root and rubbed against a stone to produce a fine powder. The baby licks a tiny amount of this powder daubed with honey from the mother's fingertip. Like all Ayurvedic herbs and roots, the curative effects inherent in them are linked to the Sanskrit names the seers bestowed them. Vacha is derived from the noun *vak*, meaning "speech." This remedy—similar in its properties to the herb calamus—is said to bless the child with a sonorous voice, as well as a wondrous faculty for learning the Vedas, and the ability for excellent communication. The popular expression of the child being born with a "golden spoon in its mouth" originated from these ancient Vedic practices.

An astrologically benevolent time is sought once more between the 11th and 41st days following the birth for the child's name bestowal ceremony. Initiating his or her formal entry into the tradition of Hinduism, the father whispers the name of the child into his or her right ear. Next, the necessary hair-shearing ceremony is observed during the day of the full moon at a temple. Here, the child's head is cleanly shaved in a ceremony that occurs between the 31st day and the fourth year of its birth. In Ayurveda, the hair is considered a secondary vital tissue relating to the Kapha dosha and is a direct result of the bone marrow tissue and central nervous system of the body. The shearing of the first hair brings the Kapha dosha within the child into a state of harmony while strengthening the nervous system and bone tissue.

Hinduism's yogic tradition informs that at the spiritual level, the exfoliation of the worn tissues for new ones helps us to shed attachment to the physical body and therefore to embrace the infinite, conscious Self. The first solid food, which consists of nourishing sweet rice, is fed to the child in a food celebration ceremony. In my tradition, the Guru who is seen as a physical, emotional, and spiritual nourisher is generally invited by the families to serve this role. In this way, the child grows in an environment where there is a unified understanding that food is nourishment, not only for the physical body, but also for the mind, and spirit. Every year, during the Holika Full Moon that generally follows the vernal equinox, I perform the food ceremony, *annaprasana*, to nourish the children of the world. In this offering I cook rice with milk, ghee, and sugar in the early morning sun and serve it to the river with the appropriate mantras and mudras so that the powerful energy of its waters may carry the nourishment to the new born children. I offer particular prayers for mothers and children who are poor, hungry, or emaciated. Sanctified by the purification of the vows of a renunciate bestowed on me by my tradition, these offerings are said to possess the undeterred ability to reach their intended destinations. Many of my disciples bring their children so I can feed them their first solid food. Usually, these special occasions are punctuated with the children's smiles and cackles of contentment.

During the first, third, or fifth year, the ceremony of ear piercing is held for both girls and boys. The purpose of this rite of passage is to endow the young person with the spirit of health and wealth. Girls are adorned with gold earrings, bracelets, and anklets, while the boys are given two gold bobs for their pierced ears. Gold represents the vital sun, as well as Lakshmi, Goddess of Prosperity. In many Vedic rituals, before the gold is offered it is placed in water, which represents the moon. Brought together in ritual ceremony, sun and moon are invoked within the person to achieve the balancing of both energies within. The two beacons in the sky are also symbolic of the left and right breath in the body, as well as the male and female genders.

The close bonding of mother and child has been of the utmost priority in the traditional home. With her bare hands, the mother breast-feeds, bathes, and massages her child every day. She is entirely available to her children's needs and handles them with care and confidence, which helps them to develop a strong inner sense of identity and security. Statistics have shown that Indian children develop remarkable sensory-motor skills at a very early age compared to children of modern cultures. This is largely due to their close body contact between mother and child.

MAGICAL REMEDIES FOR INFERTILITY

> From Him come hymns, songs and sacrificial formulas, initiations,
> sacrifices, rites and all offerings. From Him come the year, the sacrificer
> and the worlds in which the moon shines forth, and the sun.
>
> —Rig Veda

Long before, modern medicine discovered chromosomes, hormones, and proteins the ancient vaidyas recognized that plants rich in vitalizing energy (jivaniyagana) and milky sap (kshiri vrksha) would keep female hormones in good vigor and balance. They knew that a woman's body would need the five sacred foods produced by the mother cow—milk, cream, butter, ghee, and yogurt—to strengthen her fertility. According to Vedic thought, the cow's production of milk, dung, and urine symbolizes the cosmic power of life, giving fertility to the humans in the like the rain clouds of the monsoon provide fertileness to the earth. And the occurrence of both nourishments is linked to the turn of the lunar wheel. As mentioned earlier, fertility depends on nature's fruitfulness and moisture. When depleted, sterility and dryness is bound to set in. A classical remedy called *phalaghrita* (essence of the fruit with ghee) consisting of three ancient myrobalans, fruits, mixed with medicinal ghee is used to produce bountiful ojas in women. This popular remedy is used to nourish and aid the fertility of young women who are looking to conceive, or restore reproductive health to those that have suffered setbacks with their pregnancy. Besides, while imbibing this subtle yet powerful remedy, the mother-to-be may envision the rasa of the child she longs for—gender, appearance, mental disposition, and so on. Phalaghrita has been known to help the mother fulfill her desire for a son or daughter while it protects her and her child from untoward influences, ensuring their joy, strength, longevity, and prosperity. Like all Wise Earth Ayurveda remedies that you are now learning to prepare through the transcendental act of sadhana, its effect melds the energy of the physical plane with the greater powers of nature.

INFERTILITY: PHYSIOLOGICAL CAUSES

A woman's infertility may stem from a variety of physiological factors. These include age, a lack of proper development in the reproductive organs, narrow vaginal passage, unhealthy ovum produced by the ovaries, severe anemia, obesity, thyroid malfunction, stagnation in the blood, excess bodily fluid, vaginitis, vaginal acidity, vaginal stenosis, intercervical obstruction, cervical fibroids, ovarian tumors, tubercular endometritis, and chronic cervicitis. Poor nutrition may also contribute to the loss of fertility. Eating foods which are incompatible with your metabolic type, eating unwholesome foods, or eating frequently are counter productive to both virility and fertility.

Emotional and psychological factors also play a significant role in infertility. The rapid increase of feminine depression, stress, fear, anxiety, nervousness, and sexual immorality in our society has had a great impact on fertility. The breakdown of family and community, and the rise of marital or familial disharmony have added to the increasing lack of emotional and psychic support women now experience. Indeed, a woman's inability to get pregnant may also be caused by infertility in her spouse. Common factors contributing to male infertility are unhealthy sperm, faulty transportation of the sperm to the uterine cavity, obesity, weak constitution, anemia, hypothyroidism, hydrocoele, obstruction in the genital tract, and inadequate coitus. Emotional factors like stress, depression, fear, and anxiety also contribute to male infertility. Stress related habits in males and females alike such as excess drinking, smoking, and excessive sexual activity and work are also major deterrents to achieving pregnancy.

WISE EARTH HERBS FOR WOMEN'S FERTILITY

Among Ayurveda's greatest remedies for infertility—and an all around restorer for women's reproductive health—is the herb shatavari, which literally translates to "100 husbands," inferring that it has the virility power of 100 husbands! One of the main Ayurvedic rejuvenatives for women, this herb contains unusually high amounts of plant-derived estrogens, making it a healthy choice for women who want to become pregnant, or for those who are nursing. Shatavari nourishes and cleanses the blood and the female reproductive organs, and is also excellent for menopausal and postmenopausal women.

Gokshura is an important tonic for infertility, and has been used in Ayurveda Medicine for thousands of years as a rejuvenative for both the female and male reproductive systems. Owing to its calming effect on the nervous system, it is a highly beneficial tonic in the treatment of stress, which as you know, can interfere with fertility.

Brahmi, or gotu kola, is well-known in Ayurveda and has a wide range of beneficial effects. Regular use helps to strengthen connective tissue and the walls of blood vessels, including the somniferous tubules which manufacture sperm. Improved circulation due to the use of gotu kola will ensure adequate blood supply and nutrition to the male organs and also help to strengthen erections and sexual desire.

Many fertility herbs used by Native American women may be traced back to India and China—where the crone forms of these herbs may still be found. Chaste berry, black cohosh, Siberian ginseng, and gotu kola are a few of the fertility herbs that are most effective. Chaste berry, for instance, has been used in traditional medicine for thousands of years. In recent times, it has been increasingly accepted, even by conventional Western Medicine, as an effective treatment to promote hormonal balance and health. Chaste berry helps the pituitary gland in the brain stimulate the ovulation process and has been shown to improve production of progesterone and high prolactin levels, both of which can inhibit ovulation and the production of prolactin—a deficiency which according to medical science makes it difficult to conceive.

Black cohosh has been used for thousands of years by Native Americans and some forms of the herb have also been used in Traditional Chinese Medicine. It is used for a variety of complaints, but has become well-known in the West for its beneficial effects on hormone functioning due to its phytoestrogenic properties. Black cohosh is also used by herbalists to prevent miscarriage.

Siberian ginseng is a highly respected Chinese tonic that has been used for thousands of years for a wide variety of ailments. Its Ayurvedic crone counterpart is ashwagandha, which is most beneficial in both women and men for the treatment of infertility related to stress. Both Siberian ginseng and ashwagandha can be used effectively for restoring the body's vital energy and promoting its overall systemic functioning. Siberian ginseng is well-known for supporting sexual functioning and promoting fertility, and is often recommended as an aphrodisiac. Used regularly, Siberian ginseng can regulate the menstrual cycle, improve hormonal balance, and tone the uterus to improve the ability of the fetus to implant after conception.

WISE EARTH REMEDIES FOR INFERTILITY

Approach the following remedies with the same sadhana understanding that these remedies—in and of themselves—will not cure your problems. However, they will help to awaken the necessary tissue memories that may be shut down, thereby aiding you to remember your innate power of fertility. You may use these preparations for three months or so. In Ayurveda, no remedy can be taken as a permanent diet in your life.

For the following remedies, follow the directions from page 110 on how to make a soft pill or paste. Take them twice daily, once after breakfast and then again after lunch for up to three months. These remedies are most effective when you include the appropriate healthful Wise Earth Ayurveda food recommendations for your metabolic type set out in Appendix Two.

GHEE & TRIPHALA FORMULA (FOR ALL TYPES)

1 teaspoon ghee
1/2 teaspoon triphala powder

SHATAVARI & ASHWAGANDHA FORMULA (FOR ALL TYPES)

1 teaspoon shatavari powder
1/2 teaspoon ashwagandha powder
1 teaspoon aloe vera gel or ghee

SHATAVARI, DASHAMULA & LICORICE FORMULA (FOR VATA TYPES)

1 teaspoon shatavari powder
1/2 teaspoon dashamula powder

1/2 teaspoon licorice powder
1 tablespoon ghee

Follow the Vata nourishing foods recommended in Appendix Two.

SAFFRON, SHATAVARI & ALOE VERA FORMULA (FOR PITTA TYPES)

1/2 teaspoon saffron thistles
1/2 teaspoon shatavari powder
1/2 teaspoon ashwagandha powder
1 tablespoon aloe vera gel

Follow the Pitta nourishing foods recommended in Appendix Two.

TRIPHALA, GINGER & HONEY FORMULA (FOR KAPHA TYPES)

1/2 teaspoon triphala powder
1/2 teaspoon shatavari powder
1/2 teaspoon ginger powder
1 tablespoon aloe vera gel

Follow the Kapha nourishing foods in Appendix Two.

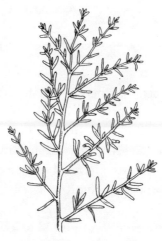

Figure 10.2 Shatavari Shrub

Shatavari shrub is an under-shrub with numerous branches and succulent, tuberous roots that produce four saponins called *shatavarin* (1 to 4). Its roots, leaves, and their different extracts possess many pharmacological properties.

Chapter Eleven

WOMEN'S SEXUALITY: THE WAY OF LOVE

I am Happiness, unfettered and free
No other happiness exists apart from me
Love is not toward others
Nor can I love myself
For I am Love.

—*Advaita Makaranda*

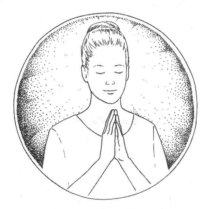

Figure 11.1 Woman in Prayer Pose

Sexuality is more than the act of being passionate, craving intimacy, filling empty space or striving for "the right partner." The fact is that most sexual activities do not result in a relationship of any consequence, or the birth of a newborn. Indeed, the majority of women who have sex have no such intention. In fact, more than 30 percent of American couples seek divorce because of infidelity. A staggering 78 percent experience some form of discomfort, disease, and illness, relating to their sexual activity.

The act of sexuality is inherently connected to love. What is the nature of love? The Vedas tell us that love has far greater meaning than attraction and intimacy between two people. According to the *Bhagavata Purana*, the way of love is called *bhakti marga*, devotion to the Divine. Love is the richest, most cherished goal of a person who recognizes the self to be a spiritual being. Among avatars, the *Bhagavata Purana* gives the greatest importance to God Krishna who reveals Himself as the archetypal lover. He established the idea that each one of us has a direct and subjective connection to attaining the Divine through devotion. Mirabai, a great female saint of 16th century India, who was enraptured with love for God Krishna, deserted her kingdom and family to follow the path of divine love. The act of love is not merely an emotional, intellectual, or psychological response, but evokes a higher meaning, that of achieving the gentle spirit of inner harmony. Love is humanity's *para-dharma*, its greatest purpose.

As a Vedic monk, I transcend the plane of desire to the higher consciousness, devoting my life to spiritual development and enlightenment. Hence, all of my activities transcend the physical and transform each and every action into celestial love. Many of my disciples who are married and have taken to the spiritual path also observe the path of bhakti marga. They live in celibacy and practice blissful fulfillment. Like the yogis and yoginis before them, they have sublimated and gone beyond the physical practice. However, you do not have to be a saint or ascetic to start your transcendence into the path of celestial love. Let the full moon dance of Shiva and Shakti remind you of your inherent quest for unity, union, and oneness with the Divine. In other words, immerse yourselves in selfless love to attain the Divine. Let every act of love be made whole with this sacred intention. Let your partner be a symbol of the deity. As in the Hindu tradition, let the act of love be a puja, a ritual ceremony to honor the deities. In this way, you may harvest the phenomenal power of pleasure, gaining access to your treasure trove of the deep emotional intimacy and sharing that you seek without pain, humiliation, and hurt.

WOMEN'S SEXUALITY

This way of approaching love and being in love can withstand the most horrendous and challenging forces of life and bring a sense of unity to all couples, indeed, to the whole of humanity. As a woman, you are inherently connected to the sacred interworkings of love on every plane of consciousness. At a physical and emotional level, we conserve vital energy by discriminative use of our sexuality. The excellent health of our vital tissues, from plasma to ovum/sperm, is called ojas. Also referred to as *bala*—youthfulness, vigor, and vitality—ojas provides stability and nourishment to the muscle tissues, moisture to the skin, and mental clarity. When ojas is healthy and plentiful in the body, the internal organs and external senses perform in good health. Healthy ojas is made from a wholesome lifestyle; the quality of our nutrition and foods, activities and work, and the state of harmony in which we function. Our glow of health, virility, fertility, reproduction, regeneration, and good health in general all depends on a healthy supply of ojas. Ayurveda informs that the most significant loss of ojas can come from indiscriminate and excessive sexual activity. Ojas is the cosmic food that nourishes the sperm and ovum. It serves a crucial role in reproduction, as it safeguards the sperm and ovum and supplies them with the energy and potency needed during conception. Although there are numerous medical causes cited for infertility and other reproductive ailments, these conditions all have their root in the vitiation of ojas.

According to Wise Earth Ayurveda, the union between male and female is fundamental to the feeding of the female artava, ovum. This nourishment is then transformed into life supportive essence, safeguarding the procreative energies of the female. The biology of sexual union is that the sperm, shukra, feeds and nourishes the artava, hence replenishing the female hunger in order to procreate. However, as you may know, even simple biology has its basis in the cosmic. Life itself depends on ojas. The good health of a child depends entirely on the shukra and artava condition of the parents. When the condition of shukra and artava are malnourished, anemic, weak, and exhausted, the female loses her fertility and the male his potency. As a result, he can no longer bring nourishment or fulfillment to the female and even though more children can continue to be born, the ojas that safeguards their excellent health and stamina of body, mind, and spirit will be dramatically diminished.

Jen and Jon were married for a year before making a conscious decision to get pregnant. After trying for two years, they were unsuccessful and were strongly considering taking fertility drugs when they came to see me before a satsanga in Massachusetts. Both hard working professionals in the computer industry, they shared very little caring time with each other. They would bring their work home and continue to labor long after the workday had ended. Their stress levels were visible. The first thing they said to me was that they had come to see me but could not stay for the satsanga due to their hectic work schedules. They wanted to know if Ayurveda had a nontoxic form of fertility drug they could use instead of the conventional treatment. I told them to consider shifting to a more reasonable work schedule and spending the necessary time to build their mutual ojas. With a synchronized look of puzzlement in their faces, they retorted, "Ojas! What's that, is it a therapy?" "You may call it that if you'd like; it's the 'therapy' of mating," I answered. They were quite amused but were eager to learn more about ojas. So I persuaded them to stay on for the satsanga and accommodated them along with the other couples in the audience by exploring the meaning of ojas and the practices that help build ojas.

CONSCIOUS MATING

Firstly, I noted, we must be clear on our purpose for wanting to bring a child into the world: the image of the child must be clearly envisioned by both parents prior to the start of this noble endeavor. To achieve this goal, you must be prepared to pause and set out the necessary time for conscious mating. To bring a physically, emotionally, and spiritually healthy child into the world, the female must be physically, emotionally, and spiritually fed, nourished, and nurtured with the attention and the shukra of her male. For this you have got to stop bringing work home, and spend caring time with each other without unnecessary intrusion. This couple's lives had become so rushed, so stressed, so motivated by material success that it had left little time to do the joyful, fulfilling, and simple little things that feed the spirit and that bond mates together. Responding to the energy of the couples in the room, I decided to teach them the practice of the Shiva-Lingam Mudra (this practice follows on pages 196-197) during the satsanga, wherein partners immediately bond energetically.

At the end of the session, nine other couples rushed up to see me as I was leaving the hall. With tears welling in all the eyes around me, I knew that something deep inside them was already touched and the shift to a salubrious act of mating had begun. Two months later, I received a sweet note from Jen. She was pregnant. "We have been dedicated to the practices you've taught us and now look forward to leaving work and spending our evenings and weekends together walking, talking, laughing, cooking, eating and making love...I think it's a baby girl."

Incredibly, by just slowing down, spending caring time together, and choosing the auspicious mating times in accord with the Vedic calendar, the Shakti of both mother and father was flowing, and there was no stopping it.

SHAKTI MUDRA: HONORING FEMININE SEXUAL ENERGY

In this book, Shakti Mudra is recommended only for women to help restore their vital energy to the womb and bring its rhythms in balance with lunar energies. This is an especially excellent practice for women who are looking to conceive, or have had a miscarriage, abortion, recent divorce, disillusionment with love, or problems relating to their reproductive health. This mudra enhances a woman's sense of self, reinforcing her femininity and self-esteem. Done on a daily basis, this practice will help to revive memory of the Shakti power within, strengthen Shakti prana, and heal the womb space.

THE PRACTICE: SHAKTI MUDRA

- Sit in lotus pose or a comfortable posture in a quiet space in your home or outdoors, facing east.
- Bring the palm of your hands together and then separate them slowly.

- Place the tips of your ring fingers and little fingers together.
- Rest the thumbs into the palm of your hands by bending them, and fold the other two fingers over the thumbs.
- Breathe deeply into the pelvic area and breathe out slowly, tracing the exhalation from the base of the perineum, circulating it through the uterus and belly.
- Maintain Shakti Mudra for approximately 15 minutes.
- Take a deep breath and make a commitment to a life of non-hurting.
- Engage your spouse or partner, and follow this mudra practice to fortify your Shiva-Shakti energies. Like Amanda and Joseph whose story you are about to read, a couple in New York who vigorously took to this practice, you too can immediately begin to redirect your love toward absolute healing.

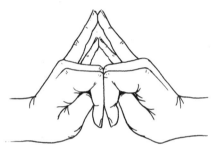

Figure 11.2 Shakti Mudra

A SACRED BOND

Amanda and Joseph, both professional New Yorkers in their early 40s, were having marital difficulties soon after the honeymoon was over. Apparently, Joseph was flirting with the concept of an "open marriage" and had not come clean on this important issue with Amanda until months into the marriage. A misguided and unhealthful concept, many people of all ages have unfortunately taken to practicing "open marriage," and have sexual partners outside of the marital union. Coming from a rich spiritual background, Amanda felt that it was hypocritical and unfair of her spouse to enter the marriage without letting her know about his sexual desires. Moreover, Amanda had envisioned marriage as a sacred bond between two people and as such felt it had to be monogamous.

I first met Amanda at a conference in New York. She had patiently stood in a long cue and waited to talk to me after my presentation on Shakti & Women's Sexuality. In a hurry to get to my next venue, I invited her to ride along with me in the taxi. She appeared in a fragile state and her hands were practically shaking by the time she entered the cab. Obviously heartbroken, she stifled back the tears and began telling me her story. She and Joseph were very much in love with each other and shared many interests. Her only grievance was his sexual orientation. I recommended the Shiva-Shakti Mudra practice for her, and gave her the contact number of one of my students in the area that would be willing to sit with her and guide her practice. As we left the taxi, I gave her a hug and invited her to bring her husband to a workshop I was presenting that coming weekend in the nearby Berkshire Mountains.

I was glad to see that both Amanda and Joseph came and stayed for the entire weekend workshop. They appeared harmonious with each other as they entered the hall, cutting a very elegant and handsome figure. There were many couples in the audience of nearly 200 participants, so I decided to teach them the mudras and mantras for strengthening relationships and trust. During the Shiva-Shakti practice, I noticed that Joseph was crying, and that Amanda was hugging and consoling him. At the end of the seminar, Amanda introduced Joseph to me and he confided that he was moved by the practice that Amanda was doing at home. When he realized how hurt she was by his "open marriage" idea, it made him recognize the sanctity of marriage and feel ashamed of himself. He was now eager to learn the spiritual ways of love, bhakti marga, and promised that he would work together with Amanda to cultivate respect for his marriage. Amanda and Joseph continue to apply these teachings in their daily lives. Amy, their precocious 7-year old daughter, is a testament to their love. This fortunate couple had learned that love when practiced with sacred intention transforms the act of sex into yoga, celestial love.

THE DANCE OF SACRED UNION

A primal dance of nature, sexual union is a necessary means of replenishing both male and female energies, except for those couples who have sublimated their passions into celestial love. Vajikarana—the limb of Ayurveda that deals with virility, says that the vital life-forming essence of ojas and the subtle life-generating fire, tejas can only grow between the couple after a long period of this cosmic dance. Just as a mother feeds her baby with her own milk over a period of time, the male feeds his female partner with the essential, cosmic nutrients of his sperm. When preserved within a monogamous union, both ovum and sperm, continuously replenished, gain progressive strength until they join to become a new life. From this bonding, the future seed sprouts with prowess and brilliance, seasoned by the esteem and love infused within the threads of the sacred material spun over a long and integral period of the relationship. When the new life is born, its genetic composition is influenced by the parents' intentions and actions long before cohabitation and, quite decisively, from the time of union between sperm and ovum.

You too may come to learn the wisdom against the indiscriminate and lawless indulgence of sexual intercourse. Men must transcend their reptilian ancestry, which tends to disconnect their genitals from their intelligence, and learn how to use their sexuality in sacred ways. From the beginning, women have made ideal teachers for this education, and need to once more guide their men into wholeness. Practiced without dharma, life-forming nectar turns to poison. Life springing from a union of that nature is generally plagued with uneasiness and sorrow. When the potentially blissful dance of sex is reduced to a blistering tedium—a hop from one partner to another, devoid of esteem, dignity, and universal rhythm—chaos and sorrow for all involved are certain to follow. Disregarding the rhythmic vibrations of nature and indulging in sexual misconduct are certain to incur the loss of love, happiness, and the impoverishment of faith and trust.

Our intentions are an essential prelude to all activities, especially sexual inter-change. Practiced as an entirely physical action, without allegiance to bhakti marga, sexual involvement becomes emotionally and physically depleting and deprecat-ing. A sure way to transmute ojas and tejas into poison and bile, indiscriminate sexual practices are primal violations against love, happiness, and the essences of Self. To quote an old Ayurveda saying about when sex is performed without proper intention and regard for human esteem, "At once, one crumbles as a dry, sapless, worm-eaten and decayed piece of wood at the merest touch." Hmmm! Lit-erally, this may be truer than we know given the galaxy of "new" diseases being discovered every day that relate to human reproduction. It certainly is true for the spirit. In violating this privileged spirit, our ability to truly love becomes dimin-ished and, after some time, we chance losing it completely.

THE COSMIC STORY OF WOMAN & MAN

> *The purpose of yoga is to unite these two principles so that Shiva and Shakti become one within the self.*
> —*Yogachudamani Upanishad*

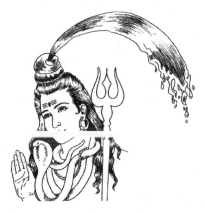

Figure 11.3 Head Pose of Lord Shiva

India's ancient masters revered the magnificent nature of the goddess and recognized her nature in every woman. They wrote their vast knowledge and research of sex in copious manuals such as the *Kama Sutra*, the *Ananga Ranga*, and *Koka Sastra*. They saw how the lunar wheel correlated with the fertility cycle of the female and understood the underlying magical mysteries and requisite qualities that contributed to sexual compatibility. They set out the astrology, astronomy, and physiognomy on this epic affair and even developed specific yoga postures for sexual enjoyment. To aid attraction between the sexes, they concocted aphrodisiacs, remedies, and charms for both women and men. Unfortunately, much of this knowledge has been used over the years as a mere physical tool to promote promiscuity.

Women play a pivotal role in the enlightenment and upliftment of a moral society. Their power grows from their investment in preserving the sacred ways of nature. It is this power that makes women the greatest educators, guides, instructors, and nourishers for their men and children. At this axial time in the history of the earth, it is imperative that women reclaim and resume their roles as nurturers, healers, and the healed.

The genesis story that follows is a metaphor for knowing the pure nature of the masculine and feminine energy, necessary to be evoked once more if we are to re-establish the relationship of love and harmony between the genders. The archetypal symbol for absolute consciousness, Shiva, also represents the masculine force of the universe. Shiva sits on the summit of the A-Ka-Tha Triangle (A: Creator; Ka: Preserver; Tha: Destroyer). This form holds the combined energies of Brahma the Creator, Vishnu the Preserver, and Shiva the Destroyer. These three cosmic energies forming the A-Ka-Tha Triangle symbolize the three forms of consciousness—truth, beauty, and purity. "A" also stands for solar energy or masculine force, "Tha" for lunar energy or feminine force, and "Ka" is a combination of both lunar and solar energies necessary to sustain the creation. The same triangle created by these three energies exists in the first chakra, *muladhara*. Here, Shiva is in the form of *Svayambu lingam* and Shakti is in the form of *kundalini*, the serpent coiled around the lingam wherein the primordial masculine and feminine energies are held in their potential form. As our consciousness grows, the sleeping serpent awakens and her divine energy of Shakti rises up through the narrow passage in the spinal column to embrace Kameshvara, her magnificent beloved. Turning the petals of all the chakras in her ascension, Shakti takes the form of Kameshvari. As you will see, this journey sets the pace for the fulfillment of human desire and development of human consciousness. The union of the divinities, Kameshvara and Kameshvari, where the masculine folds into the feminine, is the pure nature of the moon. Here, the two energies are poised as one circle of consciousness—*unmanifest*, whole, and complete. The moon transcends all genders. She is the guiding beacon of consciousness, silently witnessing the affairs of her creation.

A metaphor for the physical and cosmic union between woman and man, ancient tantric art depicts Shiva-Shakti as half male, half female. Chandra, the moon, is both masculine and feminine in nature and refers to the conjugal rite of female and male energies—yin and yang, lunar and solar, intuitive and rational. The full moon dance of Shiva and Shakti symbolizes the quest for unity, union, and oneness with the Divine. Once the genders coalesce, both feminine and masculine energies combine. Like in the sensual and loving acts of the gods and goddesses, this union is the basis of the universe's primeval desire seeded within the sperm and the ovum. Kameshvara and Kameshvari, the presiding deities of the moon chakra, are Shiva and Shakti in the form of the primeval desire, *kama*. As Kameshvara, Shiva is said to boast the most magnificent male form in the universe. He sits in Divine embrace of his beloved, Kameshvari, the most beautiful female of all the worlds.

As the projectile energy of Kameshvara is responsible for the rising upward of cosmic energy into consciousness, Kameshvari's energies extend outward, giving birth to the creation. Her Shakti-filled womb expands in the shape of the full moon, as she spills out her fertility to produce life. "When you have a goddess as the creator, it is her own body that is the universe. She is identical with the universe...She is the whole sphere of the life-enclosing heavens," recalls Joseph Campbell. Shakti has many essences, but its central meaning is Kameshvari's energy—the primordial feminine healing energies of a woman.

To reclaim these precious gems, you must re-examine and discard the conditioned mind. In modern society, almost all of us grow up with set ideas, doctrines, convictions, prejudices, and belief systems that generally oppose our direct experience, knowledge, and intuition. In Western culture, women are conditioned to hide their creativity and sexuality, and men to disdain, fear, and/or abuse it. Exercising our sexuality nowadays is tantamount to cutting out the heart to fulfill base desire. Indiscriminate use of our sexuality diminishes ojas. To start reclaiming your innate rights to the essence and idea of what it feels like to be a happily fulfilled woman, encourage your mate to join you in the Shiva-Lingam Mudra practice on the following page so that together you may pursue Divine Love. May you blossom and bond in significant ways with each other. May your path be that of bhakti marga.

SHIVA-LINGAM MUDRA: ENHANCING THE SACRED IN YOUR SPOUSE

Shiva-Lingam Mudra may be practiced by both genders, individually and together. Together you and your spouse may begin the practice of bonding by transforming your relationship into one of divine love. The Shiva-Lingam Mudra practice helps to integrate feminine (lunar/Shakti) and masculine (solar/Shiva) energies in each one of us, and also creates an indelible bond between couples. Linga literally means "attribute," or "sign of Shiva." As in all forms, figures, statues, and idols representing the Divine in the Vedic pantheon, the sages conceived these sacred symbols as a necessary form of worship since they recognized that most people need a visible, tangible form to gain access to the intangible, invisible, infinite Spirit.

The practice of Shiva-Lingam Mudra brings the reproductive organs, nervous system, and breath into a state of balance, thereby strengthening vitality and virility in the body. This mudra is also a meditation intending to calm the mind and expand intuition. A vital practice for strengthening prana and making you aware of the rhythms of your subtle body, this practice brings about a deep state of calm within the body and harmony within yourself and your relationship. The *Linga Purana* tells us that the linga is Shiva's cosmic pillar, which emerges from the base of the earth, Shakti, and stretches far into the sky. In other words, Shiva cannot stand without the support of Shakti. This pillar of infinity emanates the cosmic sound, OM. The lingam is a sign of pure consciousness.

Together, if you regularly cultivate this simple practice, you will begin to acquire insights into your own natural rhythms and how they correlate with your partner. Almost immediately, you will find yourselves moving in sync. Physically, mentally, and spiritually you will create a seamless flow between you.

Note: If you're doing this mudra alone, you may practice only the first part as the remaining practice requires a partner.

THE PRACTICE: SHIVA-LINGAM MUDRA

PART ONE:

- Retreat to a quiet place in your home or outdoors and sit facing each other either in a comfortable cross-legged position on pillows or upright in straight-backed chairs.
- Bring your left hand to the chest, palm facing upward with the fingers together.
- Make a fist with your right hand and place it securely on the left palm.
- Extend the right thumb upward. The right hand is a metaphor for your solar breath and the left hand for your lunar breath. The particular configuration of this mudra integrates the energies of Shiva and Shakti within you.
- Close your eyes and meditate on God Shiva, the source of consciousness. Visualize him in the form of a translucent crystal pillar, lingam, sitting firmly on a base of solid gold, Shakti.
- The woman should visualize her spouse as the lingam, Pure Consciousness.
- The man should visualize his wife as Shakti, the Formidable One.
- Hold the mudra for five minutes or so, and then release it. The second part of the practice that follows will help you create and seal an indelible bond with each other.

PART TWO:

- Shift your position slightly closer to face each other, and continue your mudra practice by interlacing your hands, using the right hand of the male and the left hand of the female.
- Bring your left hand up to chest level with palm up. You may brace your elbow into your waist for support.
- Make a fist with the right hand with thumb up and rest it into the outstretched palm of your wife's left hand.
- Breathe slowly and concentrate on merging your rhythms.
- Hold the mudra for five minutes or so, and then release it.

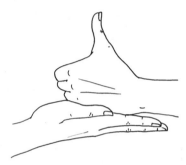

Figure 11.4 Shiva-Lingam Mudra

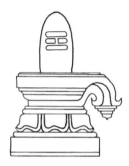

Figure 11.5 The Linga on a Base

This practice will evolve over time and should not be rushed. Gradually, you will find your energies becoming integrated within, and moving outward to express a spirit of unity and harmony with all things. Visualizing Shiva and Shakti is a significant practice for many couples who have come to me for assistance. It restores vitality and virility and evokes the spirit of bestowal to women. Men will find that the gentleness and confidence they gain from this beginning exercise will pave the way for further practice.

THE FORGOTTEN DHARMA OF SEXUALITY: SEXUAL COMMUNION AS A SADHANA

The ancient science of Vedic astrology, health, wealth, virility, vitality, and spiritual virtues were developed to help humanity live, work, and play in accord with divine energies. Dharmas are the unwritten codes of proper conduct inherent in all life. India is weaned on the tradition of dharma handed down from the rishis of ancient times. These universal values belonging to all humans protect us with resplendent grace when we are guided in all activities by the spirit of goodness, wholesomeness, honesty, compassion, cleanliness, and reverence to the greater energies of the cosmos. When we honor these subtle, invisible, intangible cosmic laws that protect the family, we safeguard our energy of Shakti. When dharma is ignored and neglected, it brings a ton of misery in our lives.

The dharma of sex is a spiritual education. Like all education, you have to invest time and energy to educate your men and children. Men have always depended on women for their education in the ways of sexuality. If your spouses are not willing to listen, just do what you have to do to nourish the sacred within yourself.

All life seeks union in many ways. One of the deepest forms of sharing is through the sadhana of sex. Even the saints and sages, who have sublimated the normal physical urges of sexuality, seek to form a union—not with another person—but with God. The yoga of life is union, and the cosmic intention in human sexual activity is the bonding of two people who henceforth walk the path of bhakti marga as one in and with the universe.

The tradition of sexual interplay, primarily for the continuance of life through procreation, has been observed as a sacred duty to all species. Foreplay and the various other activities involved in the happy dance of sexual intercourse and its aftermath have always been a beautiful and enriching part of this numinous duty. When sexual communion occurs during a harmonically auspicious time, the moral and ethical laws of society and nature flourish. The opposite holds true when sexual activities are performed during an inauspicious time of the year. Disregarding the timely and necessary conditions for sexual activity creates chaos, disease, unhappiness, and poverty.

Auspicious Times & Conditions for Cohabitation
- Primarily during the early and late winter periods, with the following days being the most auspicious: 8th, 14th, and 15th day of both the light and dark phases of the moon.
- During the spring, early fall (rainy season), and autumn, sexual intercourse should occur only on the three auspicious days cited above.
- After a purifying bath in a cool, clean, sheltered place.
- After prayers are observed and honorable intentions declared.
- Early evening is considered the best time for sexual union.

Postures During Sex
Certain positions are considered disharmonious during sexual activity. These postures create disequilibrium and often times disease. When a woman assumes the prone position during sex, the Vata dosha becomes aggravated. When she lies on her right side during sexual activity, the Kapha dosha becomes displaced and obstructs the opening of the uterus. When she lies on her left side, the Pitta dosha becomes constrained, resulting in excess internal heat, which in turn, incinerates

the sperm and ovum. The best posture is for the woman to lie comfortably on her back in a relaxed position, with her male partner lying on top of her. In this way, your sexual posture emulates the cosmic accord of Shiva—the pillar, and Shakti—the base.

Progeny: Conceiving a Son or Daughter

Harmonic timing and circumstances relating to sexual activity has nothing to do with social conventions and religious dogma. True cognizance of nature's rhythms is required to fully understand why timing and intentions are so vital to wholesome sexual activity. Far from the denial and suffocating strictures of neo-religious social dictates regarding sexuality, harmonic sexual relationship is an expression of the universe itself.

To conceive a son, sexual intercourse should be convened on the 4th, 6th, 8th, 10th or 12th days following the first day of the woman's menstrual cycle. For instance if the menstrual cycle began on the 5th of the month, the 4th day from the beginning of the cycle will fall on the 9th day of the month, the first auspicious day for cohabitation to produce a son. The 10th, 12th, 14th, and 16th days of that particular month will be the remaining auspicious days pertaining to that particular menstrual cycle.

To conceive a daughter, sexual intercourse should occur on the 5th, 9th, and 11th days following the first day of the woman's menstrual cycle. Note that the 7th day is considered inauspicious.

All the other days are considered harmonically inauspicious times to conceive children. Negative results may ensue in the physical, emotional, and spiritual health of both parents and child when conception occurs outside of these times.

Inauspicious Times and Conditions for Cohabitation

- During dawn, dusk, midnight, or daylight.
- On the evening or day of the anniversary of a parent's death.
- On the evening or day of the full moon.
- On holy days.
- During the astrological passages of a planet from one sign of the zodiac to another (consult a Vedic astrologer for details).
- During the summer season.
- Without the observance of prayers or clarification of intentions.
- Before taking a bath and in unclean circumstances.
- When there is excessive sexual activity. (Overindulgence may lead to pain and diseases, i.e., asthma, fever, jaundice, and venereal diseases.)
- During a woman's menstrual cycle, especially on the 1st, 2nd, and 3rd days. (Conception during this time poses a serious threat to the child's life.)

Part Five

WOMEN'S SACRED

TRANSITION

INTO WISDOM

Chapter Twelve

LIGHT ON MENOPAUSE

My phenomenal passage through the clinch of death helped me to understand my cosmic right to transcend disease, despair, and death—as we do millions, perhaps trillions of times through the cycle of our rebirths. This journey has given me a limitless womb that would "give birth" to millions of children.

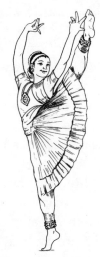

Figure 12.1 Dance of Light

Menopause is an oasis of lightness wedged between the phases of fertility and wisdom. Contrasted to the negative stereotypes surrounding menopause in the popular culture, the Vedic tradition honors all stages of a woman's life. First though, before we examine the light on menopause from the standpoint of traditional wisdom, let me briefly share with you my own menopausal journey.

Coming into this particular age symbolizes inner freedom, a freedom that I have come to own and cherish. On this very day, I have entered my 53rd year and having lost my womb at the early age of 21, I am yet to experience any negative symptoms of menopause. As you can see from the Inner Medicine healing practices in this book and from the extensive work I do at large in Wise Earth Ayurveda, you too can experience this state of profound joy as a result of the incredible inner freedom that can be claimed at menopause.

I was an eager soul from the start. It seems that everything in my life happened prematurely and intensely. At two years of age, I made a bid to return to the higher ethers, but survived near fatal diphtheria thanks to the brilliant persistence and care of my father. At the age of 10, I started my menarche, a jumpstart in expending the procreative energy of my womb. At 18, I made another attempt to reunite with my beloved Shiva—this time through ovarian cancer. As you know, I did heal; evidence that we can all heal and that we do heal. We are in a state of continual refinement, eventually to heal the body/mind/spirit into Absolute Consciousness. When we realize that healing is a natural part of our human destiny, we are better able to take control of its process. Immediately after I came out of my profound passages of healing, which included 12 surgeries, several rounds of radiation therapy and chemotherapy, a battery of prescribed drugs, and a complete hysterectomy, I had a sense that my karma with cancer was finished. Somehow, I knew I would never experience the predictable medical aftermath anticipated by my doctors. Directly after my hysterectomy, I was informed by my kind gynecologist that I would experience surgical, or "artificial" menopause. As he put it, some time in the next year or so, I would join half the world's population of women with menopause, the "inevitable symptoms" of which would be hot flashes, irritability, night sweats, depression, and so on. To forestall this frightful eventuality, immediately after surgery he handed me a prescription for Premarin (the most commonly prescribed estrogen that is named after a horse, since it's derived from the pregnant mare's urine).

Before leaving the hospital, I threw it away. I knew that I would never have the experiences he told me about. Perhaps, it was innocence that came from my unshakable faith in the Divine Mother that guided me all along. After I left the hospital with barely any prana left in my body, I did know one thing—that my journey in this life had only just begun. Cancer, like all deep diseases, is a rite of passage, an instrument of healing to help us reconcile or extinguish a set of karmas. I had finally completed the major cycle of my existence wherein I had finally snubbed out the aged, inured karmas that had kept me alienated from the profoundly simple knowledge that I am One with the Mother Consciousness.

Although my gynecologist could not have known of the extent of my rebirth and transformations yet to come, I remember his kindness as he held my frozen hands in the post-operative recovery theatre and with great compassion squeezed and rubbed them to give me warmth. Tearfully, he consoled me, "You may not regret it now, but as you grow older and feel the need for having a child of your own you will mourn this loss."

AWAKENING TO POWER

I was 21 years old then and I knew I was forever changed. The loss of my physical womb had already transcended into the manifestation of my cosmic womb.

It was on that specific day that I was awakened to my Shakti—the power of the Mother within. I knew that the "loss" of my womb foretold far greater stories. Before cancer I had already recognized that my path would not be the blissful one of marriage and bearing children. Long before I recognized my purpose, I knew I was constructed in such a way as to be a fruitful emissary of the Mother Consciousness. My phenomenal passage through the clinch of death helped me to understand my cosmic right to transcend disease, despair, and death—as we do millions, perhaps trillions of times through the cycle of our rebirths. This journey has given me a limitless womb that would "give birth" to millions of children.

Over the last 30 years, this realization has become a munificent reality as I work with, nourish, and educate women and children all over the world to understand their inner healing power. The recognition of my ability to heal and to help others help themselves to heal has provided me with the indelible knowledge that the Mother Consciousness is always at work within us. Indeed, through her grace we are capable of recognizing ourselves as her instrument. Once awakened to this fathomable reality, I knew I was Mother—in the same way as you will one day discover that you are Mother. I am one with Mother. You are one with Mother. We are all One Mother. It is only a matter of being awakened to discover who you are. My journey through cancer awakened me.

My early "coming of age" has also served me well in my spiritual path. In my Vedic tradition, women were not initiated into the lineage of the sages. This is not because they were considered spiritually inferior, but because menstruation, desire for motherhood, and spousal bliss would make them extremely vulnerable to the austerities and rigorous sadhanas that monks in my tradition must observe. However, in the last decade or so, a handful of India's great seers who are awakened to the Mother Consciousness have given this initiation to women. Even so, the few young women I know who are in their menstruating years and are granted their initiation to this path experience many challenges.

At the age of 32, I received my initiation from His Holiness, Swami Dayananda Saraswati on the bank of the sacred Ganges River. Twenty-four years after my "menopause," I was prepared to own my path and destiny as a *Swamini*. Once more, I was primed early to take my role, since ojas had flown open the inner gate to my Shakti energies. By this means, the seed of wisdom spilled out and broadcast itself for the growth of consciousness in many generations to come.

At the juncture of menopause, the essence of ojas that once propelled the juices of reproduction now convert into inner wisdom, the subtlest of ojas' energy. Although our karmas may be different, each and every woman of all cultures has the innate ability to reclaim their autumnal energy of the Shakti, and retrieve their matured ojas. To do this we must necessarily shift our focus on menopause as a transition into ascending lightness, instead of descending darkness.

A NEW LOOK AT ANCIENT WISDOM

The native women of my culture see this period as a harbinger of deep spiritual fortitude, a time to start loosening the grip on competitive partnerships with the world and to go within to commune with the greater power. According to Wise Earth Ayurveda, menopause marks the cusp of time when the physical essence of ojas matures into emotional wisdom. Physiologically, menopause marks one of two natural major transitions in a woman's biological life (the first being menarche, which we will explore in later pages) as they move from the time of life dominated by Pitta into the arena of Vata, symbolic of the autumnal time of life.

For most women, this process manifests fully somewhere between the ages of 45 and 51, with perimenopause having begun 15 years or so earlier, when the body's ojas had reached its prime. During the final stages of menopause, there is a cessation of the menstrual cycle. As we age, ojas—the autoimmune essence necessary to promote healthy growth, reproduction, and birthing—retreats at the same rate. As a result, a woman's ability to give birth closes down.

In my tradition, at the age of 60 a woman reaffirms her marital vows with her husband in a beautiful ceremony called *shashtyabda purti* when she claims her age of wisdom. This ceremony is usually attended by her children and grandchildren. The rite of shashtyabda purti is an affirmation that the procreative Shakti has matured into the wisdom-croned Shakti, a natural development in the maturing of the Shakti energy within all women. This is the juncture when the active physical and emotional womb gains complete closure and the woman may now progress into her spiritual womb.

Native women eagerly awaited this time of life as it meant the beginning of reprieve, reflection, and inner peace. Gently anticipating this golden time, savoring the idea of life untethered when we may finally release or decrease yesteryear's activities of grooming and nurturing the children, caring for the men, caring for the hearths, homes, and fields. Nothing in the world would have enticed a native woman to fetch the burden of youth for another decade or so, by pushing menopause farther into the vision of her future, even if she had at her disposal the chance for biomedical intervention to do so.

Before modern medicine and longer life spans, bringing children into the world and nurturing them was considered the primary focus in marriage. The "midlife crisis" was unknown in earlier cultures. Moreover, all native cultures honoured their women elders. The Alaskan Yupik and Australian Aborigines emphasize the contribution and wisdom of their elders by honoring them with rituals while they are still alive. In Judaism, when a woman's potent blood stops flowing, it is believed that the life force stays within to make her wise. Her wisdom is celebrated in a ceremony called *simhat hochmah*, where she becomes a crone and may walk with the *Torah* (traditionally carried by men), symbolic of the wisdom she now possesses. In the Hindu culture, at the age of 48, both women and men are inaugurated into life of vanaprastha ashrama celebrated by a special ceremony. In this tradition, a woman does not walk her crucial rites of passages alone, she is upheld by her husband as the goddess of the home, and supported by him through her growth into wisdom.

Symbolically, the retreat into the deep forest is the quest for gathering spiritual wisdom. More than symbolism, in days of yore, men, women, and couples literally retreated into the sanctuary of the forest to spend the rest of their lives there in the cultivation of inner freedom.

For the Hindu, life is a sacred journey in which each landmark marking major biological, emotional, and spiritual phases is consecrated through sacraments, called samskaras. As noted earlier, sixteen rites of passage are observed throughout one's life, beginning with the ritual observances that accompany conception and birth, and closing with last rites and ancestral ceremonies after death.

These rites serve to cultivate habitual imprints of security in the higher mind and motivate family and community into a shared relationship of invoking the blessings of the Mother. In these proactive communities, family and friends gather with their priests to perform the necessary rituals for the protection of each person in the community during important junctures of their lives.

Although we may recognize menopause as a major physiological and psychological transition, we are yet to own its spiritual implications. Medical intervention and takeover of women's reproduction arose as a direct result of women buying into the culture of youth-oriented typecasts. Targeting the middle-aged woman is a huge business for the medical and pharmaceutical industry. By the year 2010, it is estimated that almost half of the woman in the world will arrive at menopause. But unless women recast their roles to assert their authority over their own reproduction process, they will continue to be prime targets for the medical conglomerates and drug cartels. Meanwhile, the wearing away of the Mother Consciousness has served to heighten the fear, anxiety, and paranoia in our internal and external environments, causing a slow and steady erosion of women's confidence and security in themselves. At this critical time, women must re-envision themselves as wisdom carriers and not as aged women frightfully struggling to grasp onto their youth and outwardly body perfection. No amount of therapy, beauty treatments, cosmetic surgeries, hormone replacement therapy, workouts, diets, and willpower can bring us into the golden light of our wisdom. Instead, we must take pause.

THE ART OF TAKING PAUSE

We need to take a brief pause at the beginning and end of the day, a longer pause every week, and an even longer one at the end of every month. During seasonal transitions, birthdays, anniversaries, pregnancies, births, and in the crucial times of our menstrual cycles—when the appropriate pause *must* be observed—we are likely to re-enter the hallowed space of self and re-examine our lives, purpose, reality, karma, and goals. Then we can move along incrementally and remain present with all things.

The major challenge for women is that we have knotted ourselves so firmly into the awkward, rhythmless, dissonant, societal system that we can barely breathe—much less think of breaking free from it. Over the years, many of my female disciples have approached me with the same concern: "As a mother and family person, how do I take time for myself?" Taking contemplative, reflective time can be done with your family members. This pause has to do with creating the space in your home and heart that allows the family to naturally ease into calmness from the moment they arrive home. Clear the center of your living space, spread the floor with quilts, lay on it with your family members, bring them together in conversation, and do one or two brief spiritual practices of your choice or tradition that honors your family's collective entry into tranquility.

Almost all the female sadhakas of the Wise Earth School have emulated the sacred space of Wise Earth by recreating it in their kitchens and homes, implementing the Mother's energetic embrace to hold the family together in harmony. As a symbolic locust, set up a small altar in the shared living space and place a ghee lamp or a beeswax candle there to be kept lit while the family convenes. Like many of my disciples do, you may place a photograph of your guru on the altar. In my tradition, the Guru whose *darshana*, potent blessing, helps us to see the truth, is regarded as the perennial elder in our lives. You may also place a photograph of a family elder or ancestor on your altar.

Until we take the small pauses at important junctures along the way we will end up quite unprepared as we butt headlong into the big pause—menopause. For optimum and healthful entry into menopause, you would want to begin observing the sadhana practices set out in this book while you are still in your early 30s. For some women, the condition we call perimenopause, or the period of hormonal imbalance that leads up to menopause, may start as early as in their late 20s or 30s. This is the time when menstrual cycles start to respond erratically by becoming lighter or heavier, shorter or longer than usual. Most women begin to notice their hormonal levels fluctuating in their 40s. For the majority, perimenopausal symptoms occur three to five years prior to menopause.

MEDICAL INTERFERENCE

With the introduction of non-native hormones into our bodies, noxious chemicals into our food sources, and the tampering and intermingling of the genetic codes of a multitude of species, we are facing a growing miasma of new reproductive diseases which are directly linked to both the cause and result of women's hormonal dysfunction. Girls as young as seven years of age are starting their menarche; an increasing number of women are unable to carry their pregnancies to term; a growing incident of infertility in both women and men exist; menstrual cycles are bombarded with difficulties; and perimenopause and menopause have become protracted. Not to mention the endemic reality of sexual and domestic violence against women. Indeed, it appears as though a woman's rites of passage throughout her life are continually expanding to usurp more than 75 percent of her length of years. At this rate, we must examine the process and the end game of being given longer life terms by "institutions." In other words, women are now experiencing a growing number of "false hormonal transitions" accompanied by manifold layers of "new" reproductive disorders.

Recent studies have shown that an alarming number of women are having anovulatory cycles starting as early as in their mid-30s, which means that these women are menstruating but do not ovulate. As a result, the body is not able to produce progesterone during the ovulation cycle. Depletion of progesterone in the body creates an imbalance between progesterone and estrogen levels necessary to maintain good reproductive health in women. This imbalance of estrogen dominance in the body may explain why women are experiencing the side effects of depression, fluid retention, migraines, urinary tract infections, and a rise in PMS symptoms. This growing problem may also account for postpartum depression syndrome and infertility in women.

Studies have shown that the progestrogens used in birth control pills contribute to the alteration of the natural hormonal cycle. But birth control pills are just a few symptoms of a more insidious disorder, which is the medical and scientific tampering with a woman's sacred, cyclical, biological, and hormonal reproductive ability. The decrease of progesterone in the body may also play an active part in rapid bone degeneration or osteoporosis, a condition that is plaguing millions of women.

Although menopause is a biological marker for the natural process of aging, it does not have to be a time for midlife crises, or fear, anxiety, unhappiness, and decaying health. We simply need to emulate our wise female predecessors and reclaim our Shakti power and its natural rhythm of joy. Women in the rural villages of India have been the subject of studies by researchers because they exhibit little or no characteristic indicators of menopause such as hot flashes, vaginal dryness, mood swings, insomnia, bone fractures, and osteoporosis. Similarly, research observation conducted on the Mayan women of Mexico showed that they do not demonstrate any of these symptoms in their menopausal transitions. In fact, in these cultures women have lower levels of estrogen than American women, which inadvertently helps them to enjoy a smoother passage into midlife. Besides, these women share a striking similarity in their preserved sense of joy. By contrast,

American women have become habituated to higher levels of estrogen in their bodies, which makes them more susceptible to experiencing menopausal symptoms. I believe that if the Mayan or rural Indian women were to move to the big cities and became urbanized in their life habits, they would begin to experience many of these warning signs allied with menopause.

But there are ways that you can keep that sense of peace and stillness with you, even when you relocate to an urban area. Take the example of Palavi, a woman in her late 50s. She told me that two years after moving from the small, easygoing village of Gujarat to the polluted city of Mumbai, she began experiencing severe hot flashes, night, sweats and insomnia for the first time since she had started her menopause at age 42. Although she had a difficult time adjusting to life in the city, she felt she had to stay on in Mumbai to support her husband who had been relocated there for business. Palavi came to Wise Earth to learn how to reclaim tranquility in her life amid the chaotic ambient conditions of urban life. Along with using the Vata nourishing foods set out in Appendix Two, she faithfully adhered to the womb nourishing lunar practice of Uttara Vasti. Within three months her symptoms completely ended. You too may learn to keep the pure essence of the rural serenity close to you even in the midst of urban city life.

MENOPAUSE & LONELINESS

At a deeper level of spirit, menopausal challenges relate to loneliness. A woman who has fulfilled the rhythm of her womb with conscious and loving care, noble sensual satisfaction, and with the children she desires, has less chance of being lonely in her midlife years. Being happily married and bearing children, however, are not the only means to fulfilling the rhythm of the womb. Although it's not the usual karma for most women, the conscious transformation of feminine desires can also fulfill the womb by sublimating them into a higher purpose of taking the ascetic path, wherein you may serve humanity and educate and care for all children. To remove loneliness, we must eliminate the distance we have created from the Mother Consciousness. The loneliness we experience in the womb generally matures and rises into the space of the heart where it may have a devastating effect on the evolution of our joy and consciousness.

Being a mother means being true to the Mother in all of her forms, beginning with your own birth mother. One out of every four Western women I have guided has a terrible relationship with her mother. Until we heal the love between mother and daughter, it will be challenging for women to reclaim the Mother within their own wombs. It is wise to remember that we inherit the rhythms of our mothers' health. As a Spiritual Mother to many women with cysts, tumors, and cancer, I have noticed that their diseases are often related to the condition of the maternal uterus during pregnancy. Women, in particular, can benefit by discovering the links between their health issues and those of the women in their family, going back as many generations as they can trace. I have noticed repeatedly that women who have troubled relationships with their mothers also have deficiencies in their Shakti prana and cannot connect with the purifying energy of the Mother Consciousness. Anger and hurt are two of the most debilitating emotions; these sentiments block the natural flow of Shakti prana to your womb, and seal off positive flow of energy to your brain. Communication then becomes difficult and prevents you from moving forward. However, like Serena, whose healing story you are about to read, you too can heal the deep rift with your mother and together begin to laugh and heal and enjoy a fulfilling relationship with each other.

SERENA'S STORY

During the years when I was still presenting Wise Earth Ayurveda workshops in the United States, I met Serena when she attended a women's workshop I presented in New York. She was just 32 years old and had recently discovered she had a fibroid tumor the size of a large grapefruit in her uterus. I asked her, as I always do when helping women to resolve their health issues, about her relationship with her mother. "We haven't seen each other for seven years," she told me. "She's an alcoholic and had been diagnosed several years ago with bipolar disorder. She has been on and off Prozac for 10 years or more." As part of a noninvasive regimen to help her reduce the tumor, I suggested to Serena that she must reconnect with her mother and spend some time talking to her about any maternal and reproductive challenges she may have had in her life. I knew this would be a difficult step for her to take, but persuaded her nonetheless by letting her know that she would have a much healthier and gentler relationship with her mother if she realized the phenomenal role her mother plays in shaping her health legacy and memory.

She returned to see me about a month or so after I first met with her. She was eager to share news of her reunion with her mother and the discoveries she had made. She learned that Jeanne, her mother, had great difficulties with the birthing process of her two children. Because of complications with two previous pregnancies, her mother had to have a partial abortion before becoming pregnant with Serena some months later. Jeanne had just recovered from the emotional roller coaster of her previous unfortunate pregnancies, and felt unsupported by her husband when she became pregnant. She definitely did not want to have another child.

She tried to abort Serena by throwing herself down a flight of stairs. Fortunately, she did little injury to herself and was unsuccessful in aborting the fetus. On hearing this untoward news, Serena said that she felt like a dagger had been thrown through her heart. At first, she was too stunned to respond. She couldn't muster the tears to mourn her unwanted beginnings and unloved entry into Planet Earth; instead she felt her heart freeze. But Jeanne's tearful emotions in pouring out her shameful truth thawed out Serena's heart. Much to her surprise, she found herself consoling her mom. Once this secret was aired, Serena felt lightness floating through her while in her mother's arms. Finally, the darkness between mother and daughter had lifted. They noticed the fineness of the afternoon air on Jeanne's kitchen patio as the sun shone through the clouds to meet their moment of bonding. They hugged each other and wept happy tears.

Once Serena understood her mother's pain and fears, they were able to break the cycle of separation and pain they had caused each other. Jeanne reassured her after the guilt of exposing this secret was "off her chest," that she had never had any regrets in bringing Serena into the world. With Jeanne's new found ability to show love to her daughter, and with Serena's understanding of her mother's plight, they have formed a formidable bond with each other and now spend a great deal of time making up for lost affection. Maternal anger abated, Serena's health was on the mend.

Serena was able to connect her maternal ancestral memories with the condition of her own womb. In combination with her mother's help and the Wise Earth Ayurveda sadhana practices she had adopted, she turned the corner in her healing process and within a few months after her reunion with Jeanne, she decided to have the fibroid tumor surgically removed. It is now some 12 years later, and from Serena's recent note, she reported she is happily married and has a 5-year old child. She says she feels completely healed.

Serena has also influenced Jeanne's healing. Jeanne has just celebrated her ninth year of sobriety and has successfully weaned herself off her intense bipolar medications. Frequently, Serena accompanies her mother to her Alcoholics Anonymous meetings. By addressing their shared vulnerabilities, they have been able to redirect their desire toward cultivating a rich family relationship filled with love and fulfillment. Serena and her family enjoy getting together with Jeanne on occasion at her country house, in upstate New York. Like so many woman, Serena has installed Wise Earth Ayurveda practices in the center of her and her mother's lives, and continues to fortify her Shakti prana with Uttara Vasti each month following the new moon.

Remember that before you can begin to turn your course toward the light, you first must *want* to move beyond your anger toward your mother and other female forbears. Should you have trouble communicating with your mother, you may want to start the process of recovering your maternal trust and love by following this simple method for dissolving anger. When your mind moves toward rage say to yourself, "Do not go there. An angry thought is a toxic thought. Anger at my mother is anger at myself. I'm disappointed at my own lack and deflecting this karma onto my mother." After enough years of practice, the mind begins to check itself, so that you can renegotiate angry thoughts.

WISE EARTH AYURVEDA & MENOPAUSE

In Ayurveda, menopausal symptoms are caused by an imbalance of the three bodily humors, which creates toxicity, ama, and disturbs the tissue metabolism. Of the three humors, Vata plays the key role in menopausal symptoms because it rules the declining phase of our lives. Likewise, the mid-phase is ruled by Pitta and the early phase by Kapha. Vata accounts for about 80 percent of bodily challenges.

The primary emotional symptoms of Vata are nervousness, increased worry, anxiety, memory loss, and depression. Accompanied by a serious reduction of estrogen, these symptoms can easily escalate to insomnia, constipation, fluctuating blood pressure, feelings of excessive coldness after hot flashes, heart palpitations, dryness and thinning of the skin and hair, brittleness in the mucous membranes and bones, joint and muscle aches, bone fractures, and osteoporosis. Pitta types may experience pronounced hot flashes with spells of heavy bleeding, migraine headaches, night sweats, irritability, loose bowel movements, skin rashes, acne, inflamed muscles, tendonitis, bodily malodor, and urinary tract infections. Kapha types may exhibit abdominal heaviness, lethargy, listlessness, weight gain or water retention, breast swelling, yeast infections, sleepiness, and crying spells.

The primary recuperative therapies of Ayurveda called Pancha Karma are paramount to restoring hormonal balance. They also help to maintain your natural beauty and grace. Explore the warm and wondrous rejuvenative treatments set out below for your home care. Generally, Ayurvedic routines for all body types crossing midlife include a warm Vata nourishing course.

- Healthful nutrition that nurtures Vata (See Appendix Two)
- Ample and regular rest
- Nourishing Ayurvedic home treatments
- Daily herbal oil massages
- Sadhana exercises such as yoga, tai chi, and walking

In the next chapter, we will explore the rejuvenative Wise Earth Ayurveda Full Moon Practices for women who are in their perimenopausal and menopausal phases, from ginger compresses that revitalize the Shakti prana in the womb to the soporific treatment of Pichu, which calms the mind and emotions. First though, we will examine your specific imbalances as they relate to your experience with menopause. To get to the root cause of your symptoms, we will need to identify your imbalances as they relate to each dosha. In so doing, you will become familiar with the physical and emotional causes of your disorder and therefore make choices that inform both your constitutional needs and your condition.

Keep in mind that menopausal symptoms are largely Vata induced and therefore a Vata nourishing program will need to be followed by all constitutional types to achieve balance. However, the exercise below will help you to better understand your symptoms so that you may fine tune your healing course based on your personal constitution during this Vata phase of life.

Simply follow the Wise Earth Ayurveda Menopause Score Charts. Here's how to score your symptoms relating to each dosha: add up the check marks you made for each dosha at the end of each category. Whichever category received the highest score is the dosha in most need of support and balancing. If your score is equally high for two categories, focus on supporting the two doshas indicated.

WISE EARTH AYURVEDA SCORE CHARTS FOR VATA, PITTA & KAPHA TYPE MENOPAUSE

SCORE CHART FOR VATA TYPE MENOPAUSE

CHECK VATA SYMPTOMS YOU ARE EXPERIENCING:

I.	My menstrual periods are scanty, irregular, or missed	❏
2.	I have hot flashes followed by coldness	❏
3.	I have insomnia	❏
4.	I am anxious and tend to worry all the time	❏
5.	I am forgetful or confused	❏
6.	I am losing weight	❏
7.	I am frequently constipated	❏
8.	My blood pressure fluctuates	❏
9.	I suffer from vaginal dryness	❏
10.	My hair and skin are dry	❏
II.	My nails are brittle and hair is thinning	❏
12.	I have frequent urination	❏
13.	I feel pain in my joints and muscles	❏
14.	I suffer tension headaches	❏
15.	I tend to have bone fractures	❏
16.	I forget to eat	❏

Table 12.1 Score Chart for Vata Menopause

TOTAL SCORE _____

SCORE CHART FOR PITTA TYPE MENOPAUSE

CHECK PITTA SYMPTOMS YOU ARE EXPERIENCING:

1.	I have spells of heavy bleeding	❏
2.	I have severe hot flashes and night sweats	❏
3.	I have fiery dreams	❏
4.	I am irritable or angy most of the time	❏
5.	I feel burned out	❏
6.	I have abdominal tension and bloating	❏
7.	I have loose bowel movements	❏
8.	My blood pressure goes up	❏
9.	I suffer from skin rashes, acne	❏
10.	I have foul body odor	❏
11.	My muscles are inflamed	❏
12.	I suffer from tendonitis	❏
13.	I have foul smelling vaginal discharge	❏
14.	I have urinary tract infections	❏
15.	I tend to have diarrhea	❏
16.	I crave spicy, hot, and oily foods	❏

Table 12.2 Score Chart for Pitta Menopause

TOTAL SCORE _____

SCORE CHART FOR KAPHA TYPE MENOPAUSE

CHECK KAPHA SYMPTOMS YOU ARE EXPERIENCING:

1.	I feel abdominal heaviness	❏
2.	I have mild hot flashes	❏
3.	I have watery, romantic dreams	❏
4.	I feel heavy and lethargic	❏
5.	I gain weight easily	❏
6.	I am water retentive	❏

7.	I feel listless and unmotivated	❏
8.	My blood pressure goes dowm	❏
9.	I oversleep	❏
10.	My breasts are swollen	❏
11.	I have crying spells	❏
12.	I suffer from yeast infections	❏
13.	I have excessive whitish, vaginal discharge	❏
14.	I suffer migraine headaches	❏
15.	I have mentsrual spotting	❏
16.	I crave ice cream and sweets	❏

Table 12.3 Score Chart for Kapha Menopause

TOTAL SCORE _____

Understanding Your Scores

If your score is greater than seven points (total points being 16) on any of the Score Charts you are most likely experiencing a menopausal disorder. As a general rule, you will be following a Vata nourishing program, which is presented on the following pages. You will also be following the recommendations for the dosha category that came up with your highest score. For example, if your highest score came up in the Pitta category, you will be observing the healing diets and regimens for both Vata and Pitta, with more emphasis on the former.

INNER MEDICINE REMEDIES FOR MENOPAUSAL CHALLENGES

The time I came closest to experiencing any symptoms of menopause is when I was in India for a few years studying at the ashram and had no access to brown rice or any unrefined grains. During this time without my staple food of brown rice, I could feel my body having to work harder and harder to ward off impending warm flashes and night sweats. Immediately on returning to my sanctuary in the Pisgah Mountains I was able to have ample servings of brown rice—long, short, and medium grain. Within two weeks of feasting on brown rice porridges, soups, and *kichadis*, I was thriving. Except when I am fasting, I eat one whole grain of my choosing every day.

Healthful, nourishing foods and herbs have an extraordinary healing effect on the body and mind, especially when they are used in harmony with seasonal rhythms. Like the body, nature moves through specific transitions and changes. Spring is the time of childhood filled with Kapha energy, summer is the time of adolescence brimming with Pitta energy, and autumn is the time of menopause overflowing with Vata influence—the descending phase of years and energy.

Some of the most healing foods for midlife symptoms are the Vata nurturing sweet whole grains; in particular, brown rice, barley, and root vegetables. Root vegetables like wild yams, burdock, and sweet potatoes add the necessary earthy energy to the body and give it extra stability. Fruits high in boron such as apples, peaches, grapes, dates, and raisins, are excellent replenishers of estrogen. Pomegranate juice, coconut water, and lime are also refreshing aids. Mung beans, soya beans, almonds, hazelnuts, honey, and good quality yogurt, cream, and milk are all considered Vata enriching foods to be used frequently. Seaweeds like agar-agar, hiziki, kombu, arame, nori, dulse, and kelp are an amazing source of minerals (calcium, zinc, magnesium) for the body. Both kelp and dulse contain L-tyrosine and iodine, which we need to bolster the body at midlife. Following are the simple Inner Medicine remedies that will help you transition with ease through the menopause maze.

Most Vulnerable Times for Menopausal Symptoms
Challenging Time: 2:00-6:00 (morning and afternoon)
Challenging Seasons: Early fall (rainy season) and autumn
Challenging Moon Phase: Last phase of waning

Vata Nourishing Foods Best For Menopause
- Organic cow's milk, yogurt, butter, and ghee
- Whole grains (brown rice, millet, kamut, barley, and spelt)
- Wild yams
- Burdock root
- Parsnips
- Sweet potatoes
- Squashes
- Green plantains
- Golden and red beets
- Artichokes
- Asparagus
- Summer squashes
- Green beans
- Coconut water
- Lime juice
- Fruits (pomegranates, apples, peaches, grapes, dates, and raisins)
- Soya and mung beans

- Nuts (almond and hazelnut)
- Seaweeds (agar-agar, hiziki, arame, dulse, kombu, nori, and kelp)

Simple Food Steps to Alleviate Hot Flashes
Imbibe one or more of the following foods or tonics daily for six months during menopause:

- Eat a small amount of brown rice. (Take with meals or as morning porridge.)
- Drink half a glass of coconut water with the juice of half a lime in the summer, or all year long if you live in the tropics.
- Drink half a glass of pomegranate juice. (Also good for jaundice.)
- Drink warm organic cow's milk with 10 strands of saffron before bed. (You may also use almond milk.)
- Take half a teaspoon of castor oil in one tablespoon of lime juice with a pinch of rock salt daily. (You may also rub castor oil on the tummy before bed.)

WISE EARTH HERBAL REMEDIES FOR MENOPAUSE

Ayurveda's most nourishing herbs for menopause are aloe vera gel, shatavari, ashwagandha, kapikacchu, triphala, dashamula, brahmi, gotu kola, vidari, saffron, and amalaki (a natural antioxidant containing Vitamin C). As I noted previously, menopause disorders are directly connected to a greater energy of hormonal imbalance in the body, which has an adverse impact on the bodily humors, and in particular, the Vata dosha. For this reason, the food recommendations and herbal remedies provided for Vata Type in this chapter may be used by all metabolic types for any disorders relating to menopause. The menopause remedies which follow are to be taken once daily after breakfast for mild symptoms, and twice daily—after breakfast and again after lunch—for severe symptoms. You may use the remedies for a maximum period of six months. The times of day most suitable to take each remedy are indicated in each formula.

Note: For severe symptoms in all metabolic types, predominately use the Vata type menopause remedies, teas and food recommendations, set out below.

WISE EARTH REMEDIES FOR VATA TYPE MENOPAUSE

In addition to the vulnerable times for menopause presented earlier, Vata type may also experience difficulties during the following period of time.

Cyclical Timing for Vata
Challenging Time: 2:00-6:00 (morning and evening)
Challenging Seasons: Rainy season and autumn
Challenging Moon Phase: Late phase of waning cycle

ASHWAGANDHA, SHATAVARI & HONEY PASTE | SERVES TWO

1/2 teaspoon ashwagandha powder
1/2 teaspoon shatavari powder
1/2 teaspoon vidari powder (ancient relative of wild yam)
1/4 teaspoon ginger powder
1 1/2 teaspoons honey

Combine the four powders in a small bowl and add honey. Mix into a paste and take it twice daily, once after breakfast and then again after lunch for three to six months. Chase with half a glass of warm water.

SAFFRON & SHATAVARI MILK | SERVES ONE

1 cup organic milk
10 strands saffron thistles
1/2 teaspoon shatavari powder
1 teaspoon ghee

Bring the milk to a boil. Remove from heat. Stir in the powders and add the ghee. Drink an hour or so before bed. Take for a period of three to six months.

Ayurvedic Herbal Teas for Vata Type Menopause
Some of the most effective herbal teas for menopause are basil, cardamom, cinnamon, cloves, comfrey, chamomile, ginger, hyssop, lavender, lemon balm, lemon verbena, licorice, marshmallow, orange peel, peppermint, rose flower, orange peel, peppermint, raspberry leaves, rosehips, saffron, and spearmint. Use one tablespoon of dried herbs to one and a half cups of water. Use the tea infusion method shown on page 111. Drink two to three cups of tea per day.

WISE EARTH REMEDIES FOR PITTA TYPE MENOPAUSE

Note: For severe symptoms, use the Vata Type Remedies on the previous page in addition to the following. In addition to the vulnerable times for menopause presented earlier, Pitta type may also experience difficulties during the following periods of time.

Cyclical Timing for Pitta
Challenging Time: 10:00-2:00 (morning and evening)
Challenging Seasons: Spring and summer
Challenging Moon Phase: Mid-phase of waning cycle

The menopause remedies for Pitta types that follow are to be taken once daily after breakfast for mild symptoms, and twice daily after breakfast and lunch for severe symptoms. You may use these remedies for a maximum period of six months. The times of day most suitable to take the remedy are indicated in each formula.

SHATAVARI & GOTU KOLA PASTE | SERVES ONE

1/2 teaspoon shatavari powder
1/4 teaspoon gotu kola powder
1/4 teaspoon brahmi powder
1 1/2 teaspoons aloe vera gel

Combine the three powders in a small bowl and add the aloe vera gel. Mix into a paste and take it twice daily—once after breakfast and then again after lunch for a period of three to six months. Chase with half a glass of warm water.

FENNEL, CORIANDER & SHATAVARI MILK | SERVES ONE

1 cup organic milk
1 teaspoon fennel seeds
1/2 teaspoon coriander powder
1/2 teaspoon shatavari powder
1 teaspoon ghee

Bring the milk to a boil. Remove from heat. Stir in the seeds and powders, cover and allow to stand for five minutes. Strain the herbal milk and add the ghee. Drink an hour or so before bed. Take for a period of three to six months.

Note: In addition to the herbal teas for menopause listed on page 218, Pitta type may also use blackberry leaves, coriander, chrysanthemum, elder flowers, hops, jasmine, lotus, passion flower, violet, and wild cherry bark.

WISE EARTH REMEDIES FOR KAPHA TYPE MENOPAUSE

Note: For severe symptoms, use the Vata type menopause remedies presented earlier on page 219, in addition to the ones on the following page.

In addition to the vulnerable times for menopause presented earlier, Kapha types may also experience difficulties during the following period of time.

Cyclical Timing for Kapha
Challenging Time: 6:00-10:00 (morning and evening)
Challenging Seasons: Early winter and late winter
Challenging Moon Phase: Early phase of waning cycle

The menopause remedies for Kapha types which follow are to be taken once daily after breakfast for mild symptoms, and twice daily—after breakfast and lunch—for severe symptoms. You may use these remedies for a maximum period of six months. The times of day most suitable to take the remedy are indicated in each formula.

SHATAVARI & TRIKATU PASTE | SERVES ONE

1/2 teaspoon shatavari powder
1 teaspoon trikatu powder
3/4 teaspoon honey

Combine powders and honey. Mix into a paste and take it twice daily, once after breakfast and then again after lunch for a period of three to six months. Chase with half a glass of warm water.

Note: In addition to the herbal teas for menopause listed on page 218, Kapha types may also use blackberry leaves, chicory, chrysanthemum, dandelion, elder flower, eucalyptus, hawthorn berries, hibiscus, jasmine, nettle, pennyroyal, sage, and sassafras.

Chapter Thirteen

HEALING OSTEOPOROSIS: RECLAIMING STABILITY & JOY

*As aging women, we become much more susceptible to receiving
and sensing the underlying energies of our society. In subtle
and profound ways, we sense the pervasive vibration of cruelty
and savagery, and the horrific crimes against the animals, and
in particular, the maternal energies. These disturbing energies
create a huge void within the heart, a sense of helplessness that is
the single most powerful emotion that impacts our ability to heal,
age naturally, or to heal into death.*

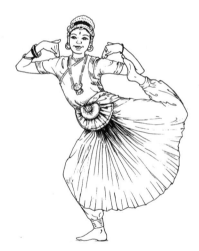

Figure 13.1 Dance of Shakti

More than 100 million women worldwide are affected by osteoporosis. Most women are taken by surprise when their doctors inform them that they have it. In the past, osteoporosis was diagnosed after a bone had been fractured or broken. Only recently has bone density awareness become available to the public. As life-style habits change across the world and more people take to living in urban areas, there is a dramatic decrease in the natural outdoor activities we once performed in the sun-drenched lands and fields. In blatant contrast, we now spend 90 percent of our days in homes, offices, vehicles, and shopping malls.

The present way of life has a devastating effect on the health and well-being of our bones. Osteoporosis literally means porous bones, or bones which are pierced with tiny cavities like that of a petrified sponge. This bone-thinning condition can rapidly accelerate the body's normal bone loss, which makes it a challenging condition to reverse.

As in all physical manifestations of a condition, osteoporosis also has its roots in the emotional and psychological body. In fact, osteoporosis is a condition that literally relates to strength and support in the body and the sense of security in the mind. It occurs more frequently in women who have psychologically not come to terms with the absolute and personal reality of their own aging, death, and dying.

Material security is also important to the aging woman. Most women in the present culture are yet to develop in themselves a solid sense of security along with the ability to support themselves financially, whether or not they may work for a living. Osteoporosis can be prevented or slowed down through healthful nutrition and rejuvenating practices, since the body is constantly recycling its vital tissues, creating new tissues while it discards the old. Besides, doing what we need to do to bolster self-confidence and self-security (emotional and financial) are very important considerations in the cultivation of strong and healthy bones. Simultaneously, building healthy bones and reversing bone loss is the key to treating this condition.

At a physical level, osteoporosis is directly linked to the volley of hormonal imbalance in our bodies reinforced by the habits of modern culture. Women in the rural, dairy-producing villages of Guyana live to ripe old ages without any incident of osteoporosis. On the other hand, 80 percent of their counterparts who have relocated from these villages to various cities in North America and have lived there for more than five years are now experiencing signs of osteoporosis. Women in rural Asia also have a low incident of osteoporosis. The primary reason for this is that their daily lifestyles—although demanding—provide ample outdoor exercise, which allows them to maintain strong bones. Besides, they nourish themselves in a pill-free culture with unprocessed foods that consist largely of grains, vegetables, and fruits. In short, they have preserved their kinship with Mother Nature.

In contrast, we live in a Western culture that is constantly pushing drugs and advertising pills touted to be the "new and improved" versions of potentially damaging chemical based medications. Fosamax, for example, is a synthetic drug that was introduced in 1994 as the miracle bone mass builder. But although Fosamax is capable of building bones, the bone that it builds has nothing to do with the body's bone tissue and its intrinsic memory of development. In other words, the bone crystal that this drug generates is static dead matter that does not respond to the body's natural environment or requirements. Like all synthetic drugs that have nothing to do with the human memory and its inter workings within its vital tissues, these medications are certain to cause harm and additional suffering. In a study published by the *New England Journal of Medicine* in 1996, it is reported that some women who have taken this drug have suffered serious damage to their esophagi.

Not all damaging drugs from the major pharmaceutical companies are derived from synthetic sources; many are extracted from plants and animals, as is Premarin, which is also touted as somewhat of a cure-all for a number of mid-life disorders, including osteoporosis. Although, the mare does carry the cosmic memory for power and virility, her urine derivative, used in this drug, has no relationship to the memory of a woman's reproductive well-being. In fact, Premarin has been proven to generate dark side effects. It also renders the reproductive organs more susceptible to cancer.

However, at a personal level in the heart of all aging women, this affliction has to do with much more than physical nutrition and medicine for aging women. It is yet another subconscious response to the breakdown of maternal humanity that plagues the feminine psyche. How does killing or discarding millions of foals while savagely mistreating their mother mares fare in the Mother Consciousness of it all? This way of savagery is how the pharmaceutical industry stewards its horse farms to produce Premarin. Aging has to do with the natural growth of maturity with the objective of reclaiming the inner peace and the wisdom necessary to complete the earthly journey and prepare for the rising of the soul into the spirit world. Naturally, age does bring a slow and gradual deterioration of vital tissues, including bone and marrow.

MATERNAL SENSITIVITY

As aging women, we become much more susceptible to receiving and sensing the underlying energies of our society. In subtle and profound ways, we sense the pervasive vibration of cruelty and savagery, and the horrific crimes against the animals, and in particular, the maternal energies. These disturbing energies create a huge void within the heart, a sense of helplessness that is the single most powerful emotion that impacts our ability to heal, or age naturally—to heal into death. In other words, our joy is being systematically robbed from us and we need to get it back.

Every minute, someone in the United States suffers a fracture as a result of osteoporosis, with more than 70,000 hip fractures and as many wrist fractures every day. There is hope, though. This Inner Medicine guide does show you how to maintain strong and healthy bones and increase their density through healthful, nourishing, and meditative practices that can increase your maternal strength so that you may avoid harmful drugs or hormones. According to Ayurveda, osteoporosis occurs as a result of malfunction in the deeply imbedded vital tissues of *asthi* and *majja*. Due to the loss of density, the skeletal system becomes brittle, giving way to bone fractures and a compressed spinal column, which descends the posture and causes discomfort and pain in the spine and back. As a deficiency disorder it is dominated by the air humor of Vata; when this condition worsens it can quickly impact other organs and functions of the body. Difficulty breathing, constipation, anxiety, nervousness, forgetfulness, physical and emotional instability, lower back pain, degenerative arthritis, loss of height, insomnia, bladder and kidney weakness, frequent urination, and dental problems are some of the conditions that may accompany osteoporosis. Feelings of loneliness or helplessness may set in as most of our culture's women are not ready for these final phases of life.

Risk factors for osteoporosis are: Vata constitution; age; genetic predisposition; hormonal imbalance; difficult menstruation; poor nutrition; hyperactivity; erratic sleep and eating schedules; and lifestyle habits (smoking, drinking alcohol, heavy use of antibiotics and anti-inflammatory drugs). To test your risk factors, complete the Wise Earth Ayurveda Score Chart for Osteoporosis below. If your score is greater than seven points (total points being 16) you should see your physician and have a baseline test done to determine your bone status. The bone results are expressed as "T-Score" referring to the trabecular, or spongy part of the bone.

WISE EARTH AYURVEDA SCORE CHART FOR OSTEOPOROSIS

SCORE CHART FOR OSTEOPOROSIS

CHECK OSTEOPOROSIS SYMPTOMS YOU ARE EXPERIENCING:

1.	I am genetically predisposed to osteoporosis	❏
2.	My body frame is slight and delicate	❏
3.	I suffer severe back pain	❏
4.	My back is hunched	❏
5.	I suffer bone fractures	❏
6.	I have asthma or difficulty breathing	❏
7.	I am frequently constipated	❏
8.	I am anxious or have anxiety attacks	❏
9.	I am forgetful, or confused	❏
10.	My skin is thin and transparent	❏

11.	My nails are brittle or I have major dental problems	❏
12.	I have frequent urination or incontinence	❏
13.	I feel pain in my joints and muscles	❏
14.	I suffer nocturnal leg cramps	❏
15.	I feel financially insecure	❏
16.	I am insecure about my future and feel helpless	❏

Figure 13.1 Score Chart for Osteoporosis

TOTAL SCORE _____

NOURISHING FOODS & HERBS FOR OSTEOPOROSIS

Wise Earth Ayurveda shows you how to increase your bone density through wholesome nutrition, nature's herbs, healthful activities, and nurturing home therapies without drugs or hormones. Osteoporosis is directly connected many of the same causes arising from an impairment of the Vata dosha that contribute to menopausal disorders. For this reason, you may use the herbal remedies for Vata menopause set out on pages 218-219, in addition to the specific osteoporosis remedies that follow.

Some of Ayurveda's most nourishing herbs for restoring excellent hormonal balance in the body are shatavari, ashwagandha, triphala, dashamula, brahmi, gotu kola, saffron, and amalaki. Common herbs excellent for boosting the hormonal system are nettles, horsetail, Siberian ginseng, black cohosh, black haw, dandelion root, echinacea, hawthorn berries, ginger, milk thistle, motherwort, raspberry leaves, sage, and valerian. You may prepare any of these herbs singly or combined as teas by using one tablespoon of herb to two cups of boiling water. Allow to steep for 10 minutes or so before straining and drinking after meals. You may add a dab of honey to your tea, if so desired.

To counter osteoporosis eat foods that are high in calcium (organic dairy foods, leafy vegetables, green vegetables, and beans), Vitamin D, (organic dairy foods), and trace minerals manganese (found plentifully in pineapples, oatmeal, cereals, and nuts) and boron (found in fruits, soya beans, nuts, and honey).

For the purpose of clarity, I will refer to the component parts (vitamins, minerals, and so on) of ingredients and foods for osteoporosis. However, I do recommend that you use the whole food rather than supplements. Avoid refined foods, iodized salt and refined sugar, excessive caffeine, alcohol, antibiotics, and anti-inflammatory drugs.

In detail I recommend:

- Dairy foods (organic cow's milk, yogurt, butter, and ghee)
- Whole grains (brown rice, millet, kamut, barley, spelt, and wheat)
- Cereals (especially oatmeal)
- Leafy greens (collards, kales, lettuces, Swiss chard, bok choy, spinach, beets, and greens
- Brassiac (broccoli, brussel sprouts, and cabbage)
- Beans (urad, black, gram, soya, mung, aduki, lima, pinto, red, and chickpeas)
- Fruits (pineapples, oranges, apples, pears, peaches, grapes, raisins, and dates)
- Nuts (almonds, peanuts, and hazelnuts)
- Seaweeds (agar-agar, hiziki, arame, dulse, kombu, nori, and kelp)
- Honey

OSTEOPOROSIS REMEDIES FOR ALL METABOLIC TYPES

Cyclical Timing for Osteoporosis
Challenging Time: 2:00-6:00 (morning and evening)
Challenging Seasons: Early fall (rainy season) and autumn
Challenging Moon Phase: Late phase of waning

GINSENG, BRAHMI & SHATAVARI PASTE | SERVES TWO

1/2 teaspoon ginseng powder
1/2 teaspoon shatavari powder
1/2 teaspoon brahmi powder
1/4 teaspoon ginger powder
1 1/2 teaspoons honey

Combine the four powders in a small bowl and add honey. Mix into a paste and take it twice daily, once after lunch and then again after dinner for three to six months, especially during the rainy season and autumn months. Chase with half a glass of warm water.

DASHAMULA, TRIPHALA & SHATAVARI SOFT PILL | SERVES TWO

1/2 teaspoon dashamula powder
1/2 teaspoon triphala powder
1/2 teaspoon shatavari powder
1 teaspoon ghee

Combine the three powders in a small bowl and add the ghee. Roll into two soft pills and take one after lunch and then again after dinner for three to six months, especially during the rainy season and autumn months. Chase with half a glass of warm water.

SIMPLE REMEDIES FOR WOMEN'S OJAS, HEART & SPIRIT

The following women's tonics may be used frequently with the lunar sadhana home therapies for women (set out in Chapter Fourteen) intended to help restore excellent health—maintain good reproductive health, hormonal balance, and a healthy heart follow. The Heart Tonic may be taken to maintain good heart health and as a restorative tonic after a hysterectomy, miscarriage, or abortion (take the Heart Tonic once daily for two to three months following the incident).

HEART TONIC | SERVES ONE

1 1/2 glasses of warm water or cow's milk
1/2 teaspoon turmeric powder
1/2 teaspoon Arjuna powder

Mix the powders in warm water or milk and drink after breakfast for a period of one to three months.

The Ojas Tonic which follows is a classical Ayurveda remedy that helps to remove toxicity from the body, restore the downward-flowing air of apana vayu necessary to keep the body's evacuation in order, and maintain good health of the joints, muscles, and bones.

OJAS TONIC | SERVES ONE

1 1/2 glasses of warm water
1/2 teaspoon triphala powder
1 teaspoon aloe vera gel

Mix the powders in warm water or milk and drink one hour or so before bed for a period of three to six months.

The following tonic is another classical Ayurvedic remedy that helps to strengthen Shakti prana that circulates the womb and restores hormonal balance to the body.

It is also an excellent tonic for removing mental fuzziness. Another Ayurvedic oil, brahmi oil, can be put on the forehead morning and before bed for mental clarity.

SHAKTI PRANA TONIC | SERVES ONE

1 1/2 glasses of warm water or organic cow's milk
1/2 teaspoon shatavari powder
1/2 teaspoon ashwagandha powder
1/2 teaspoon brahmi powder
1 teaspoon honey

Mix the powders in warm water or milk, add the honey and drink after dinner for a period of three to six months.

The following Virility Tonic is an excellent Ayurvedic remedy that helps to strengthen and restore hormonal balance to the body. It is also a classical Ayurvedic aphrodisiac and fertility tonic for women. Besides, Wise Earth Ayurveda shows you how to balance your hormones during menopause with grains, vegetables, herbs, and spices in addition to the wondrous Pancha Karma home therapies.

VIRILITY TONIC | SERVES ONE

1 1/2 glasses of organic cow's milk
1/2 teaspoon shatavari powder
1/2 teaspoon vidari powder
1/2 teaspoon wild yam powder
10 strands of saffron thistles
1 teaspoon ghee

Mix the powders and saffron in warm milk, add the ghee and drink after breakfast for a period of three to six months.

HEALING SALVE FOR VAGINAL ATROPHY | ONE APPLICATION

1 tablespoon sesame oil
10 strands saffron thistles
a small ball of cotton gauze

Using a small double-boiler, warm the sesame oil for a few minutes and add the saffron to it. Remove from heat and allow it to sit for two minutes. Dip the cotton gauze in the saffron oil and gentle insert it into the vaginal passage. Retain for one hour or so while resting. You may use the remaining oil to rub on your forehead and belly. You may also use the Ojas Tonic internally to improve the condition of vaginal atrophy. Take as directed.

REGENERATING NEW HORMONES: RECLAIMING JOY

Ultimately, we in our mid-years must relearn how to increase our ojas and cultivate our joy—take to lifestyle habits that will increase inner security and therefore our bone density. Every day, I recommend taking a 20-minute walk in the park on level ground except in cold or inclement weather. Bask in the sunlight for a half hour each day and take in ample light and prana. During the spring and summer, you may increase your outdoor hobbies such as gardening, drawing, or sketching in nature. You may join in community group activities for crones and engage in gentle exercise such as yoga, tai chi, dancing, or practicing light weight-bearing exercises. Avoid strenuous physical activities, and walking on uneven, wet, and slippery grounds. Wear good quality walking shoes or sneakers. Do not hesitate to ask for the company and the arm of your husband, friend, or your grown children if you feel distracted or ungrounded while walking.

Since a primary cause of osteoporosis is hormonal imbalance, it is vital to maintain a state of hormonal wellness, especially after menopause. In making a commitment to living healthfully, you will continually replenish your supply of ojas. Like the honeybee, you have the prowess to sublimate your ojas power so that you can transform your hormones into youthful ones. In other words, you do not need a prescription for the troublesome Hormone Replacement Therapy (HRT) simply because you have entered your menopausal years. As Rebecca did, you too may be able to avoid taking HRT. Here is her story in her own words:

I began menopause four years ago with an outpouring of heavy bleeding and extreme pain in my abdomen and uterus. I was diagnosed with adenomyosis, a condition also called 'internal endometriosis' wherein the uterus wall was expanded, thickened, and swollen with blood. My physician suggested an immediate hysterectomy to stop the bleeding. I did not want to have surgery, but my physician insisted that I take HRT to boost my hormones and out of desperation, I agreed. Within a month, I began to pile on weight and was irritable all the time. My cravings for sweets and junk foods grew, while my sleep patterns were riddled with fiery and violent nightmares. I knew I had to get off HRT but was afraid to without alternative treatment.

I had read about the Wise Earth School in Yoga Journal, and decided to go there to study with and meet Mother Maya. During my initial evaluation, Mother advised me that my constitution, which is predominantly Pitta, had been out of kilter for some time and therefore caused my painful experience with menorrhagia, which I had for many years prior to the start of menopause. She also informed me that I was coming into my Vata dominant time, which starts around age 52. She recommended that I do some of the Pancha Karma recuperative therapies for women when I returned home. I also learned the vital knowledge of healthy and wholesome nutrition along with the Shakti Mudra and Bhramari Breath Meditation practice that served to relieve my discomfort instantly.

After leaving the school I cleared out the excess storage from my home and revamped my entire kitchen. There I prepared nourishing meals from whole grains, organic vegetables, and beans, and prepared my Inner Medicine remedies with my own hands. The more I used my mortar and pestle, the stronger my heart became. I love the smells of the spices and herbs as I prepare them. Mother has opened a whole new healing vista of tantalizing aromas, sights, and sounds that make me want to sing. I devoted 30 minutes a day to my mudra and meditation practices and took brisk walks in the early morning sun. Within a few weeks of beginning the Wise Earth Ayurveda program, I was beginning to shed the weight I had gained on HRT. Finally, I was able to sleep and feel vibrant and energized after so many years of suffering. After three months of staying on the program, I was able to completely wean myself off HRT.

Because of the wisdom I learned at Wise Earth I have been able to uncover the roots of my own ancestral pain and shed light on my menstrual challenges. Now, I am finally free from the burden of the rage, bleeding, and pain I have carried for so long. I understand that it was not necessary for me to take HRT, or any other medical drugs for that matter. By learning how to nourish my inner health I am now at peace with myself. I look forward to reclaiming this rich time of my maturing life.

You too can reclaim your sense of joy and walk your journey on the earth with vibrancy. Just remember that your female body possesses a self-organizing intelligence that can adequately compensate for the diminishing hormones in your mid-years. Whereas the estrogen and progesterone levels in the body decrease after menopause, other organs are capable of producing hormones that may recompense the reduction of these hormones, keeping your bones in stable condition. When in good order, pineal glands, adrenal glands, breasts, liver, and body fat are capable of producing hormones to compensate for the natural reduction of estrogen and progesterone after menopause.

The adrenal glands, in particular, play a significant role in how we respond to everyday situations and assimilate our perceptions and experiences. The adrenals, which sit directly above your kidneys, are two thumb-size glands that act as the body's "shock absorbers." Stress is one of the major suppressors of healthy adrenal function. Anger, anxiety, worry, nervousness, fear, depression, insomnia, exhaustion, chronic pain, long-term illness, and malnutrition are the dominant factors that may contribute to adrenal dysfunction. Major hormones produced by the adrenals are adrenaline, cortisol, and DHEA, (dehydroepioandosterone). DHEA is an androgenic hormone produced in the adrenal cortex, gonads, and brain. Low levels of DHEA in the blood may be an indicator for various degenerative diseases. The correct balance of cortisol and DHEA in the body is necessary for maintaining good health. Studies have shown that when there are sufficient levels of DHEA in the body, this hormone helps to increase the serum levels of both estrogen and testosterone (the hormones associated with sexual impulses). It has also been proven that DHEA aids in stimulating bone formation and calcium absorption, thus acting as a natural prevention for osteoporosis. DHEA also produces a by-product that can stick to estrogen receptors and thereby hinder bone re-absorption. When in a state of balance with cortisol, both hormones act as a constructive buffer for the body's autoimmune system by protecting ojas while strengthening its resistance to harmful pathogens, bacteria, allergies, and viruses. DHEA is also known to lower bad cholesterol and improve cardiovascular function.

Cortisol—the hormone which is organically released in the body when a person is under stress—is also produced by the adrenal gland. Studies have shown that people living with chronic stress tend to have a dramatic increase of cortisol hormone in their systems. As a result, calcium absorption in the body is decreased and bone formation can be suppressed. Depression is also linked to the increase of cortisol, which—when in a state of equanimity in the body—plays an active role in its energy preservation and emotional wellness. This hormone also controls the production of glycogen in the liver for storage of glucose, a necessary fuel for maintaining physical energy and emotional stability. Cortisol helps the liver to convert amino acids into glucose and fat cells into fatty acids in the blood that may be used as fuel for producing energy.

Hormonal deficiency or imbalance is directly connected to the existence of ama in the body and the impairment of the bodily doshas, in particular, Vata. Pitta and Kapha doshas also have an active role in hormonal imbalance, and therefore in osteoporosis: Pitta, because our mid-life phase is generally ruled by its energies, and Kapha because it controls the early growth phase of life when the fortification of ojas, responsible for our excellent hormonal health, starts to take shape.

If you are symptomatic, or you are already on HRT and seek a non-hurtful, natural way of treating osteoporosis, you will find a plethora of wonderful herbal remedies and practices in this book that will help you to achieve much more than balanced hormones. If you do not feel comfortable weaning yourself off HRT and simply want to get rid of the horrible side effects from it, you may use these Inner Medicine recommendations, knowing that you will be cultivating a deeper level of awareness within to help remove the factors that cause your disease.

In all cases, to bolster your hormonal system and bring it in a state of balance, you may use the same Wise Earth Ayurvedic nutritional and herbal remedies for PMS in accord with your constitutional type. These recommendations are set out in Chapter Seven. You may also use the herbal recommendations for restoring excellent hormonal balance in the body mentioned earlier in this chapter under the heading *Nourishing Foods & Herbs for Osteoporosis*. I also recommend strengthening your potent "Queen Bee" memory through *The Practice: Bhramari Breath & Sound Meditation* presented on pages 55-56.

Part Six

LUNAR SADHANAS: WOMEN'S SHAKTI NOURISHING PRACTICES

Chapter Fourteen

WOMEN'S REVITALIZING MOON SADHANA PRACTICES

Sharanagata dinarta paritrana parayane
Sarvasyarti hare Devi Narayani namo'stu te.

Salutations are to you, O Narayani—you who are intent
on saving the distressed and the dejected who take refuge
under you. O you, Devi, who remove the sufferings of all!

(Narayani is Goddess Lakshmi, consort of Lord Vishnu)

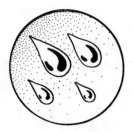

Healing is a sacred thing. It is a goddess-like quality.

FULL MOON CYCLE: WOMEN'S REVITALIZING PRACTICES

The moon is the most intoxicating symbol of a woman's innate rhythms. The native women of yore faithfully observed the lunar rhythms to ensure their womanly wellness, recognizing that the rhythms of the womb emulate the lunar cycles, which are sourced in the Mother Consciousness. Every month the moon courses through 16 phases in its waxing cycle from new moon to full moon, each phase bearing significant impact on your Shakti energy. Your health and well-being are invariably linked to the turn of the lunar wheel since the lunation cycle sets the cadence for your life force, biorhythms, and desires. The rising moon stands for the Goddess Lalita's resurrection—symbolic of the woman's menstrual cycle. When you live by the lunar wheel, her waning cycle relieves you of emotional, physical, and psychic excesses. As the waxing cycle matures, you may replenish your immunity, sensuality, and strength as the moon swells into roundness. Recharge your Shakti energy from the regenerative power source of the lunar cycles by learning to live in harmony with the movement of Goddess Lalita and her lunar deities. In so doing, you feel perennially revived in body, mind, and spirit.

LUXURIOUS SADHANAS IN THE WAXING MOON CYCLE: SEASON OF NURTURANCE

New Moon to Full Moon

Vedic women celebrated the awesome splendor of the full moon as a time of fullness and completion, purnima. The full moon affords limitless opportunities for women to beautify themselves, exercise their sensuality, and reap abundance. As noted earlier, the beginning period of the full moon is the natural cycle for ovulation and the most potent time of nurturance for women. The rituals and ceremonies performed during the waxing cycle help to nourish the spirit, strengthen the Shakti energy, and revitalize the memory of abundance.

Shukla paksha, the waxing phase, holds tremendous power to help you revive your Shakti energy. This is when the lunar cycle moves from new moon to full as the nityas, lunar deities, grow into their full healing power. The first five days of the waxing cycle that start with the new moon mark the optimum time for a woman's rebirth and renewal. During this time, women naturally seek their rebirth by releasing their profound life-making material back to the earth. As you have seen, the new moon stands for the Great Mother's act of resurrection—a metaphor for the woman's menstrual cycle. As the waxing moon gathers strength, it brings with it the energy of potency, regeneration, and rejuvenation. The full moon is therefore a crucial time for celebration. Even today, devout Hindus celebrate the significant moon cycles with the appropriate prayers, worship, fasting, feasting, vows, and offerings to the lunar deities.

Blessed with increasing moonlight and the powerful energy thrust from Goddess Lalita and her divine emanations, a woman's ojas naturally increases during the waxing phase. Her sexual vitality is once more replenished since the beginning period of the full moon is the natural cycle for ovulation and the most potent time of nurturance for women. At the full moon when ovulation is at its natural peak, neuropeptides FSH (follicle stimulating hormone) and LH (luteinizing hormone) cause the rise of estrogen levels in the body. The full moon cycle is the natural time for you to enjoy and celebrate your womanhood. Our emotional need to withdraw from the world of activity and retreat into a time of introspection happens almost immediately after the full moon.

As the moon becomes full, you receive the cooling, ojas-producing essence of the moon, which inspires ovulation and heightens your sexual impulses and vitality.

The full moon is a natural time for having sex and incorporating sadhana practices for nurturance and beautification into your daily life. Oil massage, aromatherapy, warm baths, moonlight dips in water, and the use of healing mantras and gems are the perfect practice during this time. This is also a time for sharing healthful ojas-producing foods with your beloved partner. Meals that build ojas are wholesome, organic, vegetarian foods that promote harmony in the body, mind, and spirit, foods such as: organic milk, ghee, pancakes, crepes, homemade breads, soups, casseroles, risotto, pilafs, polenta, a variety of whole and cracked grains (bulgur, couscous, brown rice, basmati rice, arborio rice), beans, pasta, fresh vegetables, salads, and desserts, such as egg-free custards, puddings, fruit pies and tarts, and strudels. Wholesome foods reinforce your spirit of abundance and celebration.

As noted earlier, the doshas' natural states are also affected by the moon phases, as well as your cycles of menstruation and ovulation. The Vata dosha is dominant during menstruation, Pitta during ovulation, and Kapha during the time after menstruation. Therefore sadhanas presented in this chapter are naturally designed to nourish and comfort the appropriate dosha during each lunar phase.

MAGICAL WATERS OF THE FULL MOON

Water is much more than a body cleanser or thirst quencher—it stands for stability, solidity, firmness, flexibility, adaptability, and movement that emulates the fluency of the mind, heart, and womb. In Vedic tradition, we bless the water every day in puja by offering the first drink to the deities. Symbolic bathing of the deity's hands and feet is done by holding a spoonful of pure water before the deity while visualizing the act of bathing their hands and feet. Water is also offered to symbolically quench the deity's thirst, before it is bathed. We may bathe the naked image of the deity, snanam, or perform a symbolic bath by using a fresh flower to sprinkle water on it. Before the blessing for the home and family in daily rituals starts, we observe *achamanam*, water sipping, by taking a spoonful of water with the left hand and pouring it to rinse the right hand, and again to sip the water.

Water is the first form of nourishment provided by the Mother to sustain the life force of the earth. Water is a conductor of awareness; it takes on different forms to help us heal. It has the ability to respond to the highest or lowest of intentions. When we are clear in our intention to nourish, nurture, and heal, water becomes the goddess instrument of lightness and can collect our disturbed emotions and cleanse them through its fluid vibrations—bathing then becomes a spiritual act. Indeed, this is why millions of Hindus bathe in the holy rivers of India every morning. Make your next bath an act of prayer—a fluid stroke of meditation—and in return, you will be surprised to see how quickly the goddess responds with abundant visions and blessings for healing.

THE PRACTICE: MOON BASKING SADHANA

Timing: Second evening of the full moon
Contra-indications: Menstruation; bleeding; or during mourning
Body Type: All types
Ideal Time: Late evening

On the next full moon, begin your auspicious celebration of your inner goddess by gathering your female friends and family and observing this exquisite Moon Basking Sadhana.

In Vedic practice, women convene on the second or third evening of every full moon to bathe, walk in the moonlight, or to sit together in meditation beneath the full moon. In the villages of India, women today still gather during this auspicious time to anoint one another with fragrant oils and sing songs to the Great Mother. I regularly invite women disciples at Wise Earth to observe the ritual of "moon basking" with me.

We sit around the small fresh water pond in which the full moon clearly reflects its brilliant aura. Sometimes, we congregate on one of the large outdoor decks where I set up 108 small ceramic bowls of water in a circle to collect Mother's Light. The sadhakas sit in silence and bask in the beauty of the moon mirrored 108 times in the bowls of water.

THE PRACTICE: FULL MOON BATH

Timing: On the full moon and for three days thereafter
Contra-indications: Menstruation; bleeding; or during mourning
Body Type: All types
Ideal Time: Early morning; early evening

APPROPRIATE HERBS & ESSENTIAL OILS:

Use the recommended soothing dried herbs and essential oils suitable for the Full Moon Bath—be sure to use organic quality herbs.

FULL MOON HERBS & ESSENTIAL OILS:

Rose petals, elderflowers, hops, lavender, lemon balm, lemon verbena, raspberry leaves, violet flowers, and passion flower. If available, you may use fresh seasonal herbs in your bath. If using loose herbs without a bolus, be certain to use a drain strainer to collect the roughage at the end of your bath. This may be placed on the earth or in your compost. Do not throw these herbs into the garbage.

SAMPLE RECIPE | ONE APPLICATION

1 cotton handkerchief
1/2 palmful of rose petals (organic)
1/2 palmful of raspberry leaves
12 drops of lavender essential oil

FULL MOON BATH INSTRUCTIONS:

First, prepare your herbal bolus by taking a palmful of herbs sprinkled with 12 drops of essential oil and wrapping it into a bolus in a cotton handkerchief. To make your herbal ball, tie two of the opposite ends of the cloth and then overlap the other two ends into a firm knot incorporating all four ends into a secure knot on the top of the bolus. Fill your bath with warm water and place the bolus of herbs directly in the bath. Allow it to sit for five minutes or so in the water before offering your prayers and entering the bath.

After the tub is filled and you have placed the sacred herbs and ingredients into the water, make an offering to the goddess (before you enter the bath). While facing east or north scoop a palmful of water with your right hand, and ritually wash both of your hands with the water, letting the water run off your hands and fall back into the tub. Take another palmful of water in your right hand and this time offer it to the goddess by slowly opening your hand and allowing the water to drip from the tips of your fingers back into the tub. Recite the following mantra three times as you pour the water from your hand:

Om apah upa sprishya
Unto You, I sprinkle water

Do not perform this *sankalpa,* sacred intention, if you know you'll be interrupted by your phone or your children. Once this offering has been completed, take your bath. It is important that you complete the bath without interruption once you have offered the water sacrament to the goddess. The act of preparing your tub, ritual washing of the hands, offering of water to the goddess, and finishing your bath must be done in one fluid and complete act for your offering to be received by the goddess and for her water blessings to be returned to you.

In recognizing the sanctity of water, you're bathing not only the physical body, but the mind, spirit, and ancestors as well. Strengthening your biological water element (Kapha humor) helps you to build stability and vitality of body, mind, and spirit.

VARUNA MUDRA: HAND GESTURE OF THE WATER GOD

Varuna Mudra is a potently wonderful practice during waxing moon time to increase your internal power of the water element. Varuna is the God of Water, and using this water nourishing mudra will evoke abundance, prosperity, richness, and joy. As noted earlier, mudras are powerful hand postures that garner specific energies within the body, mind, and spirit. Mudras draw on a subtle field of prana power within the body to strengthen the breath force. During mudra practice, you'll discover that the breath easily becomes gentler and softer as it energizes the system.

Varuna Mudra practice re-energizes the body and is especially excellent for relieving colds, sinusitis, mucous congestion, lethargy, hypertension, and stress relating to financial concerns and responsibilities. Seasonal practice of Varuna Mudra helps lighten emotional burdens, and builds the confidence and self-esteem necessary for letting go of the helm and delegating the workload and responsibilities to others who may be willing to pitch in and share your everyday load. This is a particularly excellent practice for Kapha types.

THE PRACTICE: VARUNA MUDRA

Timing: On the full moon; especially during spring season
Contra-indications: Menstruation; bleeding; or during mourning
Body Type: All types
Ideal Time: 6:00-10:00 (morning or evening)

VARUNA MUDRA INSTRUCTIONS:
- Be comfortably seated facing west since Varuna resides in that direction.
- Hold up your right hand at chest level with you palm facing you, and bend the "pinky" finger to touch the ball of the thumb.
- Place your right thumb securely over the bent finger.
- Place the back of your upheld hand against the palm of your left hand placed horizontally to embrace the right hand.
- Wrap your fingers around the right hand with the left thumb pressing over the right.

ABHYANGA: WISE EARTH AYURVEDA MASSAGE & OELATION THERAPY

Many people think Abhyanga is merely a massage, but it is much more. It is India's ancient practice to promote vitality, strength, and flexibility, while increasing the flow of prana in the body and mind. In Abhyanga, specific medicinal oils, decoctions, and infusions may be used to stimulate the vital tissues and positively influence mental and emotional states of mind. Indeed, Ayurveda's practice of Marma therapy was first introduced in India centuries before its counterpart, acupuncture, became popular in Asia. There are scores of Abhyanga therapies used in Ayurveda for the treatment of specific conditions, all of which are guided by specific cycles —lunar, solar, daily, seasonal. These therapies, many of which can be practiced at home, may be used to influence and correct dosha disorders, especially of a Vata kind; to cure orthopedic injuries; promote regeneration of tissues and organs; to relieve swollen tissues; and fine tune internal workings of the body.

Massage is one of the most effective therapies used to strengthen immunological function, relieve pain, reduce stress, improve the skin, strengthen the lungs, intestines and bones, improve digestion, and improve the body's circulation. Abhyanga increases bodily heat and improves circulation, causing the body to flush out its waste products more efficiently. It improves memory, concentration, and intelligence and produces youthfulness. Especially excellent for children, the stressed, aged, and infirm—these therapies benefit everyone.

ABHYANGA HERBAL OIL PREPARATION

You begin by preparing your oils. Oils are used in both Abhyanga massage and Snehana therapies to soothe and stabilize the body; they also act as carriers for nourishing herbs and substances added to them. Oils regulate the doshas of the female genital organs and provide the body with heat. They tone the skin and bodily tissues. Oils usually alleviate Vata, stabilize Pitta, and aggravate Kapha disorders. Kapha types may use less unctuous rubs or oils in their decoctions.

A wide variety of Ayurvedic oils and decoctions are used for massaging each part of the human body in accord with their metabolic type, or condition. Sesame oil is used as the dominant base for most rubbing oils, due to its warm, nutritive, and penetrating qualities. This oil is most beneficial to Vata types. Pitta types may use coconut oil, which is unctuous and cooling in nature.

Note: Store your Abhyanga oils away from sunlight or moonlight. Herbal infusions and decoctions have a very short shelf life and should be used no later than 24 hours after preparing them. These preparations should not be refrigerated.

INGREDIENTS:

1 gallon water (4 cups water for each formula)
Sesame oil (1 cup for each formula)

1/4 cup herb (for each oil formula)
Herbs: bala powder, triphala powder, dried rose buds, dried lotus root

UTENSILS AND EQUIPMENT:

1 large stainless-steel pot with cover
2 stainless-steel bowls
2 metal strainers (4 to 5 inches in diameter)
Clear glass jugs (for herbal oils)

Bring four cups of water to a boil in a stainless-steel pot. Add one cup of oil and one quarter cup of the herb of your choice from the formulas provided. Cover and simmer on low heat for four to six hours, or until all the water has evaporated. Allow herbal oil to cool, and then pour through a tea strainer into a glass jar. Cover and store in a cool place.

HERBAL OIL INFUSION (FOR ALL TYPES)

1 cup sesame oil
1/4 cup herb

Bring oil to boil in a stainless-steel pot. Add herbs and remove from heat. Cover and let steep for four to six hours. Pour oil through a tea strainer into a clean glass jar. Cover and store in a cool place.

BALA OIL DECOCTION (FOR ALL TYPES)

4 cups water
1 cup sesame oil
1/4 cup bala powder

Pour oil and water into a large stainless-steel saucepan and bring to a boil over medium heat. Mix in the powder, then cover and simmer over low heat for approximately four hours, or until all the water has evaporated. Let cool and strain through a fine sieve into the bucket. When the oil has cooled to room temperature, pour it into a clean glass jar, and place it in a cool place.

TRIPHALA OIL DECOCTION (FOR ALL TYPES)

4 cups water
1 cup sesame oil
1/4 cup triphala powder

Pour the oil and water into a large stainless-steel saucepan and bring to a boil over medium heat. Mix in the powder, then cover and simmer over low heat for approximately four hours, or until all the water has evaporated. Let cool and strain through a fine sieve into the bucket. When the oil has cooled to room temperature, pour it into a clean glass jar, and place it in a cool place.

ROSE OIL INFUSION (FOR ALL TYPES)

1 cup sesame oil
1/4 cup dried rose flower (organic)

Pour oil into a large stainless-steel saucepan and bring to a boil over low heat. Remove from heat. Add the rose flower, cover and let steep for four to six hours. Strain and use. (Rose sediment may be used in your bath water.)

LOTUS OIL DECOCTION (FOR ALL TYPES)

4 cups water
1 cup sesame oil
1/2 cup dried lotus root

Pour the oil and water into a large stainless-steel saucepan and bring to a boil over low heat. Mix in the roots, then cover and simmer over low heat for approximately two hours, or until all the water has evaporated. Let cool and strain through a fine sieve into the bucket. When the oil has cooled to room temperature, you may pour it into a clean glass jar, and place it in a cool place.

WISE EARTH AYURVEDA'S HEAD THERAPY

There are also many Abhyanga therapies for the head, since it is considered to be the most important part of the human body. The head contains four of the five sensory organs of the body and seven of the nine bodily apertures through which we interact with the external universe. On the very top of the head is the sacred shrine called the *sahasrara* chakra, through which the soul is said to enter the body at birth and leave after death.

Two of Ayurveda's most nurturing treatments for the head are:
- Pichu, an Ayurvedic treatment in which a piece of cotton cloth is soaked in a medicated oil and placed on the forehead.
- Shira Abhyanga, a therapeutic treatment in which oil is poured over and massaged into vital points on the head.

These therapies are effective for conditions such as heart disease, insomnia, mental disorders, exhaustion, migraines, weakness of bodily joints, facial paralysis, blood disorders, eye diseases, baldness and premature graying, dandruff, scalp sores, inflammation of the head, and female reproductive disorders. In fact, almost all diseases may be helped by these therapies. You will be able to self-administer most of the therapies which follow. However, massaging the full body, hip, and/or back will obviously require an able partner, or friend.

Beginning with Pichu, a profoundly effective oelation treatment that you may administer at your leisure at home, the specific healing therapies presented below require little time and preparation and will be of tremendous benefit to your overall health when done on a regular basis.

THE PRACTICE: PICHU—OELATION OF THE FOREHEAD

Pichu is an Ayurvedic treatment whereby a piece of cotton cloth, which has been soaked in a specific oil, is placed on the forehead for a period of time so the oil's healing properties can ease the symptoms of particular maladies. Pichu is a powerful Snehana, lubricating and loving therapy, and may be performed frequently at home to help maintain mental calm, emotional equanimity, and to help balance the doshas. It is an especially excellent therapy for women and children. For serious conditions, this treatment may be applied twice daily for approximately 14 days from the time of the new moon to the full moon.

Timing: Waxing moon phase
Contra-indications: Menstruation; bleeding; or during mourning
Body Type: All types
Ideal Time: Morning; early evening
Conditions and Appropriate Oils: Use the recommended oils below for the indicated conditions.

LOTUS OIL:
stiffness in eye muscles
dryness or sores on scalp
inflammation of head or face

ROSE OIL:
headaches
hair loss
pain in the eyes
poor vision

mental fatigue
nose bleeds

TRIPHALA OIL:
insomnia
physical injury
constipation
depression
hemorrhoids

UTENSILS AND EQUIPMENT:
Pottery bowl, 6-inch diameter by 3 inches deep, one-quarter filled with oil
Clean cotton cloth, 12 inches square
Clean cotton hand towel

Pour 1/4 cup of the appropriate oil into a small stainless-steel saucepan and warm over low heat for five minutes. Then pour into the pottery bowl. Fold the clean piece of cotton cloth so that it forms three even layers. Holding the cloth at either end, dip the middle eight inches of cloth into the warm oil, soaking it thoroughly. Let the ends hang over the sides of the bowl so that they remain dry. Place the bowl so that it is within easy reach during your treatment.

PICHU INSTRUCTIONS:
- Wash the hair a few hours before you administer Pichu.
- Release all stressful thoughts and details from the mind.
- Assemble the oil, cloth, and a clean hand towel onto a clean towel spread on the floor.
- Place a clean mat along side your treatment items.
- Soak the cloth in the oil and lie down before placing the cloth on your forehead, from ear to ear.
- While lying down, press down gently on the cloth using both hands.
- Use the hand towel to wipe away any excess oil from your hands and face.
- Close your eyes and rest quietly for 30 minutes.
- Rise very slowly and remove the cloth from your forehead.
- Using the hand towel, gently pat away any excess oil from the forehead.
- Clean oil utensil and wash the oil-soaked cloth thoroughly by hand.
- Move slowly for the next few hours and maintain a peaceful attitude for the rest of the day.
- Always keep the spirit of quietude with and around you.

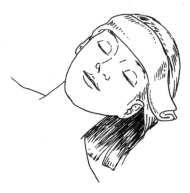

Figure 14.1 Pichu

THE PRACTICE: SHIRA ABHYANGA—HEAD MASSAGE

Timing: Waxing moon phase
Contra-indications: Menstruation; bleeding; or during mourning
Body Type: All types
Ideal Time: Morning; early evening

- Prepare a bowl of warm sesame oil and place it along with two hand towels on a table next to you.
- Sit in an upright chair, and spread one towel on your lap, and the other around your neck to catch oil spillage.
- Begin your Shira Abhyanga by following the step-by-step instructions below.

OILING THE THREE MAJOR POINTS OF THE HEAD: FIRST PHASE

Brahma Randhra: soft spot of the head
- Before commencing the massage, wash your hands thoroughly. Then, shake them and gently turn your wrists in a circular clockwise motion. Accelerate the rhythm of your hand movements until you feel a tingling sensation in your fingers. This activity allows your healing energy to flow freely.
- Sit in an upright chair.
- Part the hair in the center and pour approximately two tablespoons of oil on the Brahma randhra spot.
- Begin by massaging the oil into both sides of the head, above the ears.
- Spread the oil over the front portion of the head, while firmly rubbing the head with both hands.

Shikha: the crest of the head (the second most important point of the head)
- Bend the head forward, so that the chin touches the chest.
- Pour approximately two tablespoons of oil directly on the center of the crest. This

point is located about eight finger widths from the medulla oblongata, the place where the skull meets the neck.

- Spread the oil over the back of the head, and firmly rub the head with both hands.

Medulla Oblongata: base stem of the brain

At the center back of the head, where the skull meets the neck, is the third most important point of the head. Called the medulla oblongata, this point is pivotal to the way the brain communicates with the entire nervous system.

- Gently bend the head completely forward and pour approximately one tablespoon of oil directly on the medulla oblongata point.
- Using both hands, rub the base of the skull and the back of the neck firmly, to excite the fine capillaries of circulation and the nervous system.
- Finally, press both thumbs on each side of the medulla oblongata point and hold for a minute or so.

HEAD MASSAGE: SECOND PHASE

- Bend your head forward and downward so that the chin touches the chest.
- Bring both hands together in prayer pose.
- Place your clasped hands on the crest of the head.
- Moving your hands in a scissor-like motion, begin to decisively pound the center line of the head, moving both hands forward while pounding the head to the top of the forehead; then move the hands back again, remaining all the while on the center line of the head as you pound towards the back of the head.
- After pounding the center line of the head, take a small amount of hair, rooted directly over the three auspicious points of the head (Brahma randhra, shikha, and medulla oblongata) and twist it.
- Gently pull each one of the hair twists, beginning with the Brahma randhra point and ending with the medulla oblongata point.

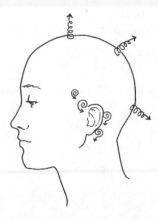

Figure 14.2 Shira Abhyanga-Head Massage

THE PRACTICE: PADABHYANGA—FOOT MASSAGE

Padabhyanga foot massage stimulates every organ of the body, and in particular a woman's womb and reproductive organs. It increases ojas and promotes a feeling of deep relaxation, inducing a feeling of total wellness in the body's entire system. Massaging the feet, considered together to be one of five "organs of action" in Ayurveda, relieves insomnia, nervousness, and dryness or numbness in that area. It also energizes the womb, reproductive organs, belly, pelvis, and colon, as well as improves overall circulation and fertility. From the Wise Earth Ayurveda perspective, the best way to heal the impairments of the womb is to lovingly care for the feet. Feet are considered the wings of the womb.

Timing: Waxing moon phase
Contra-indications: Menstruation; bleeding; or during mourning
Body Type: All types
Ideal Time: Morning; early evening

FOOT MASSAGE INSTRUCTIONS:

- Sit upright on the floor in a comfortable position so you can easily reach your feet.
- Set up a placemat within reach with a small bowl of warm sesame oil and hand towel on it.
- Bring your right foot to rest on your left knee or thigh so you can easily reach your right foot.
- Apply one tablespoon of oil to the sides of the right foot and rub thoroughly, massaging in a clockwise circular movement.
- Place your right heel in your left palm and press firmly into the ankle joint with your thumb and fingers.
- Press the tips of the toes and then pull each toe firmly.
- Apply oil to the toenails and rub them firmly.
- Use both hands to massage the "neck" of each toe.
- Stretch your right leg out and beginning eight inches above the ankles, bend forward and firmly massage the leg with both hands, gradually making your way down to the feet.
- Massage the top and bottom of the foot at the same time by holding the foot underneath with your fingers and using both thumbs to press the top of the foot.
- Repeat the same procedure on the left side, but using a counterclockwise motion where clockwise was previously indicated.

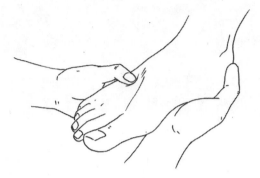

Figure 14.3 Padabhyanga-Foot Massage

THE PRACTICE: HASTABHYANGA–HAND MASSAGE

Hastabhyanga hand massage stimulates deep cognitive memories while energizing the tissues and organs of your body. Massaging the hands increases flexibility, refreshes the energy of the whole body, and strengthens the heart. From the standpoint of Wise Earth Ayurveda, the hands are the wings of the heart.

Our hands, also one of our five organs of action—energetically speaking—hold the five elements on the tips of our fingers. Earth is held in the little finger, water in the ring finger, fire in the middle finger, air in the index finger, and space is held in the thumb. Our hands are vital extensions of ourselves that enable us to touch nature and refine her within us.

Timing: Waxing moon phase
Contra-indications: Menstruation; bleeding; or during mourning
Body Type: All types
Ideal Time: Morning; early evening

HAND MASSAGE INSTRUCTIONS:

- Sit upright on the floor in a comfortable position.
- Set up a placemat on the floor within reach with a small bowl of warm sesame oil and a hand towel on it.
- Rub the right hand with a small amount of oil.
- Massage the palm of the hand by pressing with your left thumb.
- Use small circular clockwise movements with your thumb to stimulate the mound in the palm below each finger.
- Rub each fingernail with oil and massage by gently pulling on it.
- Press each finger firmly and rotate.
- Bend the fingers backward, then forward, by extending and flexing the wrist.

- Firmly shake and rotate the wrist until it is loose and has released its tension.
- Use your thumb to press the back of the hand, following through to the nail of each finger.
- Repeat the same procedure with the left hand, using counterclockwise motions where clockwise was previously indicated.

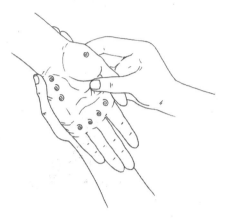

Figure 14.4 Hastabhyanga—Hand Massage

THE PRACTICE: SPECIAL HIP MASSAGE

(Requires the help of an able partner or friend).

As women, we tend to hold our grievances in our hips and thighs. Hip massage stimulates the apana air of the womb and brings the uterus into a state of contentment while relaxing the hips and legs. It increases tejas, the mellow fire that safeguards intuition. Massaging the hips arouses feelings of love and nurturing. Once love is aroused in the womb, ancestral memories awaken.

Timing: Waxing moon phase
Contra-indications: Menstruation; bleeding; or during mourning
Body Type: All types
Ideal Time: Morning; early evening

SPECIAL HIP MASSAGE: STEP ONE

- Have your partner lie on her stomach on the massage table.
- Grip the hips firmly with both hands, your thumbs on the back of the hips.
- Massage the lower back firmly, maintaining small circular motions, as indicated in Figure 14.5 on the next page.

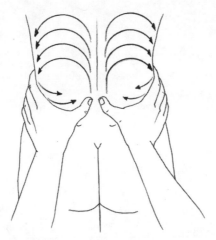

Figure 14.5   Step One: Special Hip Massage

THE PRACTICE: SPECIAL HIP MASSAGE (CONTINUED)

SPECIAL HIP MASSAGE: STEP TWO

- Have your partner lie on her left side.
- Pour one tablespoon of oil on the right hip.
- Grip the right hip firmly with both hands, your thumbs on the back of the hip, and your fingers at the front.
- Massage both the waist and hip areas firmly and steadily for five minutes, maintaining a general circular motion with your hands, as indicated in the figure below.
- Repeat the same procedure on the left hip.

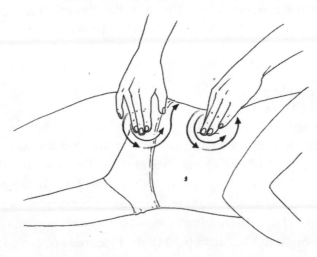

Figure 14.6   Step Two: Special Hip Massage

THE PRACTICE: ENERGIZING SHAKTI PRANA—SQUATTING POSTURE

Timing: Waxing moon phase; on the full moon
Contra-indications: Menstruation; bleeding; or during mourning
Body Type: All types
Ideal Time: 6:00-10:00 (morning or evening)

From time to time, during the waxing moon phase, you would want to keep your Shakti prana fluidly energized. A simple posture to help women under the age of 68 is the squatting posture. This posture allows you to interact with the magnetic energies of Mother Earth by drawing your apana vayu—downward-flowing prana—into rhythmic harmony, necessary for energizing your Shakti prana. You can naturally practice this pose while you are gardening, cleaning, or taking a break.

Assume a squatting posture by positioning your feet hip-width apart and parallel, and bending your knees. If you can't bring your heels flat to the floor, place a small pillow beneath the heels for support. Bend slightly forward and rest the palms of your hands on the floor. Exhale vigorously through both nostrils. After you've emptied your lungs, begin a series of gentle inhalations and exhalations while in the squatting posture and visualize Shakti prana circulating in the womb as it communes with the Mother. Continue this practice for five minutes.

As you are discovering, nourishing the Great Mother is a comforting practice that we may seek to do at any time the desire arises. One of the most auspicious times to nourish and feed her occurs the day before the full moon in the cycle of Phalguna Shukla, at the end of February into March. The full moon at this time is called the Kumbha Moon, "kumbha" literally means, "an earthen pot" signifying the womb-moon brimming with Shakti energy. Following is a wondrously nurturing act of celebration for women during the February-March Kumbha Moon.

NOURISHING THE GODDESS AT KUMBHA MOON

In the waxing moon cycle of Phalguna Shukla, the goddess is feasted on rich, creamy porridge called *pongala*. The festival of Pongal, named after the porridge, is largely celebrated in the Kerala region of India at the Attukal Temple and attracts more than one million women. Despite the massive conversion of Hindu women to Christianity in India, a multitude of Christian converts join this exquisite Goddess Mother celebration. This unifying Hindu practice is observed even in a few churches in Kerala where the sacrosanct rice porridge is offered to Mother Mary.

Ten days of celebration culminate on the full moon that comes at the end of this late February/early March waxing cycle, called Kumbha—meaning an "earthen pot, made from red clay"—a metaphor for the eternal womb of the Goddess Mother. It is hard to imagine the grandeur of this event as women from all walks of life spend the entire day devoutly preparing for this munificent occasion. On the day before the Kumbha Moon, they relinquish all other duties they may have to their husbands, children, and families. Except for the priests, guards, and service personnel, no men are allowed to participate in this ritual. One million strong, they sit in the vicinity of the temple, some in the backyards of homes along the stretch. Lining the streets for many blocks, they joyfully tend to their hearths, which are created directly on the earth.

The palpable trill of their anticipation to nourish the goddess releases abundant Shakti energy, which is experienced for hundreds of miles around the villages of Attukal Temple. Once the signal from the temple priests is given, the women light their fires and begin cooking their sublime porridge. Pongala is made from Kerala's famous hand-pound red rice, a glutinous short grain, sweetened with jaggery (unrefined sugar from the palm sugar) and boiled slowly in a new red earthen pot over an open fire largely fueled by dried coconuts.

The porridge is ready some 30 minutes later when its thick white spume trickles over the top of the pot. This devout offering is made to the goddess with the hope that she will fulfill the desires and intentions of the women. On this occasion, she is worshipped in the form of Bhagavati, the all powerful, Supreme Goddess, and Bhadrakali, the goddess in her fierce warrior appearance. In Hindu ceremony, sweet rice is considered the favorite repast of the goddess. For centuries, rural Hindu communities, especially the poor populations of farmers and villagers, have been offering sweet rice to the goddess on the sacrosanct ground of their labor, in the groves and fields, so that their efforts may be blessed and bring good health and abundance.

Timing: (For Women Only) Waxing moon phase at the end of February into the beginning of March (during Phalguna Shukla)
Contra-indications: Menstruation; bleeding; or during mourning
Ideal Time: Kumbha Moon; and the day before each full moon

NEW MOON CYCLE:
WOMEN'S REVITALIZING PRACTICES

Full Moon to New Moon
During the 14 days before the new moon—the waning cycle, krishna paksha (when the moon is in transit from full to new)—there is a dominant force of cleansing and

reorientation due to the absorptive powers of the sun at this time. The waning cycle offers ample opportunity to start slowing down, complete tasks, strengthen your breath power and life force, detoxify and cleanse, and bring the fruits of your labor to completion.

In the waning cycle following the full moon, the body, mind, and spirit also wane. It is completely natural for a woman to instinctually yearn for quietude, calm, and resolve at this time. In order to help facilitate this, you can do serene practices such as meditation, pranayama, journaling, drawing, painting, semi-fasting, and other introspective activities that lighten your emotional load and build your inner harmony.

New Moon

Taking this reflective, winding-down time is vital so you can meet the new moon with a refreshed spirit. The "marked days" around the time of the new moon are when the Supreme Goddess, along with her nityas, skillfully retreats within the womb of her moon to replenish its vitality for the next cycle. This is not to say that this phase is in any way dull. The first silver crescent of the new moon heralds a new month; a fresh beginning that is intent upon celebrating the magnificent inner force. Vedic tradition declared the new moon as a crucially auspicious time called amavasya because it signifies the goddess's emanation of rebirth. The new moon brings an end to the dark cycle when excess activities should be pared down, and cosseting within the self to conserve her energy—literally the cyclical time of the "Resting Moon," bringing with it the necessary sadhanas of "lying down." This is the optimum time to recharge and recalibrate the Shakti energy.

Like her, you too, have the precious chance to change the things in your life that bring unhappiness, lack of abundance, and coldness. You may take stock of yourself by re-examining your inner motivations, setting the motion for changing those things that do not serve you. A harbinger of rest, reprieve, and strength-gathering, the waning moon supports a natural instinct for women to absorb; and as you reclaim new life, a whole new persona is yours for the crafting.

PRANAYAMA PRACTICE

The waning phase that leads to the new moon is a time to easily reclaim your lightness by paring down activities to a minimum and intelligently using the time for introspective reprieve. The lunation cycle reflects the five natural progressions of life—birth, growth, fruition, aging, and death. The strength of the life force is eternally tied to Goddess Lalita's lunar cycle. According to the *Bhavana Upanishad*, the full monthly circuit of the moon represents the 21,600 breaths a human being would normally take in a day. Indeed, the continuum of life depends on breath. The pranayama and mudra practices set out below are especially geared to recharging the feminine life force. These practices are potent, yet gentle enough for the retiring cycle of the waning moon. Constant practice will help you strengthen your breath and Shakti prana, rebalance your hormonal system, and rejuvenate your womanly emotions and spirit.

Pranayama is a simple and effective way to extend the duration and improve the quality of your life. If you are like most people who have never practiced pranayama, your respiratory pattern probably consists of quick, shallow breaths that start and end in the chest. Think back to moments when you felt angry, frightened, or stressed, such as when you fought with a family member in which you felt you were treated unjustly, or heard the unmistakable cry of your two-year old in danger.

Of course, this physiologic reaction is the hallmark of the fight-or-flight response and is appropriate under extremely stressful circumstances. But the problem in our culture is that we cultivate shallow breathing as a bad habit that endures even under normal, far less stressful conditions. Chest breathing does not allow us to take in enough oxygen to properly feed the lower lungs, so that the cardiovascular and other biological systems cannot operate at peak efficiency. Thus, we spend much of our lives unwittingly robbing ourselves of sufficient oxygen—and the prana that comes through deep breathing—which leaves us energetically and emotionally drained. The waning moon cycle is a prime time when many emotional upheavals tend to occur. During this time, you are especially in need of rich prana to the body and mind that the following sadhanas will amply provide.

Pranayama practice induces diaphragmatic breathing, and is a simple method for transforming shallow breathing into a far deeper, more expansive form that facilitates the flow of prana throughout the entire system and revitalizes you on every level. We can instantly correct this prana deficiency through the practice of pranayama and mudra—both practices serve to quickly renegotiate and brace the vibrational forces of the body. Who would expect a simple breathing exercise or the turn of the hands to produce such wondrous results?

THE PRACTICE: DEEP BELLY BREATHING

Firstly, let's practice the art of Deep Belly Breathing, a necessary first step to gaining the full effect of pranayama practice. Many folks have forgotten what a profound joy it is to absorb quantum amounts of prana-rich oxygen daily. You can practice this conscious diaphragmatic breathing any time, even sitting at your desk or in your car.

DEEP BELLY BREATHING INSTRUCTIONS:
- Lie flat on your back on a rug, yoga mat, or any other surface that comfortably supports your body.

- Put one hand on your chest, the other hand at the bottom of your rib cage just above the belly.
- Inhale into your belly so that you can actually feel it rising, becoming round and full, while the diaphragm moves downward, allowing your lungs to fill with prana-rich oxygen. Allow the breath to travel slowly all the way up through the diaphragm, into the chest, up to the collarbones. Your chest should remain relatively stationary.
- When you have completed the inhalation, slowly exhale, and feel the belly contracting as your diaphragm moves upward.
- Continue this practice for several minutes until the mechanics begin to feel natural to you.

Pranayama is easy enough to do, once you become aware of how it differs from chest breathing. After you practice breathing from the diaphragm while lying in a tranquil posture, you can begin to incorporate this deeper, more relaxed respiration into your everyday life.

THE PRACTICE: ANULOMA VILOMA

Timing: Waning moon phase; all year
Contra-indications: Menstruation; bleeding
Body Type: All types
Ideal Time: Early morning; before bed

Anuloma Viloma is one of the most outstanding pranayama practices you may do throughout the year to balance your lunar and solar breaths, which are constantly interacting throughout your lifetime. The lunar breath is channeled through your subtle energy conduit of the body called *ida*, and flows through your left nostril. On the other hand, the solar breath courses through *pingala*, the subtle solar energy channel of the body and flows through your right nostril. Alternate nostril breathing helps you to keep both lunar and solar energies in a state of equanimity; a necessary feat if you are to maintain intelligence, memory, and health in the course of your lives.

Wise Earth Ayurveda says that once your breath is free flowing and remains in rhythm with the solar energies of the day, and the lunar energies of the night, disease can hardly take root in the body. In Anuloma Viloma practice, the classical formula for length of inhalation versus exhalation is to hold the breath for four times as long as the inhalation, then exhale for twice the length of the inhalation. Once you feel comfortable with the mechanics of the practice, you may want to silently count the seconds of your inhalation, and then try to extend your exhalation for twice that count. As you become more adept, work your way up to inhaling for eight counts, exhaling for 16. You may then incorporate the more classical techniques, which involve holding your breath between inhalation and exhalation. Begin with a ratio of 4:16:8 (so that the holding is four times the length of the inhalation, and the exhalation is twice the length of the inhalation), and work your way up to a ratio of 8:32:16.

ANULOMA VILOMA INSTRUCTIONS:

- Start with a few minutes of Deep Belly Breathing, described on pages 257-258.
- Block your left nostril with your right ring and pinky finger, and inhale through your right nostril. (See Figure 14.7 Anuloma Viloma Breath).
- Then block your right nostril with your right thumb and exhale through your left nostril.
- Continue alternating right and left nostrils for approximately 10 minutes. Be sure always to inhale through the same nostril from which you just exhaled.

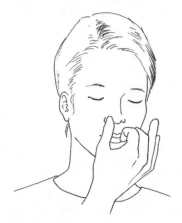

Figure 14.7 Anuloma Viloma Breath

THE PRACTICE: SHITAKARI BREATHING

Timing: Waning moon phase; all year
Body Type: All types
Ideal Time: Early morning; before bed

As noted earlier, owing to the body's natural need to claim its period of reprieve while sloughing off its attachments and burdens, the waning lunar phase can heighten emotions such as anger, angst, and frustration. To start the process of reclaiming your serenity, cooling the mind, and keeping fretful emotions at bay, you may want to add this simple, effective breathing practice to your new moon cycle of sadhanas. Shitakari breathing is easy to do and generates a deep sense of inner calm by cooling the breath and dissipating the sense of unrest. This exercise is similar to Shitali, or breath of the serpent practice, which is a powerful antidote for reducing fiery conditions of the body and mind. As you cool down your breath you'll find unhealthy emotions such as anger, resentment, and jealousy instantly dissolving.

SHITAKARI BREATHING INSTRUCTIONS:
- Sit in a comfortable upright position by keeping the spine erect and tilting the chin slightly downward. (During meditation and pranayama practice, it is strongly recommended that you sit cross-legged in lotus, or semi-lotus posture on a meditation cushion or pillow. If not possible, choose another posture that feels comfortable.)
- Start by taking a few exhalations to clear the lungs.
- Then draw the intake of breath through your mouth by opening the lips to form an "O" while slightly stretching the tip of the tongue to rest on the lower lip. Do not curl the tongue. (You'll be making a hissing sound while inhaling.)
- Hold your breath for 20 seconds or more, and then exhale through your nostrils.
- Repeat this practice 12 times.

MULADHARA MUDRA: GREAT SACRAL HAND GESTURE

This mudra practice is especially excellent for strengthening a woman's sacrum and pelvic area. The prana movement during this practice strengthens the muscle in the perineum between the anus and genital organs. Muladhara Mudra relieves pain in the lower body, menstrual cramping, intestinal spasms, coldness, nervousness, anxiety, and stress relating to fearfulness and forgetfulness. Diligent practice of Muladhara Mudra helps women to cleanse the body and release menstrual blood, thereby replenishing the Shakti prana. It is also a very good practice for women in menopause since it serves to fill the womb-space with healthy prana. Commonly called the sacral mudra, this practice also helps to alleviate bladder complaints and constipation. This is a particularly excellent practice for Vata types. This mudra comprises two hand postures, as follows.

THE PRACTICE: MULADHARA MUDRA

Timing: Waning moon phase; on the new moon; autumn season
Contra-indications: Menstruation; bleeding; or during mourning
Body Type: All types
Ideal Time: 2:00-6:00 (afternoon)

MULADHARA MUDRA INSTRUCTIONS:

- Be comfortably seated facing the south, the direction that represents earth, the element of the muladhara chakra.
- Breathe gently into the belly while holding each mudra posture for 10 breaths before releasing the hands.
- Holding up your hands with fingers stretched and palms facing at chest level, join the tips of the little finger with the tips of the thumb on each hand by curling these fingers to roughly form two circles.
- Connect the hands by allowing the joint tips to touch. The tips of the outstretched ring fingers should also be touching, roughly taking the form of an upward pointing triangle.
- Continue with the second phase of this mudra by joining the tips of your ring fingers with the tips of the thumbs and having the little fingers stretched out with the tips touching.
- Hold this mudra for 10 breaths.
- Release the mudra and continue sitting while tracing the breath through 10 cycles.

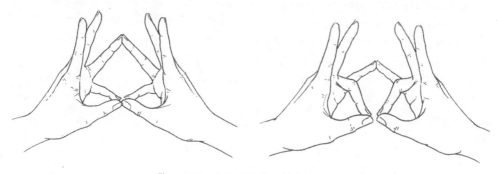

Figures 14.8 and 14.9 Muladhara Mudra #1 and #2

SHAVASANA—TRANQUIL POSE

The following practice, known as Shavasana—is a classical yoga posture which I call the "tranquil pose," (literally translated as "corpse posture"). An effortless practice to bring body, mind, and spirit into the bosom of the Mother, this practice has you "lying down," the optimum act of surrender to the waning moon. It also incorporates deep belly, diaphragmatic breathing along with a visualization that is an excellent starting point for other, more advanced breath practices. I particularly recommend tranquil posture whenever you feel overwhelmed, stressed, and exhausted. This is an especially powerful practice during the waning moon cycle when you can feel simply "blah." Even five minutes in this pose can create tremendous restorative benefits in your overall health.

THE PRACTICE: SHAVASANA–TRANQUIL POSE

Timing: Waning moon phase (especially before the new moon); all year
Body Type: All types
Ideal Time: Early morning; before bed

SHAVASANA INSTRUCTIONS:
Position your arms by your side, with palms facing up. Stretch out your legs hip-width apart and parallel. Let your body go limp and visualize your prana moving in a stream of white light, from the diaphragm to the collarbones and back. After your breath begins to move freely and silently, close your eyes and visualize your breath as a stream of translucent white light that flows from your heart and radiates to the farthest reaches of your body. Allow this moonlit breath to flood your entire being. Feel it in the tips of your fingers and toes, in the crown of your head, in each of your vertebrae, behind your eyelids, and in your throat.

Rest your mind in the serenity of the breath. Let yourself relax as fully as you can in this posture, breathing slowly and peacefully, for 15 minutes. (It's best to stay awake, but if you fall asleep in this posture, you obviously need the rest, so enjoy your nap!)

Now, open your eyes, and gently shake out your hands, arms, and legs. Look around the room, noticing what comes into your mind as you observe your familiar surroundings. Allow yourself a gradual transition to full consciousness by sitting up slowly, and taking whatever time you need before you resume your activities appropriate for the waning phase of the moon.

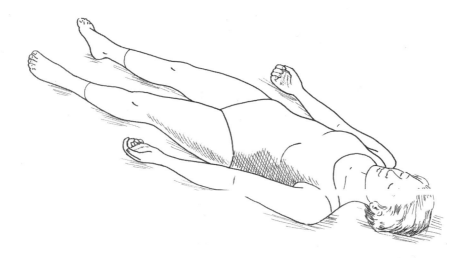

Figure 14.10 Shavasana–Tranquil Pose

STRENGTHENING WOMB ENERGY WITH GINGER COMPRESS

Timing: End of the waning phase (one week before the new moon); all year
Contra-indications: Menstruation; bleeding; fevers; or during mourning.
Body Type: All types
Ideal Time: 6:00-10:00 (morning or evening)

Ginger compresses have been used for centuries to alleviate lower back stress and to energize the kidneys, bladder, and reproductive organs. This simple therapy also encourages proper circulation in the body and restores apana vayu, the downward-flowing air in the colon and reproductive organs. A ginger compress may be applied to the body and limbs, but not to the head. Rub an ample amount of warm sesame oil on your back directly before and directly after treatment. This fomentation therapy may be applied for no more than 30 minutes.

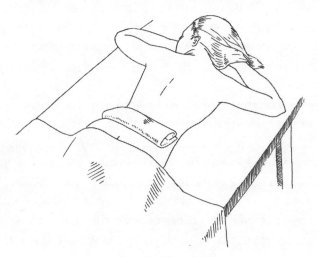

Figure 14.11 Ginger Compress

INGREDIENTS (FOR BACK ONLY):

1 gallon water
1 handful grated fresh ginger
(For entire body, use 4 gallons of water and 2 cups grated ginger)

UTENSILS AND EQUIPMENT:

1 large stainless-steel pot with cover
2 stainless-steel bowls

1 handkerchief (to wrap ginger into a bolus)
2 hand towels (for therapy)

Bring water to a boil in a large stainless-steel pot. Place the grated ginger in a small, clean, cotton pouch, secured by a drawstring. Using your stronger hand, firmly squeeze the pouch so that the ginger juice seeps through the bag and into the boiling water. Then drop the ginger pouch into the pot of boiling water. Cover and let simmer on low heat for 30 minutes. Donning protective mitts, remove the pot from heat and carefully carry it to the treatment room; let sit for five minutes before uncovering.

Spread clean blankets on the floor and place a large trivet for the pot of ginger water on one side to soak and ring the compress towel. To retain the heat, use the large towel to cover the heated towel on your back. Before lying down, prepare your compress towel by holding the ends of it with both hands, and dip the slack of the towel into the pot with the hot ginger water, without letting the water touch the ends you are holding. Twist the towel to relieve any excess water into the pot. Cover the pot to retain the heat of the water. Firmly shake the towel loose to release some heat. First test the temperature of the towel by gently placing it on your arm for a brief moment. Make certain the heat is bearable before applying the compress on your back.

Lie on your stomach on the blankets while applying the treatment to your back, exposing the area of the back to be compressed. Fold the towel and apply it directly over the kidney area on the lower back. Use your right hand and apply firm pressure over the towel. Let the towel stay on for approximately four to five minutes while you rest. When the temperature of the towel turns lukewarm, remove it and repeat the dipping and wringing procedures in the hot water. Repeat application of the hot towel on the back approximately five times or until ginger water loses its heat.

Immediately following your treatment, you'll likely experience a warm feeling expanding in your belly as though it is being lit from within. You'll be amazed to discover how quickly discomfort in the lower body disappears after the treatment. Rest for about 10 minutes before slowly rising. During the waning moon cycle, it is important to pace yourself a tad slower than you are accustomed to, gather your thoughts, examine your emotions, and write them down if you care to.

NEW MOON JOURNALING

Timing: Waning moon phase; on the new moon
Contra-indications: Menstruation; bleeding; or during mourning
Body Type: All types
Ideal Time: Any time of day or night

Journaling is a brilliant sadhana that frees the mind of its burdensome thoughts, reflecting your concerns and feelings back to you. It preserves your most private truths and emotions. Often, we are surprised by what pours out on paper because we are free to scribe the content of emotions we couldn't say aloud. Following is a simple way to begin, or continue with your journal.

Note the time and place as you begin to scribe your first entry. Do not censor yourself by worrying about grammar, punctuation, literary style, or whether or not you are "doing it right." Do not prejudge the content; whatever comes to mind is worth recording and investigating. Keep your pen or pencil moving on the page. Set yourself a time limit—30 minutes is a reasonable period. Allow your feelings and motives to float lightly on the surface of your consciousness as you record your thoughts and experiences. Try as best you can not to get caught in one endless loop of thought or feeling.

Your journal is a powerful way to witness your spiritual progress as a woman, as the rhythms of your Shakti become consonant with the Mother Consciousness. You will find yourself becoming more transparent, cultivating guileless receptivity to the sacred transmissions of the Mother.

Before you begin your journal, ask yourself these key questions:
- Do I feel comforted by the thought of keeping a personal diary to track my spiritual progress?
- What are my spiritual goals for the next three years?
- What are some of the changes I would like to bring about in my everyday life?
- How do I feel about shifting my everyday life to live in harmony with the moon cycles?
- What does my Shakti power mean to me?
- What are the new things I am discovering about myself as I begin to explore my understanding of Mother Consciousness?
- Do I like what I see?
- What desires and goals would I like to fulfill?
- What image of myself would I wish to see realized in a year from now?

Before putting pen to paper, recite the Saraswati Mantra:

Aim Sarasvatyai Namah
(ah-eem sah-rahs-wat-yi nah-mah-ha)

Saraswati is the Goddess of Wisdom, creativity, and light. Her mantra helps the mind to merge with the intuition, or buddhi. Invoking Saraswati will enable you to evoke your spirit of wisdom and objectivity while feeling refreshed, open, and ready to accept and express your thoughts on paper.

Chapter Fifteen

CELEBRATING THE SHAKTI ENERGY OF OUR DAUGHTERS

*Informed spiritual education is paramount if our girls are to
know the sanctity of their womb, heart, and soul.*

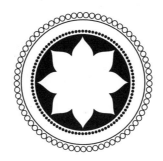

Figure 15.1 Lotus

Menarche is the first and most important transformation in the female life cycle. In the Vedic tradition, we see this as the most critical juncture to lay the early foundation for the young girl's understanding of her Shakti power as it ties in to her sexuality and fertility. The rhythm of the menstrual cycle in the spring phase of a girl's life sets the pace for how she will respond to her great, mysterious powers throughout her life. This is the pivotal juncture when she learns to either cherish or diminish the delicate force that is her maternal nature. We need to inform our girls of these noble transitory passages in their lives by guiding them into ceremony, mantras, and ancestral parables, unfolding their exclusive rights to the sacred menstrual sanctuary, instead of presenting them with only clinical education and its sanitized appendages—deodorized pads, intrusive tampons, and astringent douches.

A GIRL'S COMING OF AGE: MENARCHE

Menarche has been celebrated by most native cultures, although in the last century there has been a dramatic decline of this essential practice for young women in all cultures. Worse yet, many of these rites have been thinned out or have become perverted through ignorant, selfish, and hurtful actions of patriarchal malevolence. Unfortunately, incest and sexual abuse of young women are still prevalent in many communities around the world. This is largely due to the diminishing understanding of the significant role the female person plays in our world, fueled by the continual erosion of respect for the Mother Consciousness.

Now that we are learning the importance of these rites, we should not neglect our primordial duties to our daughters. Indeed, we have forgotten the importance of this crucial passage in our daughters' lives. In most cases, the coming of age initiation had not been observed by our own mothers. We must not continue to lose touch with the necessity of celebrating our children's most precious transition. For this, we need to celebrate their pivotal role as young women in a momentous way. When we do not, we steal away their great *menarchial* heritage and unwittingly set in motion the likelihood of moral and sexual identity crisis in their relationships. Lacking early spiritual education on the subject of their Shakti, which must be disseminated by the mother or female guardian of the girl, our young women largely find themselves in a quagmire of confusing choices and options, which only serves to diminish their understanding of their exquisite Shakti nature. By honoring the first menarchial moments of your daughters' life journeys and using this major opportunity to educate her as to the meaning and purpose of her womanhood, you become her proactive, celestial guardian on earth. Restoring the long forgotten education that we owe our girls is one of the most important tasks we can do as mothers.

A child's first formal education marks a crucial milestone in her overall development. For the Hindu offspring, education begins in a ceremony where the child writes her first letter in a tray of rice. As noted earlier, these powerful samskaras, rites of ceremony, are intended to impress upon the psyche of the child her infinite nature and purpose for spiritual advancement. Spiritual studies start before puberty in the formative years of the youth and are also consecrated with ceremony. According to the *Tarka Sastra*, the word samskara is defined as, "an indelible imprint on the memory," which suggests that when we observe knowledgeable rites and rituals that mark our transitional passages, they leave a lasting impression in our memory so that we do not stray from the path of our humanity in dharma. These disciplined rites help us to charter life's complex course by providing ample opportunities for purification of the mind and its desires, leading to a life of wholesome abundance and spiritual fulfillment.

In Hindu families, puberty rites are prominently celebrated for both girls and boys since this pivotal transitional point symbolizes their coming of age—the end of childhood and entrance into the community as young women and men. As a Hindu girl enters puberty, the ceremony of Kala Ritu is performed to acknowledge her first menstrual cycle. This ritual is called by as many names as there are languages in India. Literally meaning "the time of the season which is strongly linked to the dark moon cycle," the Kala Ritu Ceremony inaugurates a girl's coming into the springtime of her womanhood. Like the gentle seed breaking through the dense mass of the earth to reveal its fragile sprout, the menstrual seed of the young girl sprouts through her bosom into delicate breasts, as her procreative sap begins to flow downward and outward from her yoni.

Not unlike the sprout that needs to be properly mulched and protected from the early spring frost, the young girl is cosseted by her mother and held in the warm space of nurturance. She is made aware of the sanctity and delicacy of her procreative energies. The girl is informed of her budding Shakti power through playful and sometimes humorous parables, metaphors, and stories of menstruation and fertility told by her elder aunts and grandmothers. She is shown how to wear her menstrual pads, and taught how to wash them. Her mother invokes new restrictions on her daughter regarding contacts with the opposite sex. Finally, the female crones welcome her into the adult community.

THE HISTORY OF MENARCHE RITUALS

Once upon a time in India, the most elaborate rituals in a Hindu family centered on women. Pre-puberty and menarche rites were performed for the young girl that revered her source of authority in Shakti and celebrated her sexual potential. Later on, these rituals disappeared from Northern and Central India. In the South India, these rituals were challenged by massive conversion of Hindu populations to Christianity by political reformers and social activists, especially in the State of Kerala. Gradually, the plethora of rites and rituals for women deteriorated to a few negligible annotations. In Kerala, pre-pubescent girls offer rice porridge to the goddess during the festival of Pongal, while making a promise, *nercha,* to her to care for their feminine sanctity. In turn, they implore the goddess to safeguard their good health.

In Tamil Nadu, the South of India from where my maternal forebears came, you can still find semblances of traditional menarchial celebration wherein a sanctuary, *kudisai,* is constructed either inside or outside of the home. It is made from leaves and branches of mango, coconut, and neem trees, considered propitious to the occasion. The sanctuary is furbished with new clothing, toiletries, new dishes, and writing tablets. The young woman is asked to rest in seclusion, while she is served, bathed, fed, and nurtured by her mother and family elders. As you have seen, the menstrual blood is potent—packed with life-generating Shakti—and therefore the young woman is asked not to play with the animals, look at the birds on an empty stomach, enter the prayer room, touch plants, go outside alone, do domestic work, cook food, or feed her "leftovers" to the dogs. These activities are strictly forbidden. After her cycle ends, she enters the purification phase of celebration, *puniya-thanam,* which is similar to the *Goriyo* observance, described on the following page. Following her purification rites, her event is celebrated with communal pomp and ceremony. She is bathed and anointed with turmeric paste, dressed in beautiful new clothing, and receives many gifts from her mother, the family elders, and a community of friends.

Goriyo, the Monsoon Austerity Ritual consisting of purification rites for menarche, may still be found alive in many South Indian homes. This includes a fortnight of eating healthy, fresh foods which are uncooked. This rite symbolizes the young women's farewell to carefree childhood and her major transition into the responsibilities of womanhood. During the Kala Ritu ceremony, the mother initiates her daughter into a vow of chastity until she is married. She begins by teaching her about the moral, societal, sexual, and spiritual responsibility of being a woman. She teaches her about her powerful procreative energy and gives her daughter her first sari, white in color to symbolize her purity. In the stoic Hindu home, the girl may be initiated into the Gayatri Mantra, which is the most important Vedic mantra for both the male and female coming of age rituals. Finally, as you will see in later pages, the young woman is presented with the responsibility of making three major decisions of her own on that day of ceremony. She is given her first journal and is guided by her mother to write down her decisions in the form of an oath, which she then discloses to her mother. This confidence between mother and daughter is kept private between them.

A SPIRITUAL EDUCATION

Communal celebration of girls' coming of age is necessary to reclaim so that we may reinforce the physical, emotional, and spiritual education we need to provide our young people. We must concentrate on the magnificent dynamic energy of the Shakti they possess, as well as the pragmatic health care education that teaches young people how to nourish and protect their reproductive health. Informed spiritual education is paramount if our girls are to know the sanctity of their womb, heart, and soul. The understanding of their Shakti energy helps them to remember how precious, powerful, and yet vulnerable they are as women. Many young women whom I have met have confided that their first menses came as a shocking experience. At first, they were clueless as to what was happening to them. There is evidence of the growing need for young women to be informed about the management of menstruation before they arrive into menarche.

Physically caring for the womb and body as a whole is necessary education that should begin in the dusk of the girl's premenstrual state. Presenting physical female anatomical and clinical information is beyond the scope of this work. This information can be found in your libraries and schools. We know reproductive health education is increasing in schools worldwide, however, this education is mostly clinical in nature and does not reinforce our children's spiritual values. You cannot simply entrust your children's health solely to the educators. The primary educator of girls is the mother. You need to take firmer charge of your family's well-being by making radical changes in your homes, wherein you become proactive in educating your girls about their amazing female anatomy—physical, emotional, and spiritual. In so doing, they will learn the meaning and purpose of their massive transition into womanhood.

Healthful nutrition and harmonious lifeways must become staple education in our children's lives. For this, we must remain alert to their biological development and catch the early signs, such as: behaviors caused by changes in their hormonal system; a sudden breakout of acne; budding of breasts; or growth of hair in the underarm or pubic area of the body. Adolescence is a time when looking after health and moral values can help to build immunity against reproductive diseases. Unfortunately, there is an alarmingly high rate of gynecological health disorders and morbidity among adolescent girls, especially among the rural populations of the Third World where reproductive health education remains slim to none. Vaginal discharge is frequently the most common gynecological symptom reported by both rural and urban women in India.

As you know by now, the female power of Shakti is endowed with the most effective cosmic anatomy to safeguard, nourish, and progress life on earth. For this reason, we must not denigrate the understanding of our procreative nature—the ability to give birth to new life—in the physical, emotional, and spiritual sense. Menarche is one of the significant transitions in the collective female life whose rhythms are deeply connected to the Mother Consciousness. Every female womb is endowed with the potential power to manifest the Mother's Shakti, constructed with the subtle elements of unrivalled creative power. Each girl is created in the image of the Earth Mother thereby inheriting her procreative aptitude and replicating her prowess manifold times all over the world. Obviously, to say that the journey of a woman is different from the journey of a man or any other species is an understatement. Her gender role is fashioned in the power of Shakti. In short, she is naturally powerful. In this unparalleled journey, menarche marks the auspicious juncture when the Shakti starts to blossom within the female person.

COMING OF AGE AROUND THE WORLD

Once upon a time, all native traditions celebrated the rites of passage of the young woman according to their knowledge and in ways that emulated the recognition and protection of her essential prowess of creativity and abundance. In the Niger Delta Valley of Africa, the coming of age ritual for the Okrika woman is an extraordinary event. Called *Iria*, this rite of womanhood consists of elaborately painting the young women's bodies with traditional designs. Their ritual passage is supervised by the community of elder women who teach them the lessons of coming into womanhood by setting out clear instructions for their daily habits and feminine lifestyle. After an elaborate celebration, they run a race pursued by young men led by the eldest male leader who symbolizes the mythological protector armed with sticks to defend the honor of the village female. By passing through this rite, the young women are ready to enter their sacred roles as childbearing emissaries of the Great Mother.

In Mexico, girls observe their Quinceañera—coming of age—on their 15th birthday. On this day, they dress in long white gowns, receive gifts from their family and friends, and attend a special coming of age mass held in a Roman Catholic religious service. They are serenaded with live music and as the day ends their parents declare them ready to begin dating boys.

In the Yanomami culture of Brazil, as the young girl reaches puberty, she is sheltered behind a screen of leaves where she is cared for and fed by the female elders for a week while she is introduced to the new and sacred reality of her life. At the end of this time, she is looked on as a young woman who is ready to be married.

The Native American Apache's coming of age ritual is celebrated as a somber event wherein the pubescent girl is transformed into the White Painted Woman, who performs a four-day long ceremony in which she recreates the sun-generated birth of the Apache people. Symbolizing her emergence into the Great Apache Mother, the young girl is showered with cattail pollen and informed about the power of her fertility and sexuality by her crones. To conclude her rite of passage on the final day, the girl dances from sunrise to sunset to invoke the Great Mother's grace for the welfare of her people. The ceremony ends with the elders honoring her as a "mother of her people."

Even to this day, in Bali fire-dancing is observed as a coming of age ritual. Girls as young as 11 years old learn the art of fire dancing by watching the elders dance around a fire. The ability to walk or dance on fire is believed to earn the participant great spiritual powers. In India, Fiji, and around the world people still walk on heated rocks and stones to test their spiritual faith. The male spiritual elders in Hawaii, Kahunas, have been known to dance on piping hot lava to show their spiritual prowess.

THE FORCE OF SHIVA

Before we may reclaim our menarchial rites—and therein the essence of the feminine powers of Shakti—let us briefly explore the ancestral traditions of the masculine energy, or Shiva force. As noted earlier, to attain absolute harmony, we must embrace the intertwining energies of Shiva and Shakti as inseparable, each one playing a pivotal role in the power of the whole self. Together they form the one firm foundation of our transcendent universe within and without. When we recognize the true nature of our Shakti energy, we realize that our anatomy as women is cosmically programmed to perform in transcendental ways. Because of the dynamic difference between the Shiva and Shakti energies, the initiation practices and intentions for each gender is uniquely patterned after the precise energies of Shakti and Shiva.

Fortunately, the Vedas have preserved and maintained the rituals for *upanayanam* (a boy's coming of age rites) in pristine condition. As noted, the Shiva energy exists in its greater potential in the male and therefore requires its own set of specific conditions and circumstances. When a Hindu boy reaches the age of seven he becomes eligible for his upanayanam. His initiation is centered on the formation of a formidable relationship to his father necessary for his manly development. For this reason, the ceremony starts with the ritual to wean him away from attachment to his mother. Thereafter, his initiation can only be completed by the family's Guru. Following the ceremony of a Hindu boy, he becomes a full member of the spiritual community in accord with the rites of passage consigned to the societal status to which he is born, or has inherited from his ancestral lineage. In a ceremony administered by a priest, a coir string, known as *Janev*, is sanctified in front of the ceremonial fire, before it is tied in a loop and worn by the boy. The thread is hung around a boy's left shoulder to his right waistline for *Brahmins*, and from his right shoulder to his left waistline for *Kshatriyas*. This string marks the official start of the young man's spiritual education. He is taught to recite a specific mantra that can be heard only by those who have already gone through the ritual of upanayanam. The ceremony varies from region to community, and includes recitation of Vedic mantras.

The upanayanam is similar in intention to the *Navjot* ceremony of the Zoroastrians and to *B'nai Mitzvah* in Judaism. Generally, the boy's Bar Mitzvah occurs when he is thirteen. Later on in Judaism, the girl's coming of age initiation called the *Bar Mitzvah* or *Bat Chayil* was also introduced. In progressive synagogues the ceremony for girls is often called confirmation and usually takes place later, at the age of 15 or 16. These were recognized as the ages when the youngsters were obliged to fully observe the commandments and to participate in the rituals of the community.

VEDIC RITES OF THE FEMALE

Although it may appear as though the rites of passage for the young men in native cultures are celebrated with more elaborate rituals which have been better preserved than those for girls, this is not so. In a young woman's coming of age rites, elaborate concentration is placed on her completion of these rites through the *Vivaha*, or marriage ceremony. Unlike the boy, a girl's menarchial initiation evolves in two stages: firstly, the Kala Ritu is performed to celebrate her coming of age under the care and guidance of her mother. In the first rites, the mother plays the cardinal role since she is considered to be both mother and Guru to her daughter. In the second phase, the girl's fertility rites are honored as she comes of marriageable age. Through the Vivaha rites—an elaborate marriage ceremony involving seven steps or ritual passages—she finally completes her initiation as a young woman. In this ceremony, the bride is weaned from her mother's care as her husband steps in. By right of his cosmic nature in Shiva, he is meant to serve the fulfillment of her fertility and assume the perennial role of nourishing her Shakti. Through her husband's loving care, she brings closure to her initiation. The husband becomes her Guru. Clearly, marriage is more than a love affair, sexual alliance, or a carefree relationship. It is guided through specific and sacred rites of passage to ensure a lasting love and friendship between a young man and young woman.

REVIVING THE RITES OF PASSAGE FOR OUR DAUGHTERS

Celebrating menarche is an important thread in the reweaving of the healing man-dala of feminine life. Whether or not your culture has preserved any part of the wondrous rituals to elevate and protect the spirit of your children, it is impor-tant that you recast a set of practices in keeping with your ancestral history that embrace, honor, and nourish the Shakti force of your daughters. You may begin to knit strongly back together within the community of women. In so doing, you may start by gleaning as much universal knowledge as you may need from the Vedic rituals I present at the end of this chapter. At this profound juncture of time, reviving the extraordinary rites of passage for both our sons and daughters is extremely necessary. To safeguard the young, it is of significant import to pre-serve the Shakti energy by instilling its sacred principles through initiation of the Mother Consciousness into the minds and hearts of young people. Because the female child carries the active energies of the Mother Shakti within her, it is even more crucial to re-enact these sacrosanct practices for her.

Over the years, I have been overwhelmed by the daunting stories I hear from mothers of girls from many cultures who feel helpless about shaping the destiny of their children. I have met with hundreds of young people who feel lost and confused, mired with hopelessness and stress, and entirely disconnected from their parents and elders. Across social and cultural landscapes, manifold layers of pathologies beset our young people—depression, mental instability, obesity, repulsion to healthful nourishment, lack of self-esteem, identity confusion, sexual promiscuity, and suicide to name a few—all emerging from a strong repulsion to the maternal principles of life. We can trace our entire miasma of misery to one central aspect of life—erosion of the Mother Consciousness.

Our humanity depends on everything maternal: healthful nourishment; respect for the mother, and in particular, for women; passionate care for nature; compassion for all life forms while maintaining a sense of kindness and dispassion toward that which we are yet to understand. Restoring our pure nature of the Mother Consciousness must become our first priority. For this reason, I have unearthed more precious gems from my tradition to give to you a universal practice for your young women that can be initiated by mothers of all traditions. I refer to this warm and beautiful practice as the *Kala Ritu: The Menarchial Rites of Passage*, details of which are set out below.

KALA RITU: THE MENARCHIAL RITES OF PASSAGE

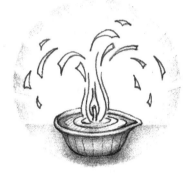

Figure 15.2 Dipa—Ghee Lamp

The compassion of the Vedic tradition that has preserved the wisdom of the body, mind, and spirit over several millennia has been known to embrace all cultures, abundantly sharing its wisdom practices and never asking others to sacrifice their ancestral and traditional ways. Indeed, very few traditions have recorded or preserved their ritual ways, but thankfully, Vedic practices are universal in nature and are therefore serviceable to all traditions.

From earliest times, Vedic women have been able to amply express their power of spirit. They have been known to conduct ritual ceremonies that concern women's issues and the rites of Kala Ritu for their daughters. These rituals are meant to invoke the fires that sustain our consciousness and memory.

Following is a simplified version of the Devi Fire Ritual you may perform to initiate your girls' coming of age. Vedic fire rituals, *yajna*, are combined with mantra and meditation to generate heat within the body to burn away physical impurities, illuminate the mind, and facilitate your communion with the celestials. The Devi Fire Ritual, the central and final part of the Kala Ritu Ceremony, is a powerful ceremony to beckon young women coming of age with loving care and wisdom. You may use this ritual as presented, or alter it to suit your understanding and needs. The important idea here is to maintain the pure intention of honoring your child's profound transition into womanhood by educating her of her rich spiritual nature.

Devi is the Sanskrit name of the Universal Mother. In guiding your young women through this powerful ceremony, you may contemplate any image or aspect of the mother within your tradition which you feel comfortable, be it Devi, Blessed Virgin Mary, Gaia, Gwan Yin, Avilokiteshvara, Nammu, Hahai'i Wuhti, Au Sept, Mawu, Ishtar, or Akua'ba. This ritual practice will help both of you to deepen your awareness of the Divine Mother and enhance your daughter's budding comprehension of her Shakti prowess and the meaning of her maternal memory. You may also observe this practice by having the young woman keep her chosen image of the Mother in mind while you guide her into recitation of the Devi Mantra, or a prayer of your choice.

Every day is the Mother Shakti's day, but Tuesdays and Fridays are the days that the seers devote to her, and the best time to make offerings to the Mother. At this time, the Mother's encompassing energy is dominant in the atmosphere and your prayers would likely be received. Considering the fact that the Kala Ritu Ceremony introduced herein is entirely renovated and reordered for your daughters, after many centuries of being lost even to Hindu mothers, it would be wonderful to encourage other mothers you know to witness these extraordinary and intelligent ritual preparations for your daughter's celebration. In so doing, they may activate this loving and informed practice for their girls when they become of eligible age.

Understanding that many of my readers may be novices to Vedic practice, I have partitioned the Kala Ritu ceremonial practice into three distinct phases, ending with the main ceremony, the Devi Fire Ritual, which has been pared down to a minimum to make it user friendly. It's worth remembering that the act of sacrifice is one of the greatest practices you can make in a spiritual life. The more effort you put into honoring your children's rites of passage, the more rewarding and productive their lives will become.

Don't be concerned about making mistakes while you are learning to perform these powerful Vedic rites. This munificent Vedic tradition is free of guilt, retribution, and punishment. Its ways are patterned after cosmic harmony, love, embrace, and empathy and has never sought to usurp any person from his or her tradition, or convert them to its own. Its wisdom-packed practices and nobility have surely touched the minds and hearts of more than half the earth's inhabitants. It is a rich culture that does not care about being politically correct; albeit Vedic stewards are very keen and precise. Alas, they tend to notice every minute detail, and will probably enjoy noting your blunders with blunt remarks and lengthy commentaries. That being said, you may celebrate your daughters' Kala Ritu with the loving practices of Kala Ritu Menarchial Rites of Passage, as follows:

Phase One: Preparation for Kala Ritu Menarchial Rites
Phase Two: Mehndi Party with Girlfriends
Phase Three: Kala Ritu Ceremony—Devi Fire Ritual

PHASE ONE: PREPARATION FOR KALA RITU MENARCHIAL RITES

Optimum Timing: Three months after the start of menarche
Contra-indications: Not during menses; non-virginal state

Immediately following the advent of your daughter's menarche, you will want to spend as much time with her as possible to educate her to the profundity of her menarchial moment. (The ceremony may start three months after the first menstrual cycle ends, but ideally, you should begin educating your child even before her menarche begins so she is prepared for its commencement.) To begin with, shop for and provide her with good quality cotton pads and show her how to use them. In my upbringing, we used pure cotton re-usable cloth and waist string, tailor made by my elder mother for the occasion. Girls were instructed on washing and caring for their menstrual cloths as a way to physically connect to the phenomenon of their menstrual blood. This, of course, may be asking a bit too much of our sanitized-minded modern women. However, whatever you do, do not use tampons or commercial and intrusive feminine products.

A few days after the girl's first cycle has been completed heralds the perfect time to introduce the young lady to the simple purification observance with healthful foods, outlined on the following page. This practice marks the end of carefree childhood and the onset of her responsibility as a young woman. The following practices of Austerity Feasting-Fast Ritual, Mehndi Party, and Kala Ritu Beautification Bath can and should be done whether or not you are planning to perform the final course of the Kala Ritu Ceremony, namely, the Devi Fire Ritual, outlined in detail on pages 283-288.

Before performing the official Kala Ritu ceremony, let us explore some of the other wholesome preparatory practices that will help to comfort and nourish your daughters.

AUSTERITY FEAST-FASTING RITUAL WITH SCRUMPTIOUS FOODS

Encourage her to observe at least a week long (pared down from the usual fortnight) of semi-fasting without cooked foods, junk foods, and animal flesh. Be her pillar of support by continuing to educate her as to the profound passage she has entered by making this fast a richly rewarding ritual instead of an ordeal. For instance, she may want to lose a few pounds, or the pimples, and look gorgeous for her once-in-a-life-time celebratory occasion. Joining her in "feasting" on healthful fresh foods will not only contribute greatly to her confidence, but in so doing, will also contribute to her inner beautification and fortification. As difficult as it may be to convince a young person to observe a semi-fast, it is the best sadhana you can engender to help her cultivate the emotional awareness that she will need at this critical junction in her life. Following is a list of scrumptious fresh, uncooked foods (get organic quality): seasonal and dried fruits (unsulphured); salads made from beans, greens, nuts, and seeds; fresh squeezed vegetable and fruit juices; and spiced milks (cow's, soya, or almond) with cocoa, cardamom, cloves, cinnamon, sweetened with Sucanat, jaggery, honey, or maple syrup.

AUSPICIOUS TIMING FOR KALA RITU CEREMONY

Once the Austerity Feast-Fasting is underway, begin contemplating the advent of celebrating your daughter's menarchial season. It is important to work in astronomical harmony with the celestials, heavens, and stars. In this way, your effort is maximized, and you can begin to see your ritual rewards almost immediately.

To ensure the date chosen for the Kala Ritu Ceremony is auspicious to this activity, contact a Vedic Astrologer, *Jyotisha*, to determine the appropriate date for the Kala Ritu Ceremony. These rites may also be performed within the first year after the onset of her menstrual cycle, but optimum timing is three months after her first cycle has been completed. This ceremony must not be conducted during the girl's cycle, or if she is not a virgin. In the latter scenario, you may guide her into observing the nurturing sadhanas for the full moon and new moon, set out in the previous chapter.

Once the date has been established, invite the women of your family, and especially the women elders, to contribute the following gifts for your daughter's big day (see following page). It is preferable to keep this affair within the maternal family, albeit you may invite your close female family friends. It is considered inauspicious for young girls who have not entered their time of menarche to join this occasion. Include her girlfriends in this momentous occasion during the colorful mehndi ritual—painting the hands with natural henna—that happens the day before the actual ceremony.

KALA RITU BEAUTIFICATION BATH

The bathing ritual that follows is a necessary precursor to the Kala Ritu Ceremony, although it stands on its own merit and may be performed as an independent practice each month after the cessation of the menstrual cycle.

Timing: Early morning, three days following the end of the first menses
(Tuesdays and Fridays are preferred days)
Contra-indications: During menstrual cycle; bleeding
Gifts to be Given by the Mother:
- A beautiful, white lacy frock, or a white cotton sari, trimmed in gold
- New white cotton underwear
- A stock of menstrual cotton pads

Prepare a warm bath and add a few drops of lavender essential oil, along with a handful of pink rose petals. Either you, the mother, or a female family elder may help the young person into the bath and afterwards gently scrub her back while chanting Vedic mantras. Alternatively, you may sing the songs of your tradition.

Directly after the bath, dry off the young woman's body and lavishly anoint her full body with a mixture of warm sesame oil mixed with a few drops of either sandalwood or lavender essential oil. Afterwards, she should be dressed in her new ceremonial frock.

FOR HER PROSPERITY:
GIFTS OF ABUNDANCE

Jewelry is the perfect gift to be given by female relatives and friends: gold, precious, or semi-precious stones, such as fresh water pearl, emerald, ruby, topaz, or sapphire necklaces, bracelets, anklets, watches, or earrings. Do not give elaborate, gaudy, faux jewelry, or silver or bronze gifts. The cost of expensive gifts may be shared by family members. A few light pieces of quality jewelry are always better than a truckload of junky gifts.

Natural beautification products such as moisturizers, facial cleansing scrubs and creams, soaps, shampoos, essential oils, hair oils, and so on, are also appropriate gifts for the occasion. Teach your girls that natural beauty is the most beautiful: to not use heavy makeup, harmful hair dyes, and chemically packed commercial cosmetics, but instead to care for and nourish their body—skin, hair, teeth, eyes, and yoni.

PHASE TWO:
MEHNDI PARTY WITH GIRLFRIENDS

A day before Kala Ritu Ceremony is the perfect time for the feet of the young woman to be decorated with mehndi. At this time, her girlfriends who have already entered menarche may help decorate and paint her feet. Unlike the bathing ritual, the mehndi party is not a necessary precursor to the Kala Ritu Ceremony, although it adds to the great fun and beautifying theme for the young woman. Furthermore, it provides a perfect opportunity for the young woman to share her big event with her girlfriends since—to preserve specific blessing energy of the goddess—the Kala Ritu Ceremony should be attended only by the mother, maternal family elders, and her close female friends. Mehndi art, historically intended only for women, may be performed as a fun loving celebration during occasions such as birthdays and holidays. See *The Practice: Mehndi Application & Directions* on page 281.

HENNA PAINTING OF FEET

Timing: Early evening before Kala Ritu Ceremony
Contra-indications: During menstrual cycle; bleeding; illness; or mourning

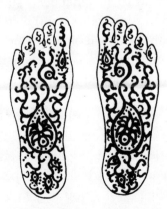

Figure 15.3 Mehndi Painting of Feet

The decorative, fun-loving art of mehndi body painting is traditionally done for brides the day before their wedding. I have taken to introducing this practice of painting mehndi on the soles of the feet of the young women during their Kala Ritu ceremony as a bridge of understanding for them to start fathoming their enormous Shakti power. Mehndi is more than the art of body painting. It is used by women to cleanse, beautify, and adorn the body. It is a beautiful and gentle way to introduce modern girls to the vast trove of ancient healing secrets that lies within their womanhood.

Hindu goddesses are often depicted in ancient drawings with mehndi tattoos on their hands and feet, dating this Indian art form back to beginningless time. It is also believed that this art originated in Egypt where it was used to beautify the nails and hair of the mummies. Its recognition may be traced back to the Mughals' invasion of India in the 12th century. The royal Rajputs of Rajasthan popularized mehndi, which was made famous by their skilled craftsmen and women who excelled in delicately painting the hands and feet of princes and princesses with fine gold and silver sticks. From then on mehndi has been regarded as a fundamental ritual practice for propitious occasions, particularly weddings.

A significant cultural practice in many communities of the world—India, the Middle East, Asia, North Africa, and Pakistan—mehndi is used to beautify, decorate, and inspire spiritual creativity, with patterns drawn from indigenous fabrics, local architecture, natural environments, and cultural experiences. In South India, motifs are predominantly culled from India's vast historic spiritual yantras, which are painted in the center of the palm before dipping the tips of the fingers in the henna to form a cap on each. In North Africa, very intricate designs are developed around nature's themes of beautiful birds, fishes, and animals. Arabic motifs like flowers, leaves, and geometrical shapes predominate in Muslim regions. Sudanese patterns are large, bold, and floral, with geometric angles.

Mehndi powder comes from the dried leaves of lawsonia inermis, a member of the loosestrife family of dwarf shrubs that bears small, fragrant pink, white, or yellow flowers that are used in Ayurveda's natural cosmetics. The green powder of the dried leaf is mixed with water, lemon juice, eucalyptus, and clove oils, and sometimes tamarind paste is introduced as a thickener. Before conical tubes were used to apply the henna, women dipped their fingers into the paste and formed the designs with thin sticks, thereby leaving the trademark of colored capped fingertips which became the most popular mehndi motif in South India.

Before getting started, review the mehndi kit and familiarize yourself with the use of the cone and preparation for mixing the mehndi paste. Practice a test run or two on yourself or on a female friend before the party begins. Using the conical tube, similar to that of icing a cake, you may begin to apply the henna on a part of your body that is not so visible. You do not want to steal the girls' thunder before their big day arrives. Show the girls how to perform the mehndi and stay close by to oversee the process without being too imposing or intrusive in their Mehndi Party. Only the girls who have already crossed into menarche can apply the mehndi to the subject, although younger girls can participate in the preparation of the mehndi and bear witness to the jubilant affair.

THE PRACTICE: MEHNDI APPLICATION & DIRECTIONS

- Cut a small hole (about one-eighth of an inch wide) at the tip of the cone to allow a thin stream of henna to flow. Be careful not to create too big a hole as it will result in too thick a flow of henna.
- Start with the soles of both feet.
- Make sure that the feet are clean and dry.
- Begin by anointing the feet with rose or orange flower water, and dry them off.
- Rub a few drops of eucalyptus essential oil on the feet while resting them on a stool with legs outstretched to expose the surface of the soles.
- Once you have applied the henna design leave it on the soles to dry for at least two to three hours, while you continue with your festivities.
- Continue to sit with your feet off the ground until the paste dries.
- Once the paste is dry and starts to crumble, carefully dust it off. The longer the paste stays on the more vibrant the orange-red hue becomes. The motif on the skin darkens over time and can last for several weeks depending on how often it is exposed to water.

PHASE THREE:
KALA RITU CEREMONY—DEVI FIRE RITUAL

Timing: Three months or so after the start of menarche
(Consult with a Vedic astrologer as to the optimum timing for these rituals)
Contra-indications: During menstrual cycle; bleeding; mourning; non-virginal state; illness

Vedic rituals are effective and universal in intention, but they are profoundly detailed procedures that require specific attention to timing, a code of behaviors, and rules—all finely meshed with harmonious dharma. If you choose to observe the Devi Fire Ritual, carefully contemplate the following procedures and review and secure the sizeable list of utensils and ingredients necessary for the ceremony. Should you desire to go forward with this potent phase of the work, you are advised to practice chanting the Devi Mantra with your daughter a few days prior to the ceremony.

Although I have pared down this ritual to make it easier for you, you will need to embrace this ceremony with all your heart to reap the abundant blessings and rewards from your efforts. In the work of the spirit, it is your sacred intention that counts the most. Therefore, if you lose your calm, mispronounce the mantras, make mistakes with your mudras, or take missteps in the process of learning to do these pujas, the goddess will be the first to understand. Indeed, she may even crack a smile, and depending on the extent of the faux pas, she may burst into hearty laughter.

At this remarkable phase of your daughter's celebration, guests should be invited to bring gifts for the young lady's special celebration. It is also customary to invite your guests to stay on for a scrumptious wholesome feast following the ceremony. Female family elders may tell positive and engaging stories and parables relating to the following themes: innocence, infatuation, love, challenges, menarche, marriage, and sexuality.

SETTING UP THE KALA RITU ALTAR

You will need the following utensils and ingredients, which should be reserved only for the purpose of performing rituals.

Necessary Utensils & Ingredients:
- An image of the Devi*
- A photo of your Guru (if applicable)
- Pure water in a new brass cup, *tirtha* cup*
- A new brass tray (12 inches in diameter)
- A new tiny brass spoon (to dip the water)
- A handful of white basmati rice (in a new bowl)*
- A handful of fresh flowers, white or pink (clip stems short)
- A garland of flowers made from white and pink roses, or carnations
- A few pinches of red sandalwood powder (in a new bowl)*
- A few sticks of sandalwood or *champaka* incense secured in an incense holder*
- Ghee (reserve a bottle of ghee to be used only for rituals and prayers)*
- Ghee lamp, *dipa**
- A few cotton wicks for the ghee lamp
- A large new bowl of fresh organic fruits, covered with a new napkin
- A small fire pot, *kund* (6" diameter)*
- A wooden board on which to place the fire pot
- Pine kindling, *dhup* (tiny pieces) and camphor resin*
- A small brass ladle for the ghee*
- A few pinches of yellow sandalwood powder*
- Pure water and sandalwood essential oil for the mother's feet-washing
- A new diary and pen

* Items may be purchased at Indian grocery stores.

Choose a quiet site, preferably in the northeast corner of your home or living room to create your altar space. Spread a new cloth or sheet on the floor. Place a picture, statue, or image of the Devi where you can see her clearly. If you have a Guru, place his or her photo on the right side of the goddess. In front of the image, you may set up your earthen firepot on a clean board and tray with all the ingredients and utensils you'll need for the ceremony. Place the tirtha cup of water, spoon, sandalwood powder, basmati rice, garland, and loose flowers on the right side of tray. Go ahead and prepare your ghee lamp by inserting the cotton wick and placing a tablespoon of ghee in it. You may also insert your incense into its holder and sit it by the ghee lamp. For easy lighting dampen the tip of the wick with ghee. Prepare the firepot by putting a few pieces of kindling and half a cube of camphor into your fire pot. Do not light the fire until it is required.

If possible, perform the ritual outside, otherwise, remember to cover your fire alarm. The earth, a river, or an ocean are the most auspicious places to put your sacred ritual ashes, but you may also place them in a secluded place on the ground in your garden if necessary. The Kala Ritu Ceremony follows.

THE PRACTICE: KALA RITU CEREMONY

Follow the aforementioned directions for the young lady's bath and beautification. After being dressed in her new white frock and before beginning the puja, the daughter honors her mother by washing her feet.

WASHING THE FEET OF THE EARTHLY MOTHER:
Perform this rite in an outdoor space such as a lawn or deck. The daughter will prepare a basin of warm water with 10 drops of sandalwood essential oil poured into it. She will need a clean hand towel, a handful of flower petals, and a small plate with a dab of sandalwood paste. (To make the paste, take a teaspoon of red sandalwood powder and mix it in a few drops of water.)

- Begin the feet washing by bowing to your mother and bending forward to touch her right foot.
- Next, take the basin in both hands and pour the water over her feet.
- Then sit on your knees, or in a comfortable squatting pose to dry her feet and then decorate them.
- Use the ring finger of your right hand to dip into the sandalwood paste and place a dab of it on each of her feet, right foot first.
- Repeat the process with her left foot.
- Afterward, sprinkle the flower petals on her feet, and take another bow.
- To conclude the feet-washing rite, compose a brief avowal to honor your mother. Following is an example of the sentiments and words you may express:

Mother, I will honor you all of my life. I am grateful for all of your love and care and I will do my best to live up to the highest ideals of our tradition and my sacredness as a woman.

After the feet washing ceremony, begin the Kalu Ritu Ceremony. You may guide your daughter to the puja in the altar space you have created by seating her facing east. Seat your family members and guests behind the subject before taking your place as the ceremonial guardian of the puja. Sit facing your daughter with the firepot placed on the ground between you.

INVITING THE GODDESS INTO YOUR HOME:
Before beginning the ritual offering to the Goddess, invite your guests to utter the following beautiful Vedic invocation during this offering:

O Gods and Goddesses, I beseech your holy attention to our cause at this auspicious occasion. May a thousand streams gush forth from this offering, like milk from a bountiful, pasture-fed cow.

Now to the ceremony offering:
- With your left hand, take a spoonful of water from the bowl and pour it into the palm of your right hand. Rub your hands together and let the drops of water fall on the cloth.
- Put another spoonful of water in your right hand, intone the following Devi Mantra: "*Om Sri Devi Maa, Svaha,*" and then sip the water.
- Repeat this sacred mantra along with the sipping of water three times.
- Next, using the same procedure, wash your daughter's hands and have her repeat the Devi Mantra three times. She will then take her seat to the right side of you and hold the tray with the ceremonial ingredients in her lap. Keep the ghee lamp, incense holder, and covered bowl of fresh fruits within reach.
- Offer a seat to the Goddess in your home by inviting her with these words and a few pinches of grains:

Recite, "Dhyaayaami Samarpayaami," then offer rice to the Goddess.
Recite, "Aavaahayaami Samarpayaami," then offer rice to the Goddess.
Recite, "Ratnaasanam Samarpayaami," then offer rice to the Goddess.

(We meditate upon you, O Goddess. We invite you to sit upon the jewel studded throne we have prepared for you.)

You may repeat this procedure for inviting the Guru into your home, as well. Close your eyes for a few minutes and visualize the Goddess sitting on a gem-studded throne, beautiful, smiling, and full of grace while waiting to be honored as your guest in your home.

WASHING THE FEET AND HANDS OF THE GODDESS:

Recite, "We now humbly bathe each of your lotus feet and gently wash each of your precious hands, O Goddess"

- With your right hand, offer a spoonful of water by holding it before the image of the Goddess for a moment, and then placing it into the brass cup.
- Chant the following mantra while visualizing yourself bathing the sacred feet of the Goddess:

Paadayoh Paadyam Samarpayaami.
We now humbly bathe each of your lotus feet, O Goddess.

- With your right hand, offer a spoonful of water by holding it before the image of the Goddess for a moment, and then placing it into the brass cup.
- Chant the following mantra while visualizing yourself bathing the sacred hands of the Goddess:

Hastayoh Arghyam Samarpayaami .
We now humbly bathe each of your precious hands, O Goddess.

OFFERING WATER TO QUENCH THE THIRST OF THE GODDESS:

- With your right hand, offer a spoonful of water by holding it before the image of the Goddess for a moment, and then placing it into the brass cup.
- Chant the following mantra while visualizing the Goddess receiving the water in her hand and sipping it:

Om Bhur Bhuvah Suvah Aachamaniyam Samarpayaami.
In all three worlds, we humbly offer you fresh, pure water for sipping.

BATHING AND GARLANDING THE GODDESS:

- While ringing the small bell with your left hand, pick up a flower with your right hand, hold the stem between your ring and middle finger, and dip it into the tirtha water before sprinkling it on the image of the Goddess.
- Repeat this sprinkling three times while visualizing bathing the Goddess with this intention in mind:

O Goddess, we now bathe you with the pure water from the sacred river, Ganges.

- Recite the following mantra during the symbolic bathing of the Goddess.

  Om Sri Devi Maa, Samarpayaami.

- Next, have your daughter place the garland around the Goddess's neck (if a statue), or over her picture.
- Using the ring finger of your right hand, dip and rub the fingertip into the bowl of red sandalwood powder and place it on the third eye region of the Goddess's image. Keep this intention in mind:

  O Goddess, please accept this fragrant sandalwood powder.

- Take a few pinches of rice and a handful of flower petals and pour them with your right hand in front of her image, keeping this intention in mind:

  We now offer this unbroken rice, and for the fulfillment of our devotion, we offer fresh blooming flowers, O Great Goddess.

OFFERING INCENSE TO THE GODDESS:
- Light the incense and secure it in a holder.
- Use your right hand to circle the incense three times over the entire image of the Goddess. At the same time, ring the bell with your left hand. On the third time, raise the incense holder higher over the Goddess and ring the bell louder. Keep this intention in mind:

  We offer this fine incense for your pleasure, O Goddess.

- To complete this round of your ceremony, offer the Goddess water, a flower, and a pinch of rice again.

OFFERING LIGHT TO THE GODDESS:
- Light the ghee lamp and offer it to the Goddess.
- As with the incense, circle it three times over the Goddess with your right hand while ringing the bell with your left hand.
- On the third circling, raise the ghee lamp higher over the Goddess, ring the bell louder.

- Keep this intention in mind:

  O Great Goddess, the friend of devotees, see this lamp offered which is lit with pure ghee and which provides abundant auspiciousness.

- To complete this round of your ceremony, offer the Goddess water, a flower, and a pinch of rice again.

OFFERING FOOD TO THE GODDESS:

- Uncover the bowl of fruits while chanting the mantra below.

  Om Amritamastu Amritopastaranamasi Svaha.

- Circle a spoonful of water over the fruits with your right hand as you ring the bell with your left hand.
- Afterwards, affix a flower between your middle finger and ring finger with the flower facing inward, then with a gentle wafting motion of your hand direct the aroma of the fruits toward the nose and mouth of the Goddess.
- Repeat this motion three times while reciting this mantra:

  Om Sri Devi Maa Svaha, Om Sri Devi Maa Svaha, Om Sri Devi Maa Svaha.

- As you complete your ceremony, toss the flower in your hand at the feet of the Goddess and with it, the offering of your heart.

Properly installed in your home the Goddess becomes present in your heart. Pleased with your efforts, she blesses you, your guests, and your daughter on her auspicious occasion.

FINALIZING THE KALA RITU CEREMONY WITH THE DEVI FIRE RITUAL:

Your daughter now takes her place in front of the firepot facing the Goddess; you may sit to her right to assist her in completing this ceremony. The intention of the Devi Fire Ritual is to secure the Goddess's blessings in your daughter's life, and for her to take her menarchial vow by making her affirmations. She is presented with the responsibility of making three major decisions of her own on this day, in the presence of the Goddess.

- She begins by chanting the Devi Mantra 16 times, as follows:

  Om Sri Devi Maa.

- Shielding her mouth with her right hand, she then whispers her three decisions into the right ear of the Goddess. This must be done quietly so that her intentions are not heard by anyone else, including the mother.
- Afterwards, she lights the firepot (already prepared with kindling and camphor).
- With her right hand, and using the ghee spoon, she pours a tablespoon of ghee into the fire.
- Use a flower to sprinkle water over the fire three times in a clockwise manner while keeping your attention poised on your major occasion.
- Throw a few flower petals into the fire.
- Allow the kindling to blaze into a contained fire. As the offering burns, look directly at the Goddess's face and again recite the Devi Mantra 16 times. Focus on the three important decisions you have just made in her presence and to fulfill your desires; safeguard your physical, emotional, and spiritual health; and provide you with abundant prosperity and wisdom. You will know when she is pleased with your efforts. Sometimes, she smiles. Sometimes, she winks.
- While the flame is still burning, carefully guide your guests to the flame and have them take the Goddess's blessings by extending both hands in an open prayer pose a safe distance over the flame, scooping the energy of the Goddess's light toward their faces.
- You then present your daughter with the gift of a new diary and ask her to write down in her own words the oath or the three decisions which she has made to the Goddess.
- While she is scribing her oath, you may disperse the fruits as *prasadam*—blessings from the Goddess—to each of your guests.
- Invite your guests to remain in quiet contemplation of this magnificent affair while your daughter is writing her first menarchial journal entry.
- After noting her vow, she then discloses it to her mother by quietly sharing it with her. She gives permission to her mother to remind her of her affirmations if she should transgress them or forget them. She also makes a promise to her mother to confide in her or to seek her help with any major challenge she may encounter while she is unmarried. This confidence between mother and daughter is kept private between them forever.

You have now successfully completed the Kala Ritu Ceremony. Close family elders may help with the conscientious clean up of the altar and ceremonial space, as you escort your guests to another room where gifts may be given to your daughter. Afterwards, you can enjoy a wholesome feast together, before bringing closure to the gathering. Be sure your guests keep the focus alive on the young woman's special event.

A YOUNG WOMAN'S MENARCHIAL TIME CULMINATES INTO FERTILITY

Seven Steps to Fulfillment: Saptapadi

After a young woman's menarche rites end, her fertility rites begin. Within seven to nine years after the onset of menarche is considered the ideal time for marriage in the tradition, although this timing has been perverted by socio-economic priorities. During this time the girl may continue her academic education and hone her feminine skills, while the mother becomes the official Guru for her daughter in all ways. A suitable husband approved by the family has to be found first. In my tradition fertility rites are observed with lavish nuptial celebrations conducted with a pantheon of ceremonial rites, 13 altogether. Each ritual is rooted in Vedic wisdom, signifying specific aspects of the couple's life to follow after marriage.

In Hindu tradition, Vivaha, the marriage ceremony marks the final set of rites that bring closure to the young woman's menarche. This closure may be accomplished by sanctifying the Shakti of her womb through a ceremony that is intended to initiate her natural power of fertility. In reality, the Vivaha rites mark her entry into the weighty stage of her life where she can contemplate her amazing maternal power as it ripens into fertileness. She contemplates her fresh, new authority to bring life through her. As noted earlier, it is the husband who becomes the initiator of her womb. According to Hindu dharma, he is the only being who is sanctioned to perform this rite. In other words, the Vivaha ceremony blesses and initiates her fertility rites.

The Vivaha is regarded as a sacrament and not a contract. In the Vedic view, it is a sacred bonding of two souls joined as one consciousness for the duration of life. Steeped in rich cultural metaphors and spiritual symbols of the Vedas, Hindu marriage is based on the theme of magical-spiritual-social union which is intended to help ascend the energy of each partner's karma into the progressively pious content of their souls. Obviously, the ancient framers of Hinduism knew that the preservation of harmony, peace, and fulfillment of the couple's lives together is of the utmost priority. The Vivaha is meant to be a time filled with devout spiritual aspirations and noble human intentions for the harmonious and prosperous union of two compatible souls. The abundant celebrations and preparations can extend into an entire fortnight. Unfortunately, the breakdown of family and community life across the boundaries of almost all cultures has served to fracture this phenomenal conclusion to a young woman's initiation.

The next rite of passage after the Kala Ritu is a woman's marriage rites. The day before her wedding the bride is ceremonially cleaned, beautified, and decorated and her palms and soles are skillfully painted with mehndi. On the wedding morning, various ablutionary rituals are performed on both the bride and the groom in their own homes. Their bodies are anointed with turmeric, sandalwood paste, and essential oils which cleanse the body, soften the skin, and make it appear lit from within. Their elders cleanse them with an Ayurvedic bath of rose water, milk, and honey while being serenaded with Vedic mantras. A lavish wedding canopy has been erected and decorated with aromatic vines and flowers at the wedding site. In the center of it, the sacred fire will be installed by the priest.

The marriage ceremony is a complicated affair that I can't describe in detail within these pages. In brief, it begins with the bride and bridegroom facing each other while sitting directly on the cloth-laden earth. The priest ties the bride's traditional dress to the groom's shirt in a knot signifying the sacred union. The bride and the bridegroom garland each other and exchange the rings. To gain the blessings of the lord for the couple's momentous life together, the priest lights the nuptial fire by feeding it with crushed sandalwood, herbs, sugar, rice, ghee, camphor, and pine sticks. Before the fire, which represents the divine witness and sanctifier of the sacraments, the bridegroom stands facing west and the bride sits in front of him facing east. He takes her right hand and recites a mantra to the Goddess Saraswati for their happiness, long life, and harmonious bond.

O Saraswati, Gracious Goddess, rich in progeny,
You whom of all the gods and goddesses, we first serenade
May you bestow prosperity on this marriage.

For the blessings of abundance in their lives, the bride offers an oblation of parched rice into the fire for the gods and goddesses. The grain is poured into her hands by her brother, or someone acting on her brother's behalf. Taking the bride by the hand, the groom leads her three times around the nuptial fire. Both offer oblations and recite appropriate Vedic hymns to gods for prosperity, good fortune, and conjugal fidelity. Afterwards, they touch each other's hearts and pray for union of their hearts and minds. At the end of each round of nuptial fire, both the bride and groom step on a stone and offer a prayer for their mutual love to be steadfast like the stone. The bridegroom calls upon his bride as he guides her to place the tip of her right foot onto the stone:

Come, beautiful one
Come, step on the stone
Be strong like the stone
Resist all enemies
Overcome all adversities.

The exquisite marriage rituals are concluded with the Saptapadi Ceremony, the heart of the nuptials wherein the bride and bridegroom take seven steps around the ceremonial fire, agni. In the marriage ritual, these steps bear special significance as they symbolize the contiguous relationship of love and respect between the couple. With each step they take a sankalpa to honor and serve each other—altogether seven oaths are taken.

The Saptapadi Oaths, as follows:

With God as our guide, let us take
The first step to nourish each other
The second step to grow together in strength
The third step to preserve our wealth
The fourth step to share our joys and sorrows
The fifth step to care for our children
The sixth step to be together forever
The seventh step to remain lifelong friends
The perfect halves to make a perfect whole.

To conclude the Vivaha, the groom utters these evocative words to his bride:

With seven steps we become friends
Let me reach your friendship
Let me not be severed from your friendship
Let your friendship not be severed from me.

Afterwards, as a sign of absolute support to his bride, the groom stands behind her and places his hand over her right shoulder to touch her heart with this sentiment, "I hold your heart in partnership, may our minds be as one, may you rejoice in my sound with all your heart. You are joined to me by the Lord of All Creatures."

To seal the ritual vows he ties the *Mangala Sutra Dharana*, auspicious marital necklace, around his bride's neck, knotting the thread containing the religious symbols for God Vishnu and God Shiva—intended to safeguard her forever. The groom then parts his bride's hair and rubs holy red powder, sindhur, on the mid-path of her head symbolic of her married status. With this rite, the ceremony concludes with the priest offering final prayers that sanctifiy the union as being indissoluble. The groom's parents bless the couple and offer gifts of cloth and flower to the bride indicating that she has now become an important member of their family. Guests sing blissful wedding songs and shower flower petals on the couple for long life, healthy progeny, and a happy union.

Chapter Sixteen

MEDITATIONS OF THE
MOTHER CONSCIOUSNESS
IN EVERYDAY LIFE

*Lalita is the eternal reminder of the infallible truth of self—
that your conviction must remain firm amid the changing
landscape that is human nature. The necessity for you to
remain fixed to the center point of faithfulness may reveal
your true purpose as a woman.*

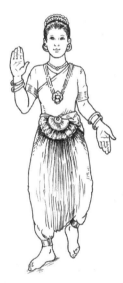

Figure 16.1 Goddess with Two Hands in Mudra Poses

Right Hand: Abhaya Mudra is the pose for granting protection and removing fear.

Left Hand: Varada Mudra is the gesture for granting boons and forgiveness.

We can each be proactive on our journey and at the same time remain true to
our nature rooted within the Mother Consciousness. Even as we effect change in
accord with the phases of our life, karma, and rebirth, we are nonetheless eternally
poised in the formless pure consciousness of the Self. In essence, we are on a womanly journey that mirrors that of Lalita Maha Tripurasundari, the central goddess
of the Sri Vidya tradition (also known as the Auspicious Wisdom tradition) of Hinduism. She is the Supreme Goddess, or manifestation of Parashakti.

Within the Sri Vidya tradition, meditation, prayer, and ritual practices play the most significant role in the everyday lives of women. Women of the Hindu culture feel immense joy and bring forth wellness and prosperity for their family through worshipping the Goddess Mother, and you too may take to remembering her and her nityas on the moon's waxing days. The myriad ritual supplications, mantras, and yantras honoring the goddess are symbolic of the milestones of your eternal sojourn. In using these potent lunar meditations, you are emulating the goddess, mirroring the ebb and flow of her waxing moon as she moves from one notch to another along her eternal journey. In so doing, you may beckon the immutable divine forces closer to you.

INTRODUCING THE GODDESS LALITA MAHA TRIPURASUNDARI

Lalita comprises the entire time and space continuum. She controls the lunar wheel of time, kalachakra, representing the entire manifestation of time and space as it appears within and without. Although the goddess is honored in manifold forms through a variety of supplications, she remains steadfast to her true Self as the Mother Consciousness.

Lalita is also known as the Red Goddess since she issues the three *gunas* and the five elements of ether, air, fire, water, and earth, which are responsible for the creation and sustenance of life. Because of this, she produces all the worlds, planets, elements, rites, sacrifices, austerities, arts, music, festivities, dances, nourishment, and cares for all of her gazillions of charges. As the wielding force of time and space, she controls the moon, sun, and fire, and moves the lunar wheel of time. As the moon remains itself, though shape shifting in accord with its phases, so too does Lalita. In the pages below you'll see that her appearance changes with the cycle of her 15 nityas also known as the "eternities." On the 16th day of the lunar cycle, called Sadakhya, the lunar deities who emerge from Lalita's womb fold back into her to produce the exquisite visage of the full moon. This phase is represented by the Goddess Mother and shows her most auspicious form as Lalita Maha Tripurasundari.

VEDIC ICONOGRAPHY

> The chakra of the letters of the Samskritam alphabet is
> based on time and so it is identical with the sidereal zodiac.
> —*Tantraraja Tantra*

Contrary to popular belief, Hinduism is not a tradition of idolatry. Vedic people do not worship lifeless sculptures, statues, and idols. Physical forms are used in temples, institutions, and homes as a means of evoking the subtle energy force within cosmic divinity. Through rich Vedic iconography, the tradition depicts detailed physical appearances of the deities demonstrating the cosmology of each and every aspect of their subtle force. These sacred shapes and forms are metaphorical in content and range from simple to elaborately intricate. In fact, every letter, word, and meaning of the Vedic language is rooted in the primordial sonic cosmology, believed to be designed by the gods from their vast knowledge of the cosmic sound. Officially called *Devanagari*, the communication form used among the gods and goddesses, *Samskritam* (commonly known as Sanskrit) is the language of cosmic evolution. For example, Samskritam alphabet contains the sum total Shakti power of all deities, each letter possessing the authority and force of specific Shakti energy, with the 15 Sanskrit vowels each representing a lunar deity.

The rishis knew that materializing the shapes and forms of energy would make it possible for the devotee to gain access to the deities' subtle field of power and divinity. Through the manifold ritual venerations provided by the seers, you may evoke their divinity. Access to these auspicious cosmic fields are granted through the richly informed supplication provided by the sages. In other words, the inaudible, intangible subtle energies of Lalita's universe can be made comprehensive to the human person and thusly be aroused through visible forms and appearances of the deity.

NITYAS: LUNAR DEITIES

In contemplating the profound series of lunar meditations set out in the pages that follow, you'll learn the core descriptions of the nityas as each aspect symbolizes a particular network of potent energy held by them. The nityas represent the 15 propitious lunar days, tithis, of the waxing moon, each possessing her yantra, mantra, tantra, and ritual venerations.

In remaining attuned to the lunar days of the waxing moon, you may witness the spiraling fields of consciousness that lie within your transformative human nature. You are all nityas of the Goddess Mother, and you too must consciously reconnect to the source of the Mother Consciousness. Lalita is the eternal reminder of the infallible truth of Self—that your conviction must remain firm amid the changing landscape that is human nature. The necessity for you to remain fixed to the center point of faithfulness may reveal your true purpose as a woman.

Like all Vedic practices, the moon rituals presented in these pages are intended for the well-being of the Self, the community as a whole, and for women from all traditions. You will discover that living in harmony with Lalita's cycles of the waxing moon will help strengthen your Shakti energy, thereby enhancing your inner vibrations and the life force necessary to awaken consciousness of the buddhi and heart. As is the intention of all Vedic archetypal forms, Lalita's physical appearances are valuable in making her subtle forms and energies comprehensible and reachable. Through the lunar meditations, set out below, which are focused on the sublime images of the Goddess Mother, you will be able to access her phenomenal Shakti within yourself. It is likely you will discover that the Shakti energy within you is more than the feminine energy of the creation. It is the Supreme Goddess herself within you. The core attention in these rich meditations is placed on Lalita's maternal abundance.

For immediate access to the Mother in your meditation, I have presented Lalita Maha Tripurasundari and her 15 nityas with their Sanskrit yantras each coinciding with the appropriate moon days. As noted earlier, yantras are sacred Vedic symbols or drawings which reveal the cosmic energy. Each nitya also has her ritual sequence, and vidya mantra, (primordial mantra that evokes self knowledge) which I have provided for your use. Vivid descriptions of the nityas are also provided in each practice so that you may visualize them in their myriad forms and colors while meditating. Since each nitya holds explicit Shakti powers, you may call upon them for the attainment of specific goals. In so doing, you may materialize the lunar deities as your perennial guides. These lunar meditations yield the most efficacious results when you practice them during their appropriate lunar day.

LUNAR MEDITATIONS: SIXTEEN LESSONS IN MOTHER CONSCIOUSNESS

The vidya mantra for each nitya is prefaced by the bija sounds (primordial seed vibrations) for the Mother Goddess—*Aim Hrim Shrim*—and followed by powerful salutations—*Shri Padukam Pujayami Tarpayami Namah* (I worship and nourish myself at the lotus feet of the deity). The Sanskrit yantras associated with specific days of the moon are placed above the names of the lunar deities. These are simplified versions of the cosmic yantra for each nitya. In these profound meditations centered on the Mother Consciousness, reciting the deities' names is of great importance since these "names" are in actuality the mantra, the subtle form, of each deity. In meditating on the goddess and her 16 prolific cosmic forms (15 nityas, and the goddess herself), you will come to see that every day is Mother's Day. Installing these contemplations as a priority in your daily life you'll discover magnificent ease and abundant gifts of the spirit coming your way.

The following series of meditations are to be practiced during the appropriate waxing days of the lunation cycle. You will need a lunar calendar to determine the time of month that each of the 16 waxing moon days occur. These meditations occur during the waxing moon cycle, beginning with the new moon and ending with the full moon. A complete rotation of lunar meditations will yield 16 meditations monthly.

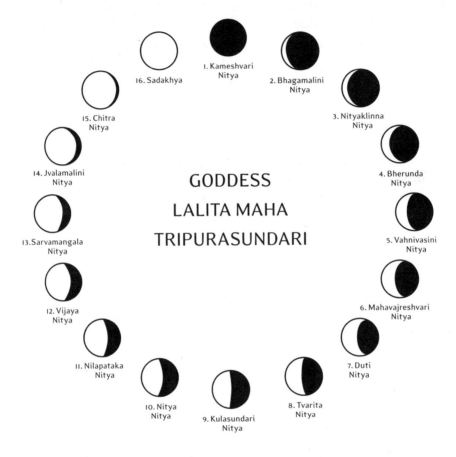

Table 16.1 Mandala of the Waxing Moon with Nityas

PREPARING FOR LUNAR MEDITATIONS

Meditations for the goddess are most effective when practiced directly before dusk or dawn. Begin your meditation practice by establishing a serene space in your home (preferably in a room situated to the north, east, or northeast) to sit, contemplate, pray, chant, meditate, or otherwise be at one with yourself—a place where you feel calm and have complete privacy. As noted earlier, a specific nitya reigns at each notch of the waxing moon cycle. Start your meditation on the day of the new moon by facing east and visualizing the specific Cosmic Yantra (Sanskrit Vowel) of the nitya you are venerating.

Before you start this process, spend some time reading the descriptions of the nityas whose power you are about to invoke into your life. Start practicing pronunciation of the vidya mantra for each deity so that it flows easily while you are meditating. Familiarize yourself with the nature of the unique Shakti power each nitya possesses. For example, the deity for the new moon—the first day of the waxing moon—is Kameshvari Nitya. Her cosmic vowel form is *AH*. Her Shakti power is the fulfillment of desire; and her vidya mantra is, as follows:

Aim Hrim Shrim
Om Hrim Kameshvariyai Namah
Shri Padukam Pujayami Tarpayami Namah

Because of the complexities of the vidya mantra for each nitya, I have provided an abbreviated version of the mantras so they are easier to use. Following is the lunar meditation presented in its generic form. Use the same instructions for each of the meditations. The necessary descriptions and information for each nitya is presented on the following pages.

Also presented at the end of this chapter is the meditation for the full moon that occurs on the 16th day of the waxing moon. At this time, the Supreme Goddess Lalita Maha Tripurasundari is celebrated in her full splendor.

THE PRACTICE: SIXTEEN LUNAR MEDITATIONS

- Acknowledge the day of the waxing moon and venerate its presiding nitya.
- Visually form an image of that nitya from the image description provided.
- Note her specific Shakti power and memorize her form in the Sanskrit yantra. Sit quietly for about five minutes until you have a concrete visualization of her in mind.
- Having captured the yantra of the nitya, recite or read her vidya mantra 108 times, keeping her unique Shakti power in mind.
- After mantra recitation, sit quietly for about 15 minutes or so, as her Shakti energy becomes aroused within and flows through you.

KAMESHVARI NITYA/FIRST NOTCH OF THE NEW MOON

The first nitya in the cycle is Kameshvari, which means Lady of Desire. She is described as having the color of ten million suns at dawn. She wears a diadem of rubies, and necklaces, waist chains, and rings. She is red, has six arms and three eyes, and bears a crescent moon, smiling softly. She holds a bow of sugar cane, flowering arrows, noose, goad, and a decorated nectar-filled cup, showing the mudra of bestowing boons. She holds the flowering arrow of desire—each of the five petals represent the five transformations of desire: longing, infatuation, arousal, enchantment, and wasting.

Shakti Power: Fulfillment of Desire; Granter of Feminine Boons
Cosmic Yantra/Sanskrit Vowel: *A* (pronounced "AH")

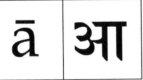

Vidya Mantra: *Aim Hrim Shrim*
Om Hrim Kameshvariyai Namah
Shri Padukam Pujayami Tarpayami Namah

BHAGAMALINI NITYA/SECOND NOTCH OF THE WAXING MOON

The second nitya in the waxing moon, Bhagamalini, whose name refers to the flowering yoni, has a remarkably weighty mantra. She has six arms, three eyes, sits on a lotus and holds in her left hands a night water lily, a noose, and a sugar cane bow. In her right hand, she carries a lotus, a goad, and flowering arrows. Around her is a host of Shaktis all of whom look like her.

Shakti Power: Flowering Yoni; Fertility
Cosmic Yantra/Sanskrit Vowel: *AA* (pronounced *"AAH"*)

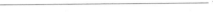

Vidya Mantra: *Aim Hrim Shrim*
Om Hrim Bhagamaliniyai
Shri Padukam Pujayami Tarpayami Namah

NITYAKLINNA NITYA/THIRD NOTCH OF THE WAXING MOON

Nityaklinna, the third nitya, has a compassionate nature, her name meaning "eternally wet." Nityaklinna's face is bathed in perspiration and her eyes move incessantly with desire. She is smeared with red sandalwood paste, wears red clothes, smiles, has a half moon on her head, and holds a noose, goad, and cup and performs the mudra for dispelling fear. She is surrounded by nineteen attending Shaktis.

Shakti Power: Giver of Ojas, Enjoyment, and Freedom

Cosmic Yantra/Sanskrit Vowel: *I* (pronounced "E")

Vidya Mantra: *Aim Hrim Shrim*
Hrim Nityaklinna Madadrave Svaha
Shri Padukam Pujayami Tarpayami Namah

BHERUNDA NITYA/FOURTH NOTCH OF THE WAXING MOON

Bherunda, the fourth nitya, is the color of liquid gold, and has three eyes and eight arms. She smiles sweetly and is adorned with beautiful ornaments on her hands, feet, arms, and waist. She carries in her hands a noose, goad, shield, sword, mace, thunderbolt, and bow and arrow. Effectively employing her mantra is said to destroy the effects of poison.

Shakti Power: Immunity Giver; Remover of Toxicity
Cosmic Yantra/Sanskrit Vowel: Long *I* (pronounced *"EE"*)

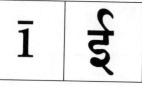

Vidya Mantra: *Aim Hrim Shrim*
Om Hrim Bherundayai Namah
Shri Padukam Pujayami Tarpayami Namah

VAHNIVASINI NITYA/FIFTH NOTCH OF THE WAXING MOON

The fifth nitya in the lunar cycle, Vahnivasini, means, "dweller in fire," which infers that she lives in the fire that devours the universe at the time of its dissolution. She appears as a beautiful young woman, the color of gold, with eight arms, dressed in yellow silk garments, and adorned with rubies. She holds a red lotus, a conch, a bow of red sugarcane, and the full moon in her left hands. In her right hand, she carries a white water lily, golden horn, flowery arrows, and a citron. She is surrounded by infinite numbers of Shaktis who resemble her.

Shakti Power: Giver of Knowledge; Remover of Ignorance of Your True Nature
Cosmic Yantra/Sanskrit Vowel: *U* (pronounced *"OU"*)

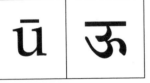

Vidya Mantra: *Aim Hrim Shrim*
Om Hrim Vahnivasiniyai Namah
Shri Padukam Pujayami Tarpayami Namah

MAHAVAJRESHVARI NITYA/SIXTH NOTCH OF THE WAXING MOON

The sixth nitya, Mahavajreshvari, is described as rose-red in color, having a compassionate countenance and wearing red garments. She has four arms, three eyes, and wears a crown of red rubies and red jewelry. Decorated with red flowers, she sits on the throne of a golden boat, which floats on an ocean of blood. Having imbibed pure grape wine, she sways from side to side. She carries a noose, goad, sugar cane bow, and flowering arrows. She is surrounded by a host of Shaktis who are dressed like her.
Shakti Power: Giver of Compassion and Joy
Cosmic Yantra/Sanskrit Vowel: Long *U* (pronounced *"OOU"*)

Vidya Mantra: *Aim Hrim Shrim*
Om Hrim Mahavajreshvariyai Namah
Shri Padukam Pujayami Tarpayami Namah

DUTI NITYA/SEVENTH NOTCH OF THE WAXING MOON

The seventh nitya, Duti, is dressed in red, with nine jewels in her crown. She has a sweet smile and is surrounded by rishis who sing her praises. She has eight arms and three eyes and appears as brightly lit as the summer sun. She carries the horn, shield, mace, cup, goad, cleaver, axe, and lotus in her hands. She is called Shiva

Duti because she makes Shiva her messenger, *duti*.

Shakti Power: Giver of Prosperity and Affluent Boons
Cosmic Yantra/Sanskrit Vowel: *R* (pronounced with a rolling sound *"RR"*)

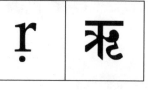

Vidya Mantra: *Aim Hrim Shrim*
Om Hrim Shivadutyai Namah
Shri Padukam Pujayami Tarpayami Namah

TVARITA NITYA/EIGHTH NOTCH OF THE WAXING MOON
Tvarita is the eighth nitya of the lunar cycle. She is called Tvarita, which means "swift," owing to the rapidity with which she grants fruit to her devotees for their spiritual work. Dark in color, she is young and as beautiful as the lotus flower. She has three eyes and four hands, holding the noose and goad. With her other two hands she displays the mudra that dispels fear and grants boons. She wears a crown of crystal with peacock feathers on its crest and sits under a banner made from peacock feathers. She is dressed in garments made from fresh, new leaves and wears anklets, waist chains, and bangles made of peacock feathers. She wears a necklace of strings of red *gunja* berries, her breasts smeared with red sandalwood powder. She is adorned with eight fierce serpents.

Shakti Power: Giver of Immediate Spiritual Rewards
Cosmic Yantra/Sanskrit Vowel: Long *R,* (pronounced *"RRR,"* a longer version of the rolling *"RR"* sound)

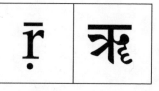

Vidya Mantra: *Aim Hrim Shrim*
Om Hrim Tavaritayai Namah
Shri Padukam Pujayami Tarpayami Namah

KULASUNDARI NITYA/NINTH NOTCH OF THE WAXING MOON

The ninth nitya, Kulasundari has twelve arms and six faces. In her right hands she holds a rosary made of coral, a lotus, a lemon, a gem-studded pitcher, and a cup. Her hand displays the mudra of exposition. Her left hands hold a book, a red lotus, a golden pen, a garland of gems, and a conch shell, and demonstrates the mudra for granting boons. She is surrounded by celestial musicians and gods. Kulasundari sits in the lion seat facing east.

Shakti Power: Unifier of the Three Phases of Reality
(i.e. Knowledge, Knower, and Object of Knowledge)
Cosmic Yantra/Sanskrit Vowel: *LR (pronounced "LRR," a short rolling "R")*

Vidya Mantra: *Aim Hrim Shrim*
Om Aim Klim Sauh Kulasundariyai Namah
Shri Padukam Pujayami Tarpayami Namah

NITYA NITYA/TENTH NOTCH OF THE WAXING MOON

Nitya Nitya is described as having the glow of the rising sun at dawn. She rules the Shaktis of the seven vital tissues of the body, and is the tenth nitya of the moon. She is dressed in red garments and is adorned with rubies. She has three eyes and twelve arms. She holds in her hands a noose, white lotus, sugar cane bow, shield, trident, goad, book, flowering arrows, sword, and skull. With her eleventh and twelfth hands, she demonstrates the mudras that grant favors, and ward off fear.

Shakti Power: Giver of Health; Guardian of Dhatus
(The seven bodily vital tissues)
Cosmic Yantra/Sanskrit Vowel: Long *LR* (pronounced *"LRRR"*)

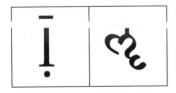

Vidya Mantra: *Aim Hrim Shrim*
Om Hrim Nitya Nityayai Namah
Shri Padukam Pujayami Tarpayami Namah

NILAPATAKA NITYA/THE ELEVENTH NOTCH OF THE WAXING MOON

Her name means "sapphire banner," and she is the eleventh nitya of the moon with skin of sapphire blue. She has five faces and ten arms, and is dressed in red garments and decorated with a myriad of gems. In her left hands she holds a noose, banner, shield, horn bow, and displays the mudra that bestows gifts. In her right hands she carries a goad, dart, sword, arrows, and shows the mudra that dispels fear. She sits on a lotus surrounded by a bevy of Shaktis who resemble her. She possesses a range of siddhis, magical powers.

Shakti Power: Giver of Magical Powers (siddhis) to her devotees
Cosmic Yantra/Sanskrit Vowel: *E* (pronounced *"A"*)

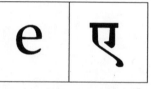

Vidya Mantra: *Aim Hrim Shrim*
Om Hrim Nilapatakayai Namah
Shri Padukam Pujayami Tarpayami Namah

VIJAYA NITYA/TWELFTH NOTCH OF THE WAXING MOON

The twelfth nitya, Vijaya Nitya, is victorious in battle and brings success in the trading of goods. She has five heads and ten arms. In her hands she holds a conch, noose, shield, bow, white lily, discus, goad, arrows, and a lemon. She wears a garland of human skulls.

Shakti Power: Bestower of Victory; Remover of Obstacles
Cosmic Yantra/Sanskrit Vowel: *AI* (pronounced *"AI"*)

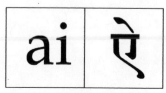

Vidya Mantra: *Aim Hrim Shrim*
Om Aim Vijayayai Namah
Shri Padukam Pujayami Tarpayami Namah

SARVAMANGALA NITYA/THIRTEENTH NOTCH OF THE WAXING MOON

The thirteenth nitya of the moon, Sarvamangala Nitya, is all-auspicious. She governs the *kalas*, digits, of the sun, moon, and fire. Her eyes symbolize the sun and moon. She has two arms and one head, and smiles sweetly as she sits on her lotus yantra. In her right hand she holds a citron and with the left she demonstrates the mudra for giving rewards. She is surrounded by seventy-six companions all of whom come from the lunar, solar, and fiery luminaries.

Shakti Power: Time Keeper; Ruler of the Kalas
(The digits of sun, moon, and fire)
Cosmic Yantra/Sanskrit Vowel: *O* (pronounced *"O"*)

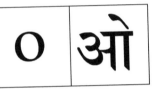

Vidya Mantra: *Aim Hrim Shrim*
Svaum Om Sarvamangala Nitya
Shri Padukam Pujayami Tarpayami Namah

JVALAMALINI NITYA/FOURTEENTH NOTCH OF THE WAXING MOON

Jvalamalini means "garlanded with flames." As the nitya of flame, she represents the fourteenth notch of the waxing moon. She has a body of flaming fire, and six smiling faces, each having three eyes. She has twelve arms. In ten hands, she holds a noose, goad, arrow, mace, tortoise, spear, and flame respectively. With the remaining two, she displays the mudras for granting rewards and dissipating fear. She is surrounded by numerous Shaktis, all of whom resemble her.

Shakti Power: Giver of Wisdom; Remover of Fear
Cosmic Yantra/Sanskrit Vowel: *AU* (pronounced *"AU"*)

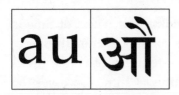

Vidya Mantra: *Aim Hrim Shrim*
Om Hrim Jvalamaliniyai Namah
Shri Padukam Pujayami Tarpayami Namah

CHITRA NITYA/FIFTEENTH NOTCH OF THE WAXING MOON

The last nitya in the moon's waxing cycle is Chitra. Her name means "variegated" and she wears a silk garment of manifold hues and colors. She has one head and four arms. In two hands, she carries a noose and a goad and shows the mudras for giving rewards and removing fear with the other two.

Shakti Power: Giver of Transformative Power; Remover of Fear
Cosmic Yantra/Sanskrit Vowel: *AM* (pronounced *"ANG"*)

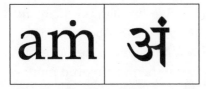

Vidya Mantra: *Aim Hrim Shrim*
Ckaum Am Chitra Nitya
Shri Padukam Pujayami Tarpayami Namah

SADAKHYA/SIXTEENTH NOTCH OF THE FULL MOON: LALITA MAHA TRIPURASUNDARI

Lalita personifies all fifteen Nitya Shaktis. As she reaches fullness in her sixteenth phase, she is known as Sadakhya, noted earlier. Through her immutable reach she endows all deities and Shaktis with pranic power. Her limitless Shakti pervades every living being. The Sri Chakra is considered the vibrational abode of the Supreme Goddess. She is the Deity of the concentric threefold circle depicted in the Sri Chakra yantra, with each nitya portraying a chakra within the legendary yantra. In the *Tantraraja* text, Shiva informs that the Supreme Goddess Lalita resides in the *meru*, centrifugal force of the universe. She is surrounded by the seven oceans containing seven islands beyond which is the kalachakra, wheel of time, which moves in a clockwise course by her will power, or Shakti. The wheel of time is divided into twelve spokes within which the planets are contained. From the meru, Lalita controls her universe with the aid of her nityas—fourteen of whom dwell on the seven islands and seven oceans. Her fifteenth nitya—Chitra—occupies the cosmic space or *paramavyoma*.

The three primary characteristics of Lalita's iconographic symbolism are auspiciousness, purity, and absoluteness. Keep these unconditional virtues in mind while meditating upon the Supreme Goddess. Lalita wields absolute power in ruling her universe. She is beyond conception, the Supreme Goddess who contains everything within her and pervades the entire universe. And yet she is the loving wife to God Shiva and caring mother of her creation. As does Shiva, the entire creation is dependent upon her for its subsisting reality. Once again, we see the unified theme of the interdependence of Shiva and Shakti. In venerating Lalita, emphasis is placed on her cosmic nature of beauty, benevolence, and maternal grace.

Mother's vast power is beyond the reach of word and concept, but you can reach her from within. In the *Lalita Sahasranama*, you are informed that access to the Supreme Goddess is attainable if you worship her with "your mental gaze turned inward"; in other words, the only place you'll discover her is within the temple of yourself. The Supreme Goddess is the source of all mudras and mantras, and therefore you may acknowledge her, worship her, and adore her through practicing her mudras and mantras. The most propitious time to do so is during the full moon.

Use Lalita's image at the beginning of this book to envision her awesome presence. In this chapter, her hands are poised in two of her much-loved mudras depicted in her iconography, Varada Mudra and Abhaya Mudra. Introduced earlier, in the latter hand gesture she gives absolute protection to remove fear from the hearts and minds of her children. Through Varada Mudra she grants boons to her charges fulfilling their desires. This mudra also indicates divine compassion. All believers seek the blessings of the Divine and pray for forgiveness. These two mudras are the most famous mudras among Hindu gods and goddesses since they confirm that our prayers for personal security and fulfillment of our dreams and wishes are being answered. Having captured Mother's awesome essence, begin to recite the powerful Shakti Mantra that follows. Through continual practice, you will gain access to the Supreme Goddess and become aware of the Mother Consciousness within and without.

Shakti Power: Contains power of all Nitya Shaktis
Cosmic Yantra/Sanskrit Vowel: *AH* (pronounced "AHH")

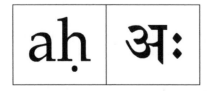

Lalita's Shakti Mantra:
Aim Hrim Shrim
Om Mantra Sarayai Namah
Om Sudhasrtyai Namah
Shri Padukam Pujayami Tarpayami Namah

Pronounced:
Oom Mantra Saa-raa-yai namaha
Oom Su-dhhaas-rit-yai namaha

Reverence to Her who is the Source of all Mantras
Reverence to Her who is the Source of Spiritual Nectar (Knowledge)

YOUR WISE EARTH AYURVEDA® METABOLIC TYPE

In each person, the five elements congregate in patterns of energy known as *doshas*, which rule the functions of the body. The teaching of the doshas is the science of *Ayurveda*, the earth's oldest extant tradition of healing, healthful living, and longevity. To some degree, every person has all three doshas in his or her constitution. Understanding the doshas helps us understand how to get and stay healthy. Western Medicine developed from investigating the microcosm, the physical world of matter and microbes. Ayurvedic Medicine, however, sprang from a deep and penetrating inquiry into the macrocosm. A holistic system, Ayurveda cures by removing the source of disease, which can only happen after you *identify* the source of the disease—not just the symptoms. According to the Vedic seers, disease is caused by living in ways that transgress nature's rhythms and by ignoring our own innate wisdom—dissonant use of the mind and senses, eating improperly, and ignoring the cycles of the seasons.

UNDERSTANDING THE DOSHAS

Knowing which dosha is dominant in your body helps you understand your physical rhythms. The doshas are classic examples of energy and matter in dynamic accord. The literal Sanskrit meaning of dosha is "toxicity" or "impurity," since doshas become visible usually when they are in a state of imbalance. The existence of doshas suggests that the human body is vulnerable to disease; in a state of balance or health, we cannot detect the doshas. In a state of imbalance or disequilibrium, however, the doshas become visible as mucus, bile, wind, and all bodily discharges. If we ignore these early signs of disorder, imbalances can quickly become full-blown disease.

The three doshas coexist to varying degrees in all living organisms, and each is formed by a union of two elements in dynamic balance. Air and space, both ethereal elements, form the dosha called *Vata*. In Vata dosha, air expresses its kinetic power of mobility, which is Vata's physio-psychological nature. Dryness is an attribute of motion and when excessive, it introduces irregularity and changeability into the body and mind. The element of fire forms the dosha known as *Pitta*. In Pitta dosha, fire expresses its transformational power, Pitta's physio-psychological nature. Heat is an attribute of transformation, and when in full force it produces irritability and impatience of the body and mind. In *Kapha* dosha, water expresses a stabilizing force. Heaviness is an attribute of stability, Kapha's physio-psychological nature. Excessive heaviness introduces lethargy into the body and mind.

Each dosha also has a primary function in the body. Vata is the moving force, Pitta is the force of assimilation, and Kapha is the force of stability. Together they are an impressive example of seemingly adversarial forces in potential harmony. Vata is the most dominant dosha in the body, since air, its main element, is much more pervasive in the world than fire and water. Vata tends to go out of balance much more quickly than Pitta and Kapha. Vata governs bodily movement, the nervous system, and the life force. Without Vata's mobility in the body, Pitta and Kapha would be rendered lame. It is most influenced by the *rajas* principle.

Pitta governs enzymatic and hormonal activities, and is responsible for digestion, pigmentation, body temperature, hunger, thirst, and sight. Pitta is a balancing force for Vata and Kapha. It is most influenced by the *sattva* principle.

Kapha governs the body's structure and stability. It lubricates joints, provides moisture to the skin, heals wounds, and regulates Vata and Pitta. Kapha is most influenced by the principle of *tamas*.

Vata, Pitta, and Kapha pervade the entire body, but their primary domains are in the lower, middle, and upper body, respectively. Kapha rules the head, neck, thorax, chest, upper stomach, fat tissues, lymph glands, and joints. Pitta pervades the chest, umbilical area, lower stomach, small intestines, sweat and sebaceous glands, and blood. Vata dominates the lower body, pelvic region, colon, bladder, urinary tract, thighs, legs, arms, bones, and nervous system.

Apart from its main site, each dosha has four secondary sites in different areas of the body. These five sites are considered each dosha's center of operation, and include various support systems for the entire body.

Each of the doshas' five sites has a specific responsibility toward the maintenance of the organism, and interact continuously with the external elements to replenish energy within the body. Thus they are energetically much more influential in the maintenance of our overall health than their mere physiological expressions would suggest. In fact, as they manifest within the physical body, they need to be continually cleansed out of the body in order to maintain harmonious internal rhythms.

Each dosha's seat is associated with organs where its energy and function are most manifested. The primary seat of Vata, for example, is the large intestine. The air of the colon also affects the kidneys, bladder, bones, thighs, ears, and nervous system. Vata's four remaining seats are the skin, lungs, throat, and stomach.

The stomach is Pitta's main seat in the body. The fire of the stomach affects the small intestine, duodenum, gall bladder, liver, spleen, pancreas, and sebaceous glands. Other seats for Pitta are the blood, heart, eyes, and skin.

Kapha's main seat is also the stomach; the water of the stomach affects the lymph glands and fat tissues. Other sites for Kapha are the heart, tongue, joints, and head. The water of the head also affects the nose, throat, and sinuses.

Since each dosha is formed from two elements, it bears the qualities of both. Vata types, for example, influenced by the reigning elements of air and space, tend to be somewhat ungrounded. Pitta types are generally fast, fluid, and fiery, patterned as they are after fire and water. And those in whom Kapha is dominant tend to be slow and methodical, since they are heavily affected by the characteristics of their main elements, water and earth. Every moment of every day, we are able to see the doshas in action through the elemental qualities we find in ourselves and the environment.

ELEMENTAL SOURCE OF METABOLIC TYPES:

VATA	Air/Space
PITTA	Fire/Water
KAPHA	Water/Earth

QUALITIES OF THE METABOLIC TYPES:

VATA (Like Wind)	PITTA (Like Fire)	KAPHA (Like Water)
dry	hot	oily
cold	oily	cool
light	light	heavy
mobile	intense	dense
erratic	fluid	stable
rough	fetid	smooth
bitter	sour	sweet
astringent	pungent	salty
pungent	salty	sour

YOUR METABOLIC CONSTITUTION

The dosha that is dominant in you determines your metabolic type. Knowing what type you are provides you with helpful tools for maintaining a healthy life of balance. It also helps in diagnosing disease. Although disease has numerous causes, including genetic, environmental, and karmic factors, irritation of the doshas is always due to ill health. The proportion to which Vata, Pitta, and Kapha exist within you is what makes your constitution different from someone else's.

Your constitution is determined at birth by the states of balance or imbalance of your parents' rhythms during conception, as well as from the particular permutations of the five elements in the sperm and ovum at the time of conception. Once you are born, your constitution remains constant throughout your lifetime, but the condition of your doshas can change according to disharmonious factors in your lifestyle and environment. The practices of sadhana can help bring back the doshas into a state of harmony and certainly can help maintain your health.

There are other clues to help you determine your own or another's constitution. For example, the Pitta type will tend to have straight hair that is reddish in color. Does this mean if you're of African descent you can't be Pitta? Of course not. The Vedic seers who developed Ayurveda were people of color and of course can be dark-skinned and light-skinned. Even if you are dark-skinned and have essentially black hair, there may be a reddish tinge to the hair; it can be kinky, but it will get prematurely gray. Pitta skin may have a reddish tone as well, and regardless of the underlying skin color, it will be oily and warm.

Pitta types are more shapely and athletic than Vata or Kapha. Their body has the shape of an inverted triangle—broad-shouldered and slim-hipped. They tend to eat spicy, pungent foods, and sweat a lot. They can be moderate in weight. Pitta can have brown or hazel eyes, or greenish ones like tigers. They may be fiery or volatile or aggressive in temperament. Their physical problems are generally related to the stomach, liver, spleen and small intestine—hyper-acidity, diarrhea, poor sight, skin rashes, liver, spleen, and blood disorders are some of the common complaints of Pitta types. Their strengths are that of good physical stamina, strong intelligence and mental focus. They also tend to be successful, courageous, and practical in their dealings.

Vata types have hair that is thin and dry and often kinky or frizzy. Their skin has a grayish hue. They tend to be thin and angular, because they're formed by the wind, like a desert plant. Their eyes are usually brown, narrow, and uneven in shape, and their skin is always dry around the eyes. Likewise, they often have dry, cracked skin. Vata types have trouble putting on weight and often seem mentally distracted. Generally their physical problems are in the lower body, the large intestine and colon, because that's the seat of Vata. They tend to develop conditions such as constipation, insomnia, flatulence, arthritis, and osteoporosis.

Their strengths are that of a strong and sensitive spirit. They strive for inner freedom and are generally environmentally and spiritually attuned. They have deep faith and are generally flexible and adaptable to life's varying situations.

Kapha types are the most voluptuous, with abundant, wavy hair. They have what I call a "moonlit" complexion, meaning that the hue is very fair regardless of color. Many dark people have translucent skin that looks as if the moon is reflected in it. Their eyelashes are long and curled, and the eyes themselves tend to be big pools. They have a cool and complacent temperament. They have moist skin that can be oily, but is always cool; their hands and feet are typically cool. The weak spot for Kapha is in the upper body: lungs, throat, thyroid, and tonsils, and they tend to be susceptible to conditions such as colds, coughs, allergies, tonsillitis, and bronchitis. Their strengths are that of physical and maternal endurance, calmness, and patience. Humility, nurturance, and fortitude are common Kapha virtues.

Once you understand these concepts, you can determine the constitution of the people around you. For example, my assistant is a Vata-Pitta type. Her skin tends to be dry. She has a strong spiritual temperament, with a deep spiritual faith. She loves her inner freedom, although she can be impatient. My mother is the rare Kapha-Vata type who is immensely patient and steadfast. My father is a Pitta-Kapha type who had a full head of abundant, wavy locks, with a quick and alert mind. He excelled in meeting life cheerfully regardless of the obstacles he faced.

The box below summarizes the characteristics of the nine different body types—Vata, Pitta, and Kapha, and the various combinations of the three doshas.

VATA

Element: air/space
Energy: cold
Texture: dry, rough
Temperament: austere, indecisive
Emotional Strength: spiritually adept
Emotional Weakness: irregularity, fearful
Body Structure: thin, angular, very short or very tall
Complexion: brownish or greyish

PITTA

Element: fire/water
Energy: hot
Texture: oily, soft
Temperament: fiery, vibrant
Emotional Strength: materially adept, visionary
Emotional Weakness: indulgent, aggressive
Body Structure: athletic, well-shaped
Complexion: yellowish or reddish

KAPHA

Element: water/earth

Energy: cool

Texture: smooth, dense

Temperament: methodical, slow

Emotional Strength: maternal, nurturing

Emotional Weakness: attachment, greediness

Body Structure: heavy, compact

Complexion: pale, clear

VATA-PITTA

Element: dominant—air/space, subordinate—fire/water

Energy: cool

Texture: sometimes dry, sometimes oily

Temperament: sometimes indecisive and sometimes fiery

Emotional Strength: spiritually inclined, goal-oriented

Emotional Weakness: irregular, fearful, and sometimes aggressive

Body Structure: thin, tall, or lanky

Complexion: brownish or yellowish

PITTA-VATA

Element: dominant—fire/water, subordinate—air/space

Energy: warm

Texture: oily, sometimes dry

Temperament: cheerful, sometimes aggressive

Emotional Strength: materially adept, goal-oriented

Emotional Weakness: ambitious, intolerant

Body Structure: moderate to thin, well-shaped

Complexion: yellowish or tan

KAPHA-VATA

Element: dominant—water/earth, subordinate—air/space

Energy: cold

Texture: smooth, dense, sometimes dry and rough

Temperament: extreme tendencies, sometimes methodical, and sometimes indecisive

Emotional Strength: nurturing, spiritually inclined

Emotional Weakness: unmotivated, attached

Body Structure: moderate to heavy (easy to gain weight, easy to lose weight)

Complexion: pale, sometimes dark

VATA-KAPHA

Element: dominant—air/space, subordinate—water/earth

Energy: cold

Texture: dry, sometimes smooth

Temperament: extreme tendencies, mercurial, irregular

Emotional Strength: spiritually adept, maternal

Emotional Weakness: isolated, fearful

Body Structure: thin to moderate (easy to lose weight, easy to gain)

Complexion: dark, sometimes pale

PITTA-KAPHA

Element: dominant—fire/water, subordinate—water/earth

Energy: warm

Texture: soft, moist

Temperament: decisive, patient

Emotional Strength: well-balanced, materially adept, vital

Emotional Weakness: possessive, indulgent

Body Structure: well-shaped, moderate to heavy

Complexion: reddish, sometimes pale

KAPHA-PITTA

Element: dominant—water/earth, subordinate—fire/water

Energy: cool, sometimes warm

Texture: smooth, dense, moist

Temperament: slow but methodical

Emotional Strength: excellent stamina, tenacious

Emotional Weakness: stubborn, lethargic

Body Structure: solid, curvaceous, and heavy

Complexion: pale, sometimes reddish

NURTURING YOUR METABOLIC TYPE

The Ayurveda principle of "like increases like" helps us nourish our individual rhythms and achieve balance in our lives. According to this principle, we are nurtured by the elements and inclinations other than those innate to our metabolic type. Just as an individual who has a predominant quality of air in his or her nature has to work on building more stability, one who is extremely fiery needs to develop more moderation in his or her activities. You should avoid the intake of things that are like your own qualities—qualities that you already have—and increase the intake of things that are unlike your constitutional attributes.

ELEMENTS THAT NURTURE THE METABOLIC TYPES

VATA: (Nurtured by fire, water, and earth)	PITTA: (Nurtured by water, air, space, and earth)	KAPHA: (Nurtured by fire, air, and space)
consistent	calm	stimulating
moist	cool	dry
heavy	substantial	warm
smooth	aromatic	light
hot	sweet	pungent
sweet	bitter	bitter
salty	astringent	astringent

NURTURING YOUR PERSONAL RHYTHMS

These balancing principles are to be applied especially during your most vulnerable seasons. Each dosha is increased in its own seasons providing increased opportunity to gain a deeper understanding of our inner rhythms. The Vata seasons are early fall and autumn. The Pitta seasons are spring and summer. The Kapha seasons are early and late winter. Follow the recommendations presented below that are most appropriate for your metabolic type, as determined in the chart in this Appendix. And keep in mind that, depending on your imbalances and seasonal demands, you may be able to engage from time to time in the nourishing regimens other than those for your own prakriti.

For Vata Type: Nourishing Quick and Irregular Rhythms
Balancing Principle: Stability
• Maintain a steady routine around eating and sleeping habits.

- Choose only the activities that create ease and allow yourself adequate time to complete them.
- Take ample rest.
- Eat wholesome, fresh, warm, moist, and nourishing foods.
- Avoid bitter, cold, fermented, stale, and raw foods.
- Buffer yourself against cold, damp, and wet environments.
- Make an effort to embrace warmth, love, healthy rituals, and routines.

For Pitta Type: Nourishing Fast and Decisive Rhythms
Balancing Principle: Moderation
- Rise with the sun and go to bed by 10 p.m.
- Plan activities ahead to avoid time pressure.
- Ease yourself out of all stressful activities and maintain only those projects that create ease.
- Eat wholesome, moderately cool, or warm, substantial, and calming foods.
- Avoid hot, spicy, oily, salty, fermented, and stale foods, as well as the use of stimulants.
- Shield yourself against hot, humid, and stressful environments.
- Make an attempt to embrace serenity and calmness.

For Kapha Type: Nourishing Slow and Methodical Rhythms
Balancing Principle: Stimulation
- Engage in stimulating physical exercise every day.
- Open yourself to new and invigorating experiences.
- Rise with the sun every day.
- Eat wholesome, light, warm, pungent, and stimulating foods.
- Avoid cold, oily, rich, and excessively sweet, sour, or salty foods.
- Buffer yourself against cold, damp, and wet environments.
- Unburden yourself of all old loads and lighten your heart.

NOURISHING FOODS FOR YOUR WISE EARTH AYURVEDA® METABOLIC TYPE

Following is a list of nourishing foods for your unique metabolic type. My upcoming book *Abundance: From Feast to Fast* provides a complete list of food recommendations and seasonal recipes suitable for your metabolic type.

NOURISHING FOODS FOR VATA TYPES

To buffer the cold, dry, and cranky qualities of Vata, take easy to digest, warm, and nourishing foods. Use fresh, organic, seasonal, and local, family farm-grown foods if possible.

The following food recommendations are the most appropriate for long-term use by the Vata type:

Avoid caffeine, refined sweets, alcohol, saturated fats, excess salt, oily and spicy foods, and commercial dairy products. Highly processed junk foods, meats, and refined foods that are packed with additives are also to be avoided. Avoid frozen, canned, stale, commercially grown, bioengineered, transgenic foods; irradiated spices; refined salts, sugars, flours, and hydrogenated oils.

Vegetables (Use Seasonally):
Sweet potatoes, yams, pumpkins, winter squashes (acorn, butternut, buttercup), summer squashes (yellow, crookneck, zucchini, patty pan), watercress, bok choy, asparagus, carrots, daikon, green beans, beets, leeks (cooked), onions (cooked), broccoli, cauliflower, and cooked leafy greens.

Fruits (Use Seasonally):
Apricots, avocados, bananas, berries, cherries, coconuts, grapefruit, oranges, kiwi, lemons, limes, tangerines, mangos, melon, papaya, peaches, pineapple, plums, rhubarb, tamarind, dates, figs, raisins, grapes, and strawberries. (Dried fruits are to be cooked before using.)

Grains (Whole, Cracked, and Cereal):
Brown rice (short, medium, and long grain), Basmati white and brown rice, Arborio Rice, sushi rice, wild rice; oats, cracked wheat, spelt, and kamut; whole wheat, spelt, or kamut berries; barley, quinoa, and amaranth.
Use Occasionally: Soft cooked millet, bulgur, rolled oats (cooked), wheat pasta, rice noodles, and couscous.

.Legumes:
Aduki, mung (whole, split), tofu (cooked), kidney, lima, lentils, and black beans.

Nuts and Seeds (Use Occasionally):
Almonds, macadamias, pumpkin seeds, Brazil nuts, peanuts, sesame seeds, chestnuts, pecans, sunflower seeds, cashews, pine nuts, walnuts, and pistachios.

Dairy (Organic):
Buttermilk, whole cow's milk cheese, cream, butter, ghee, yogurt, cottage cheese, and sour cream.
Use Occasionally: Mild soft cheeses.

Oils:
Dark sesame, light sesame, almond, olive, and sunflower.

Sweeteners:
Juice concentrates, maple syrup, dates, Sucanat, sugar cane juice, jaggery, and unprocessed brown sugar.

Herbs & Spices:
Anise, asafetida, basil, black pepper, bay leaf, cayenne, coriander, cumin, fennel, caraway, cardamom, saffron, mustard seeds, sage, nutmeg, savory, curry powder, ginger, parsley, tarragon, oregano, thyme, turmeric, cinnamon, cloves, rosemary, curry leaves, garam masala, and garlic.

NOURISHING FOODS FOR PITTA TYPES

To reduce the hot, penetrating, and volatile qualities of Pitta, take easy to digest, fresh, warm, and nourishing foods. The following food recommendations are the most appropriate for long-term use by the Pitta type. Use fresh, organic, seasonal, and local, family farm-grown foods.

Avoid caffeine, refined sweets, alcohol, saturated fats, excess salt, oily and spicy foods, and commercial dairy products. Highly processed junk foods, meats, and refined foods that are packed with additives are also to be avoided. Avoid frozen, canned, stale, commercially grown, bioengineered, transgenic foods; irradiated spices; refined salts, sugars, flours, and hydrogenated oils.

Vegetables (Use Seasonally):
Greens (kales, collards, bok choy, mustard, landcress, watercress), bitter greens (arugula, radicchio, dandelion, lettuces, endives), asparagus, green beans, artichokes, broccoli, cauliflower, brussel sprouts, cabbage, cucumbers, jicama, artichokes, karela, okra, parsnips, peas, potatoes, sprouts, sweet potatoes, yams, pumpkin, winter squashes (acorn, butternut, buttercup), summer squashes (yellow, crookneck, zucchini, patty pan) bamboo shoots, celery, black olives, and pumpkins.

Fruits (Use Seasonally):
Apples, apricots, berries, cherries, coconuts, dates, fresh figs, grapes, sweet oranges, pears, pomegranates, sweet tangerines, mangos, melons, pineapples, plums, raisins, cherries, watermelons, strawberries, kiwi, quinces, limes, and sweet dried fruits.

Grains (Whole, Cracked, and Cereal):
Barley oats, cracked wheat, spelt, and kamut; whole wheat, spelt, or kamut berries; barley, long grain brown rice, sweet brown rice, Basmati white and brown rice, Arborio rice, and sushi rice.
Use Occasionally: Rolled oats, wheat cereals, barley cereals, wheat or spelt pasta bulgur, steel cut oats, whole wheat or spelt flour, and couscous.

Legumes:
Aduki, mung (whole and split), soya, kidney, lima, lentils, black beans, chickpeas, navy, pinto, split peas, and tofu.

Nuts (Use Occasionally):
Coconut, roasted sunflower seeds, roasted pumpkin seeds, poppy seeds, and water chestnuts (cooked).

Dairy (Organic):
Butter (unsalted), cow's milk, cottage cheese, and sweetened yogurt.
Use Occasionally: Mild soft cheeses.

Oils:
Sunflower, soya, olive, and coconut.

Sweeteners:
Barley malt, maple syrup, dates, fruit concentrates (apples, pears, mango, figs, apri-

cots, grapes), unprocessed brown sugar, and Sucanat.

Herbs & Spices:
Coriander, cumin, cardamom, cilantro, curry leaves, dill, fresh basil, fennel, turmeric, saffron, peppermint, spearmint, and ginger.
Use Occasionally: Black pepper, cloves, nutmeg, mild curry powder, mild garam masala, caraway, cinnamon, and mace.

NOURISHING FOODS FOR KAPHA TYPES

To ward off the cold and sluggish qualities of Kapha, warm, stimulating, and nourishing foods should be taken during your menstrual cycle. Use fresh, organic, and local, family farm-grown foods. The following food recommendations are the most appropriate for long-term use by the Kapha type.

Avoid caffeine, refined sweets, alcohol, saturated fats, excess salt, oily and spicy foods, and commercial dairy products. Highly processed junk foods, meats, and refined foods that are packed with additives are also to be avoided. Avoid frozen, canned, stale, commercially grown, bioengineered, transgenic foods; irradiated spices; refined salts, sugars, flours, and hydrogenated oils.

Vegetables (Use Seasonally):
Greens (kales, collards, bok choy, mustard, landcress, watercress, turnip greens), bitter greens (arugula, radicchio, dandelion, lettuces, endives), asparagus, green beans, artichokes, broccoli, bell peppers, peppers, carrots, carrot tops, celery, corn, eggplant, karela, jicama, leeks, cauliflower, brussel sprouts, cabbage, okra, parsnips, peas, potatoes, sprouts, summer squashes (yellow, crookneck, zucchini, patty pan), spinach, sprouts, and turnips.

Fruits (Use Seasonally):
Apples, apricots, berries, cherries, peaches, pears, persimmons, pomegranates, quinces, and raisins.
Use Occasionally: Grapes, tangerines, mangos, oranges, limes, lemons, raisins, and strawberries.

Grains (Whole, Cracked, and Cereal)
Barley, buckwheat, millet, rye, and corn.
Use Occasionally: Long grain brown and Basmati rice, quinoa, oats, and amaranth, barley, rye, and millet cereals; rye, millet, and barley flours; rye pasta, buckwheat pasta, oat bran, corn grits, and soba noodles.
Use Rarely: Cracked wheat, spelt, and kamut.

Legumes:
Aduki, mung (whole and split), soya, kidney, lima, red lentils, black beans, chick-peas, navy, pinto, split peas, and tofu.

Seeds:
Roasted pumpkin seeds and roasted sunflower seeds.

Dairy (Organic):
Goat's milk and unsalted goat's cheese.
Use Occasionally: Spiced yogurt drinks and ghee.

Oils (Use Minimally):
Corn, sunflower, olive, and mustard.

Sweeteners (Use Minimally):
Raw honey, rice or maple syrup, barley malt, dried fruits, and citrus fruit juice concentrates.

Herbs & Spices:
Ajwain, cinnamon, hot peppers, pippali, allspice, cloves, marjoram, rosemary, anise, coriander, mustard seeds, saffron, asafetida, cumin, sage, basil, curry leaves, nutmeg, bay leaf, curry powder, tarragon, black pepper, dill, orange peel, thyme, caraway, dill seeds, oregano, turmeric, cardamom, ginger, paprika, cayenne, gar-lic, parsley, cilantro, garam masala, spearmint, and peppermint.

Aditi. free, vast space, whole; cosmic womb of creation; the Source, Aditi is sometimes depicted as the Cow of Plenty; one who feeds the celestials, humans, and spirit; the Perfumed One

Adi Rishi. "the first seer"; The Sage Narayana is considered the first *rishi* to "see" and articulate Vedic vision. The knowledge he shares is in the 16 mantras known as *Purusha Sukta*—which provides information on the cosmic anatomy and ecology

Agni. "fire"; one of the fire elements; god of the element fire, invoked through Vedic ritual, the God Agni is the divine receiver of oblations and prayers

Advaita. the doctrine of monism, according to which Reality is ultimately non-dual, comprised of One Whole principle; the vision of Vedanta

ahamkara. ego in Vedic anatomy; the "I" notion; cosmic memory recorder; located at the base of the brain where ego functions are stored

ahara rasa. ingested nutrients, before they are digested

Aham Brahmasmi. literally, "I am Brahman"—Pure Consciousness

ahimsa. "nonharming"; abstinence from harmful thought, action, or word; a significant moral discipline in Hinduism

ajna. "limitless power"; name of sixth chakra

ama. metabolic toxicity caused from poor digestion, undigested food, poor quality foods, and so on

amavasya. "new moon"; representing the lunar emanation of rebirth

anahata. fearless, non-afflicted; nature of the black antelope; symbol and name of fourth chakra

ananda, anandam. essence of reality; limitless consciousness; the state of the Ultimate Reality of self, and universe

angula. the Vedic unit of measurement that refers to the distance between the joints of each finger; this unit of measurement may be used to gauge spices, herbs, such as cinnamon sticks, and the roots of turmeric and ginger

anjali. "Prayer Mudra" of the hands clasped with palms touching; also a unit of measurement in Vedas, which refers to the volume that can be held when two hands are cupped together

ankusha. "goad"; symbol of God Ganesha's power to remove obstacles from the spiritual aspirant's path

annam. "that which grows on the earth"; food as in nature's plants, fruit, leaves, herbs, seeds, grains, minerals, twigs, roots, and barks intended to feed, nourish, and foster good health; plant life is a special sacrifice decreed by the Supreme Goddess for the benefit of her children

annamaya. earthly plane of existence; food-sheath; first depth of cosmic anatomy

annaprasana. Vedic food offering ceremony; or rites of nourishment

anubhava. personal experience

anupana. in Ayurveda, the medicinal base, like ghee and honey, used to transport and direct medicines into specific tissues of the body

apana. fourth air of the cosmos; keeper of the emptiness; preserves spirit of nonattachment; one of five bodily airs; air controlling ejection of bodily wastes

apsaras. celestial beings

arogya. "health"; the opposite of disease (*vyadhi*); excellent state of well-being; true nature of the Self

artava. "ovum"; the seventh and final tissue layer; female reproductive tissue; derived from the Sanskrit root *rtu,* meaning "season"; according to Ayurveda plentiful *ojas* in the body depends on the healthy quality of *artava* and *sukra* (sperm)

asthi. bone and cartilage tissue; fifth layer of vital tissue in the body

Atharva Veda. "Atharvan's knowledge"; one of four Vedas that deals with magical spells, rituals, and *prayogas*; source of Ayurveda (See also *Rig Veda, Sama Veda,* and *Yajur Veda*)

Atman. indwelling spirit; soul within body; Conscious Self

avidya. "ignorance"; generally refers to ignorance of the absolute reality, or of the True Self

Ayurveda. "science of life, health, and longevity"; an eight-branch holistic system of medicine considered the first medicine system in the world. It is the most comprehensive nature-based system of health and healing. Rooted in the *Atharva Veda* and *Rig Veda,* Ayurveda Medicine includes: general medicine, surgery, physiology, gynecology, psychology, pediatrics, diseases of the head, pharmacology, veterinary science, herbology, rejuvenation therapies, sexual rejuvenation, science of the subtle body, and demonology.

bhaga. one who contains all power, wealth, fame, beauty and virtues; name for the vulva

Bhagamalini Nitya. "flowering yoni"; lunar deity of the second notch of the waxing moon cycle

Bhagavan. "one who possesses sixfold virtue"; a god of the *Rig Veda,* Lord of wealth, power, and happiness

bhakti. faith, devotion

bhakti marga. path of devotion

Bherunda Nitya. golden in color, she is the lunar deity of the fourth notch of the waxing moon cycle

Bhramari. "a bee"; a traditional breath practice named after the Goddess Bhramari in which the practitioner imitates the bee and vibrates the entire nervous system, brain, and body, by buzzing the vocal chords

bija. "seed"; as in, *bija mantra*; a karmic imprint on the subconscious

bija mantra. "seed syllable"; a primordial sound, such as *aim, hrim, shrim*

bindu. "drop"; the dot placed above the Sanskrit letter "m" in a syllabic word or mantra; the nasalized sound itself; also, an energy center of consciousness in the head directly above *ajna* chakra

Brahmacharini. spiritual aspirant in Vedic monastic lineage; one whose life is devoted to the pursuit of spiritual knowledge; student of the Vedas; one whose conduct is *Brahman*, conscious and compassionate

Brahmacharya. one of the foundational practices of yoga, renunciation of the material world and devotion to scriptural study; the observance of chastity in thought, word, or action

Brahman. Absolute Consciousness, which is distinct from *Brahma*, the Creator (deity of the *buddhi*)

Brahmana, Brahmin. "evolved or mature soul"; the soul which is exemplary of wisdom, tolerance, and humility; from *Brahman*, "growth, evolution, swelling of the spirit"; also, a member of the priestly class of Vedic society

Brahma Shabda. cosmic sound

Brahmavidya. knowledge of Brahman—the Ultimate Reality

buddhi. cognition; faculty of personal wisdom; intuitive faculty; resolve of the mind; the intellect; *buddhi* is characterized by the fivefold qualities in yoga: discrimination (*viveka*), voluntary restraint (*vairagya*), cultivation of inner quietude (*shanti*), contentment (*santosha*), and forgiveness (*kshama*). Also, Buddhi-Mercury, son of Shiva; deity who rules Wednesday

chakra. "wheel"; the energy centers of consciousness located within the subtle body (There are 14 major chakras in all, seven primary chakras can be seen psychically as multi-petaled lotuses, each bearing one of the colors of the rainbow. These are situated along the spinal column from the base to the cranial chamber. Additionally, there are seven chakras, barely visible, that exist below the spine. These are the centers of karmic consciousness, the seat of all negative emotions.)

chandra-mauli. "moon-crested"; a blood vessel in the vulva which acts as a magnetic lodestone, drawing the energy of the moon to revitalize the womb

chandra-mukha. "moon-faced"; a Sanskrit name for the vagina

chapati. thin Vedic flatbread baked on a skillet and allowed to balloon over an open fire

chit. pure awareness; that which is self-revealing; transcendent consciousness, beyond all thought

Chitra Nitya. "variegated"; the lunar deity for the 15th notch of the waxing moon cycle

chitta. "mind"; "memory"; the psyche or consciousness that depends on the play of attention, as opposed to *chit*

Dakshinamurti. "south-facing form"; Lord Shiva depicted sitting under a *pipala* tree, transmitting the knowledge of the Vedas through silence to four *rishis*

damaru. "drum"; a small double-headed, hourglass-shaped drum used in Vedic rituals and meditation practices (The sound of this drum is associated with the element of space.)

darshana. "vision"; "sight"; seeing with inner or outer vision; receiving the grace and blessing of the deity, holy person or place (Gods, Goddesses, and Gurus are said to "give" darshana, while disciples and devotees "receive" darshana. This direct infusion of energy and blessing from a venerated being is a long-standing tradition and sought after experience of Hindu faith.)

Deva. "shining one"; "god"; generic name referring to Vedic gods; *devas* are powerful beings in the subtle realms of existence

Devabhasa. cosmic medium of communication used by the gods and goddesses; original name of the Sanskrit language (The proper name of the Sanskrit language is *Samskritam*)

Devi. "the shining one"; generic name for the Mother Goddess

dhal. traditional Indian bean soup

dhara. "bowl" and "womb"; inferring that the cosmic bowl of the womb is pervaded by lunar energies

dharana. "sustaining"; concentration; prolonged focus of attention on a single mental object and leading to meditation

Dhara Devi. "support"; a name of the Earth-Goddess

dharma. from *dhri*, "to sustain, carry or hold"; Divine law; right action according to the laws of nature; also, the path of righteousness, virtue, justice, and truth (Dharma is the inherent nature of the human and its fulfillment is the profound aim of human destiny)

dhatus. seven layers of vital tissues in the body responsible for safeguarding its cellular memory and immunological function

dhup, dhupam. pine kindling used in Vedic fire rituals

dhyana. "meditation"; meditative contemplation or absorption; the seventh limb of Patanjali's eightfold Yoga

doshas. bodily humors of which there are three: *Vata* (air/space), *Pitta* (fire/water), and *Kapha* (water/earth); also, *dosha* refers to the five flaws of human nature: lust, anger, greed, fear, and delusion

Duti Nitya. surrounded by *rishis* who sing her praises, she is the lunar deity of the seventh notch of the waxing moon cycle

dvani. dynamic, audible sound

Gaja. "elephant"; elephant symbol of the fifth chakra, *vishuddha*

Gandarva. "fragrant"; the name of the celestial musicians

Ganga. Ganges River originating from the head of Shiva; considered the most sacred river by Hindus; *Ganga Mata* is the name given to Goddess of the River (Each day millions of Hindus take sacred dips in this Holy River and its tributaries.)

garbha. embryo; according to the Vedas the soul enters the body along with the eightfold material for creation

garbhadhana. Vedic fertility rites or the rite of conception

Gayatri. the celebrated mantra of the *Rig Veda* imparted to the *Brahmins* at the time of their initiation into *Brahmacharya* at the age of eight. The Gayatri Mantra is considered the greatest among Vedic hymns. It is addressed to the sun-god as a form of the divine light. Gayatri is also called the Mother of the Vedas, and protects those who recite it.

ghee. purified butter, prepared by simmering unsalted butter on low heat until all the water content of the butter boils off and the milk solids remain. Ghee is considered a primary elixir of good health.

guna. quality, nature, or virtue; also the three primordial aspects of creation—*sattva, rajas,* and *tamas*

guru. spiritual teacher or enlightened person in the Hindu tradition; belonging to the Vedic lineage

ha. Sanskrit syllable representing the solar energy

hamsa. "gander"; generally translated as "swan," the breath, or life force (*prana*); a type of wandering ascetic

Hatha Yoga. "yoga of force"; the yoga of physical and mental discipline developed by the seers as a means of physical, emotional, and spiritual revitalization. Hatha Yoga consists of postures (*asanas*), internal cleansing practices (*dhanti* or *shodhana*), breath control (*pranayama*), locks (*bandhas*), and sacred hand gestures (*mudras*), all of which regulate and energize the flow of *prana* and purify body, mind, and spirit.

ida-nadi. "soothing conduit"; the lunar, feminine current flowing along the left channel of the spine

jivaniyagana. in Ayurveda, plants rich in vitalizing energy with the chromosomes, hormones, and proteins to maintain vigor and balance in the female hormones

jnana. liberating wisdom; according to the *rishis, jnana* is the last of the four successive stages (*padas*) of spiritual unfoldment

jnani. a wise and enlightened person; according to the vedas, it is possible to gain enlightenment even while still embodied—the self-realized sage who is thus liberated is known as a *jnani* or *jiva-mukti*

Jvalamalini Nitya. "garland of flames"; lunar deity for the 14th notch of the waxing moon cycle

kala. "time"; an integral aspect of the finite world; nutritional membrane for vital tissues

kalala. soft mass of the embryo in the first month of life

kalachakra. wheel of time; the time/space continuum; 15 *kalas* (phases of time); the history of eternity as it evolved from Lalita, the Supreme Goddess

Kali. "darkness"; Vedic goddess Kali, who destroys illusions; Hindus honor her as the Great Mother from whom all are born and to whom all must return (According to Vedic cosmology, we are living in the age of Kali. Kali energy is what moves through us in times of stupendous change and transformation.)

Kali-Yuga. "yoke of Kali"; the fourth and final phase of universal existence; the age of cosmic dissolution that precedes the dawn of the golden era (This period is believed to have commenced in 3102 B.C.E.)

kama. "desire"; a deity, the Vedic Cupid; also, excessive desire or lust, one of the obstacles on the spiritual path

Kameshvara. *kama*=desire; *Isvara*=Highest Lord, Supreme or Personal God; Shiva as the presiding deity of the moon chakra in the form of the primeval desire, *Kama*.

Kameshvari. *kama*=desire; *Isvari*=Supreme or Personal Goddess; Shakti as the presiding female deity of the moon chakra in the form of the primeval desire; first of the 15 *nityas*, or lunar deities; consort of Kameshvara

Kameshvari Nitya. "deity of desire"; the lunar deity of the new moon; first notch of the waxing moon cycle

Kapha. one of three doshas; biological water humor; the principle of potential energy which controls body stability and lubrication

karana sarira. causal body; the soul "form"; also called *anandamaya kosha* (sheath that masks consciousness)

karma. duty; consequences of actions; deeds performed from free will

karma yoga. "yoga of action"; the necessary performance of actions that are in harmony with one's innermost purpose, nature, and being (*sva-bhava*); a primary life practice in yoga

kichadi. a traditional repast in Ayurveda wherein specific quantities of grain and bean are combined with gentle spices and ghee into a thick wholesome porridge (Basmati rice and mung beans are generally used.)

kosha. "sheath"; Vedic term for a bodily casing, of which there are five: the food-body, breath-body, mind-body, cognitive-body, and infinity-body or Infinite Self

krishna paksha. "dark phase" of moon transiting from full to new; waning cycle

kshiri vrksha. milky sap of the plant; in Ayurveda, medicinal plants with milky sap used to cure infertility and boost hormonal activity

Kulasundari Nitya. showing the mudra of exposition, she is the lunar deity for the ninth notch of the waxing moon cycle

kundal. "coiled"; referring to the serpentine force of Kundalini

kundalini. the primordial cosmic force embedded in the first chakra; primal energy of manifestation symbolized by a coiled serpent at the coccyx of the spine (The kundalini's ascent to the crown chakra creates a temporary state of transcendence into the Absolute Reality.)

Lalita Maha Tripurasundari. "Mother Consciousness"; Lalita Maha Tripurasundari is the central goddess to the Sri Vidya (Auspicious Wisdom) tradition of Hinduism; she transcends all forms—gross, subtle, and transcendent; she is Pure Consciousness (In Vedic iconography, she is portrayed as a woman-child Goddess who delights in *lila*, play and pleasure. She is in the center of the *meru*, centrifugal force of the universe, from where she rules the three worlds and controls the wheel of time and space. She projects 15 Nitya Shaktis.)

Lalita Sahasranama. one thousand Sanskrit names of the Supreme Goddess venerating her absolute nature; name of the text with 1000 names of the Goddess

linga, lingam. "sign or attribute of Shiva"; Shiva's cosmic pillar which emerges from the base of Shakti and stretches far into the sky; from this pillar of infinity emanates the cosmic sound, OM

Maha-kala. "great time"; dissolver of time"; one of the names and forms for Shiva, Maha-kala devours time and with it all forms, and by so doing, helps the soul to transcend the nature of dualities

Maha Shakti. "Great Mother"; the feminine power of creation

Mahavajreshvari Nitya. rose red in color, she is the lunar deity of the sixth notch of the waxing moon cycle

majja. marrow tissue; sixth layer of vital tissue in the body

mala. traditional Vedic prayer beads consisting of 108 beads, or multiples of nine; forerunner to the rosary; also, a garland of flowers

mamsa. muscle tissue; third layer of vital tissue in the body

manas. the mind; mental acuity; empirical mind; seat of desire and governor of the sensory and motor organs: *manas* is characterized by desire and willpower

mandala. a circular mystical diagram, *yantra*, without beginning or end—symbolizing the infinite; a picture or group of syllables or words used in meditation to access the infinite inner realm

mandir. Hindu temple

mahabhutas. the five gross elements—space, air, fire, water, and earth

manipura. "city of gems"; third chakra; psychic center at the solar plexus which governs willpower

manomaya. sheath that masks the mind; mental plane; third layer of vedic cosmic anatomy

mantra. "mystic sound"; a sound, syllable, word, or phrase in Sanskrit imbued with significant power (When chanted, mantras help to calm the mind, harmonize the body's rhythms and evoke deep spiritual qualities. Traditionally, to be effective, mantras must be given by the preceptor through initiation.)

Mantra Yoga. the yoga of mystic sound; recital of the Vedic chants

marma. Ayurveda's vast tapestry of the anatomical reflex points of the body; junctions of *pranic* energy; vital junctures where muscles, tendons, joints and ligaments intersect; precursor system to acupuncture

masala. a traditional mixture of Indian spices

mouna. silence, a primary aspect of yoga *sadhana* practice

Maya. "measure"; the creative operative force of creation, preservation, and dissolution; the mirage that hides the Ultimate Reality; the principle of manifestation; relative reality

Maya Shakti. Mother Nature; the primordial force behind creation

medas. fat tissue; fourth layer of vital tissue in the body

mithya. interdependent; that which has its basis in something else (For example, the Creation has its source in the Absolute Reality and cannot exist without it.)

moksha. "liberation"; "release"; liberation from the cycles of rebirth which according to Vedanta, is the highest of four possible human pursuits or goals; final liberation or Self-realization

mudra. "seal"; a sacred hand gesture which evokes cosmic consciousness; moves *prana* to shift negative energy into positive vibration (Mudras are a vital and integral aspect of Hinduism's healing modalities such as, ritual, worship, prayer, dance, yoga, and Ayurveda.)

Mudra Vijnanam. the knowledge of sacred hand practices developed by the Vedic seers

muladhara. "not supported"; first chakra; four-petaled psychic center, located at the base of the spine, which governs memory

muni. an ascetic, or forest-dwelling sage, who has kinship with all creatures; also, one who practices *mouna*, silence

nada. inaudible cosmic sound or vibration

nadi. "conduit"; "channel"; according to Ayurveda, the human anatomy consists of a network of 72,000 subtle conduits or nerve channels, along which flows *prana*, the life force; of these channels, three are most significant—*ida, pingala,* and *sushumna*

Nataraja. "King of Dance"; God Shiva as the Cosmic Dancer depicts stillness and motion, spirituality and creativity, creator and the created, merging into One Consciousness; Nataraja represents the Primal Soul (*Paramesvara*), power, energy, and life of all that exists

Navaratri. A nine-day Hindu festival celebrating the Goddess Mother in her three primary forms—Saraswati, Lakshmi, and Durga. This festival occurs twice annually during the onset of the waxing moon in spring and autumn

Nilapataka Nitya. "sapphire banner"; she is the lunar deity for the 11th notch of the waxing moon cycle

nimitta karana. "efficient cause", one who is an instrument of truth

Nityaklinna Nitya. "eternally wet"; lunar deity of the third notch of the waxing moon cycle

Nitya Nitya. "eternity"; the lunar deity for the 10th notch of the waxing moon cycle

nityas. "eternities"; lunar deities representing the 15 *kalas*, or phases of the waxing moon; goddess emanations of the Supreme Goddess of the universe

ojas. "glow of health"; cellular immunity reflected in one's aura; energy produced through disciplined yogic practice, especially the practice of chastity

pada. the foot; section, stage, or path; according to *Shaiva Siddhanta*, there are four *padas* or stages for the soul to move through

padabhyanga. Ayurvedic foot massage

paramavyoma. "cosmic space"; abode of Chitra; 15th Nitya of the moon

parampara. a lineage; unimpeded succession (i.e., the Vedic parampara of the *Guru* tradition)

Parashiva. Lord Shiva as the pillar of consciousness; one of two primordial aspects of creation; Absolute Reality

Parashakti. Goddess Shakti as the basis of creation; one of two primordial aspects of creation; beyond time, space, and form

Pasupati. "lord of souls"; Shiva as Lord of the Creatures

Patanjali. Traditionally regarded as the author of the *Yoga Sutras* and of the *Brahma-Sutra of Badarayana*, one of the foundational works of the Vedanta tradition. Patanjali lived in 200 C.E. It is also the name of the Sanskrit grammarian who lived in 150 C.E.

phalaghrita. "ghee or essence of the fruit"; a classical Ayurveda remedy used to increase *ojas* in the body (It consists of three ancient myrobalans (fruits) mixed with medicinal ghee.)

pingala nadi. "tawny conduit"; the solar, masculine current flowing along the right channel of the spine

Pitta. biological fire humor; the principle which controls digestion and the enzymatic and endocrine systems

Pitri. "forebear", or "ancestor"; the ancestor plays a significant role in the daily life of the Hindu people, and in other earth-honoring traditions

Pitri Paksha. an auspicious time of year in the Vedic calendar when the *pitris*, or ancestors, are remembered and nourished with rites, rituals, and prayers

prajna. "wisdom"; liberating wisdom which gives way to Transcendental Reality

prajna-paradha. "crimes against wisdom"; going against the grain of intelligence; perverting the mind and dharma; engaging in activities known to be unwholesome

prakriti. "primary matter or nature;" active potential principle of manifestation; gross energy form which all the elements are issued; metabolic nature; nature consisting of the three *gunas—sattva, rajas,* and *tamas*

prana. life force; vital air; from the root *pran* (to breathe); first of the five airs of the body; called "ki" or "chi" in Oriental medicine; one of the three primordial conditions of the cosmos—*ojas, tejas,* and *prana*

Pranava Upasana. a form of meditation using specific *bijas,* primordial sounds

pranamaya. breath-sheath; pranic plane; second depth of the cosmic anatomy

pranayama. "breath control"; Vedic science of controlling and strengthening life force through systematic breathing practices

prayoga. Hindu sacred rites of passage

prinana. sense of joy and exhilaration

puja. Vedic ritual or ceremony

Pujari. Hindu priest, generally from the Brahmana lineage; pundit

Purana. "ancient Hindu lore"; a popular religious body of work on Vedic cosmology and theology

purnima. "full moon"; as in the full splendor of the Supreme Goddess. Lalita Maha Tripurasundari

Purusha Sukta. the youngest hymn from the *Rig Veda;* Purusha is the cosmic person, having a thousand heads, a thousand eyes, a thousand feet and encompassing the earth, spreading in all directions into animate and inanimate things

raga. classical composition and rendition in Indian music; originated from the Vedas

rajas. cosmic force of activity; one of the three *gunas—sattva, rajas,* and *tamas;* excess *rajas* causes the mind/body to become aggressive, overactive, and unstable

rakta. blood tissue; second vital tissue layer of the body

rasa. "taste"; lymph or plasma; the first of the seven vital tissues of the body; *rasa* generates the complex chain of reactions that the body experiences from its initial perception of food to the stimulation of the brain cells that excite the appetite; also "aesthetic" and "refined" beauty

Rig Veda. "knowledge of praise"; the oldest collection of Vedic hymns; the most sacred Vedic scripture (See also *Atharva Veda, Sama Veda,* and *Yajur Veda.*)

rishi. "seer" in Vedic tradition; a term for an enlightened being, a wise and psychic visionary (In the Vedic age, *rishis* lived in forest or mountain retreats, either alone or with disciples. The *rishis* are the greatest visionaries, and cosmic physicists who are the inspired conveyors of the Vedas—the vast wellspring of knowledge that informs all aspects of the Creation and the unmanifest.)

rita. cosmic rhythm; sacred order of the universe

Rudra. "wielder of stupendous powers"; "red, shining one"; the name of Shiva as the universal force of dissolution and re-absorption (Rudra-Shiva is revered as the "Terrifying One" and the "Lord of Tears")

Sadakhya. "full moon"; or 16th day of the waxing moon represented by Lalita

Maha Tripurasundari

sadhaka. one who practices *sadhana*, living in harmony with nature within and without; a spiritual aspirant

sadhana. wholesome activities practiced in accordance with the cyclical rhythms of nature; sacred practices that honor Mother Consciousness; healthful, joyous response to life

sadhu. "virtuous"; "simple"; "pure"; a holy person dedicated to a spiritual life

sahasrara. "a thousand petals"; the seventh chakra, situated in the subtle crown of the head

Sakahari. vegetarian; one who honors the life force of all beings

Sama Veda. "knowledge of chants"; the Vedic hymns containing the chants used in ceremonies and rituals (See also *Atharva Veda, Rig Veda,* and *Yajur Veda.*)

samadhi. "sameness"; "standing within one's Self"; state of cosmic union with Divine; state of true yoga, in which the meditator and the object of meditation are one (*Samadhi* has two levels: *savikalpa samadhi*—identification or oneness with the essence of an object; and *nirvikalpa samadhi*—identification with the Self, in which all modes of consciousness are transcended and Absolute Reality—which is beyond time, space, and form—is experienced.)

samana. third of five airs of the body; keeper of balance

samsara. the course of worldly life; misery created from ignorance of your true nature; living in duality; feelings of separation from the Divine

samskara. karmic imprint remaining in the subtle body to propagate rebirth; Vedic sages established a system of 16 primary sacraments intended to safeguard life in its continuum from birth through death into rebirth

sanchitakarma. "karmic bank account"; accumulated karmas accounting for recurrent births (The collective scorecard of each individual's karmas is maintained in a cosmic account that 'keeps track' of each soul's journeys through rebirth.)

sapta padi. in Hinduism, the ritual of seven steps is taken by bride and groom during the marriage ceremony (Symbolic of their eternal unification, the bridegroom leads the bride in the northern direction around the ceremonial fire.)

Sarvamangala Nitya. "all auspicious"; the lunar deity for the 13th notch of the waxing moon cycle

sat, satyam. "truth"; "existence"; "being"; that which is the Ultimate Reality; the cosmic truth

satsanga. "in the company of the sacred or real"; Vedic traditional practice of sitting in the presence of saints, sages, and enlightened beings who communicate or transmit cosmic truth

sattva. cosmic force of balance and contentment; one of three *prakriti gunas—sattva, rajas,* and *tamas*

Shakta Upanishad. text disclosing the teachings related to Shakti, the feminine force of the creation

Shakti. primeval Hindu Goddess; cosmic feminine force; power, energy; power of the Mother Consciousness

Shakti prana. the primordial feminine *pranic* force of the Shakti that flows within the genitals, womb, and belly; a specific *prana* that circulates the two lower chakras, located around the perineum and sacrum

shanti mudra. the sacred hand gesture of cosmic peace

Shashtyabda purti. a rite of passage in which Hindu women reaffirm marital vows at age 60; one of the 16 *samskaras* to mark the age of wisdom.

shatavari. Literally, "100 husbands"; Ayurvedic herb containing unusually high amounts of plant-derived estrogens used to balance the female hormonal system and strengthen virility

shirovasti. one of numerous head therapies in Ayurveda used to improve vision, and relieve mental stress and anxiety

Shitakari. a specific pranayama practice to cool the breath wherein the breath is inhaled through the mouth

shukla paksha. "light phase" of the moon when it is in transit from new to full; waxing cycle

shukra. "sperm"; the seventh tissue layer; the male reproductive tissue; Ayurveda informs that plentiful *ojas* in the body depends on the healthy quality of *shukra* and *artava* (ovum); *also* Sanskrit name for Venus

siddhi. "perfection"; "accomplishment"; "magical power"; spiritual perfection that results from complete identification with the Ultimate Reality

smriti. "memory"; "remembered knowledge"; the tradition of the *rishis* which gave way to revelation, *sruti*

snanam. "sacred bath" or ritual dip in sacred water which revitalizes spiritual energy (Every day, millions of Hindus take *snanam* in the Ganges River.)

Sri Chakra. Abode of the Supreme Goddess; Lalita's creative manifestation portraying the *yantra* and *mantra* that represent her subtle form of absolute space and cosmic vibration (According to the *Bhavana Upanishad*, the human body and the cosmic universe subsisting in time and space are both conceived in the subtle formation of the Sri Chakra.)

sruti. what is heard; cosmic revelation as heard, seen and articulated by the Vedic seers

sukshma. "subtle"; "fine"; "penetrating"

sukshma prana. subtle life force

Surya. Vedic Sun-god

Sushruta Samhita. "text written by Sushruta", Ancient Vaidya, Sushruta, is considered the forerunner in medical surgery (The world's first known surgery procedures were practiced in Ayurveda. *Sushruta Samhita* (600 B.C.E.) is the pioneering work on surgery, which is studied to this day. Hippocrates, Greek father of medicine, lived two centuries later. Also among the many other ancient authorities on Ayurveda are Charaka and Vagbhata.)

sushumna. "she who is most gracious"; central and main channel within spinal column (This channel extends from the root chakra at base of spine to the crown chakra of the head, and it is along this central pathway that the aroused *kundalini* must ascend.)

svadhisthana. "one's own base"; sacred chakra situated directly below the naval

Svayambu lingam. Shiva is in the form of the serpent coiled around the *lingam* wherein the primordial masculine and feminine energies are held in their potential form

tamas. cosmic force of inertia; natural state of the body during rest or of the universe during dissolution; one of the three *gunas*—*sattva, rajas,* and *tamas*

tantra. "loom"; a body of sacred scripture originated in the early centuries of the Common Era, pertaining to Tantrism and primarily dealing with ritual practices centering on the feminine goddess force, *Shakti*

tapas, tapasya. "heat"; "glow"; asceticism; observance of austerities and yogic disciplines to induce inner luminosity and vitality; intense disciplines imbibed by the sages, seers, and yogis

Tvarita Nitya. "swift"; the lunar eighth notch of the waxing moon cycle

tejas. effulgent, brilliant energy; the light of pure consciousness within the body; subtle fire; one of the three primordial conditions in creation—*ojas, tejas,* and *prana*

tha. Sanskrit syllable representing the lunar energies

tithi. "lunar day"; the Vedic calendar is determined by the lunar cycles, divided into two fortnightly periods, *pakshas*, and 30 lunar days, *tithis*

udana. second of five breaths of the body; rising air; universal keeper of memory and personal sound

Upanishad. "sitting near"; Vedic scriptures composed from what was seen and articulated by the celestials and *rishis* (The Upanishads expound the metaphysics of Oneness, the Whole, nondualism [*Advaita Vedanta*]. Over 200 Upanishads exist, although Vedic traditionalists recognize only 108 of them. These Upanishads are organized in eight distinct groups. Originally, Vedic texts were not written, but memorized and transmitted from teacher to pupil by word of mouth.)

Ushas. "dawn"; Daughter of Heaven, the light of dawn that illuminates the world; consort of the Sun-god, Surya; Vedic cow goddess

Uttara Vasti. one of Ayurveda's therapies used to cleanse and nourish the womb; the Sanskrit word *vasti* refers to the stomach lining of the animal, which was used in ancient times to create the first Uttara Vasti therapy bag; *uttara* means "womb"; "cosmos"; "that which is filled" (The wise perceive the womb as uttara—filled with contentment and fulfillment, carrier of life itself.)

Vac. "speech"; a feminine deity, the Mother of the Vedas (She is said to have four *padas*, aspects, human speech being one of the four padas that is known to humans.)

vajikarana. Ayurveda branch of medicine that deals with virility

vajra. "unyielding"; a thunderbolt; the weapon of Indra, Lord of the Firmament

vanaprastha ashrama. retreating into the forest during mid-life; observing a life of abstinence; one of four stations prescribed in the life of a Hindu person (In India, many couples that take to a spiritual life observe celibacy for years while maintaining a loving bond and companionship with each other.)

vandhyatva. infertility; defined in Ayurveda as associated with the Vata condition although it may involve all three doshas

Vahnivasini Nitya. "dweller in fire"; lunar deity of the fifth notch of the waxing moon cycle

varna. pure vibration; profound silence; unmanifest sound

vasana. "trait"; "characteristic"; "quality"; desire or longing (In Patanjali Yoga, the subtle subliminal imprints in the mind stamped there as a result of our actions and volitions.)

Vata. biological air humor; the principle of kinetic energy in the body, mainly concerned with the nervous system and which controls all bodily movement

vibhuti. "blessing"; sacred ash produced from the venerated fire in Hindu ritual ceremonies

vidya. knowledge

Vijaya Nitya. "victorious"; the lunar deity for the 12th notch of the waxing moon cycle

vijnanamaya. sheath that masks intelligence, and the intuitive power; fourth depth of the cosmic anatomy

vikriti. state of imbalance and disease in the body, generally caused by disharmonious habits and lifeways

vina. an ancient Indian stringed instrument (Goddess Saraswati is depicted as playing the vina.)

vishuddha. "purity"; the fifth chakra, situated in the throat; center of divine love

Vriksha-Natha. a name for Shiva, Protector of the Vegetation

vyana. fifth air of the cosmos; air of circulation

yajna. "sacrifice"; the ritual sacrifices fundamental to Hinduism (In the Vedic era, external sacrificial ritual was internalized in the form of deep meditation.)

Yajur Veda. (*Shukla Yajur Veda* and *Krishna Yajur Veda*) One of four primary Vedic scriptures containing religious texts focusing on liturgy, rituals and sacrifices, and how to perform the same (See also *Atharva Veda*, *Sama Veda*, and *Rig Veda*.)

Yama. "Lord of Death"; one who receives the souls of the deceased

Yama Damstra. period of time between November 22 and December 9, when the earth begins its northward rotation around the sun (According to the Vedas, Lord Yama actively scours the earth for souls during this time. This time holds within it an innate structure of fear and mental disturbance.)

yantra. Hindu sacred scribes, drawings, and mandalas that are made to evoke specific cosmic energies and vibrations of the deities

yoga. from the root *yuj* ("to join or unite"); spiritual discipline or mystical practice to merge body, mind, and spirit, or inner and outer universe; one of six classical schools of thought presented by Patanjali in his *Yoga Sutra*

yoni. cosmic gateway or womb; source of creation; vulva

yoni mudra. "sacred hand gesture that seals the womb"; a potent mudra to arouse Shakti's power (In Tantric Sri Vidya tradition, the goddess is invoked through 10 hand gestures.)

yuga. "yoke"; according to Vedic cosmology, there are four stages of existence in the world, each consisting of several thousand years

WISE EARTH AYURVEDA®
EDUCATIONAL RESOURCES

Wise Earth School of Ayurveda, Ltd.
P.O. Box 160
Candler, NC 28715-0160 USA
Telephone: 828-258-9999
E-mail: info@wisearth.org
Website: www.wisearth.org

Mother Om Mission
Executive Office
4255 Seton Avenue
Yonkers, NY 10466 USA
Telephone: 646-773-2330
E-mail: info@wisearth.org
Website: www.motherom.org

Punarnava Ayurveda
Dr. Ram Kumar
A-21, Parsn Galaxy
Nanjundapuram Road
Coimbatore 641 036 India
Telephone: 91-422-2311521
                91-422-4308081
E-mail: ramkumar@punarnava.com
            kavita@punarnava.com
Website: www.punarnava-ayurveda.com

WISE EARTH AYURVEDA® PROGRAM OUTREACH CENTERS

Australia & New Zealand
Katie Manitsas
Samadhi Yoga Center
36 Lennox Street
Newtown
NSW 2042
Telephone: 02-9517-3280
Website: www.samadhiyoga.com.au

Brazil
Dr. Ana Maria Araújo Rodrigues
Escola de Ayurveda do Brasil
Rua Paul Bouthilier 207
Belo Horizonte - Minas Gerais
CEP. 30315-010 Brazil
Telephone: 55-31-32279855
          55-31-32643152
E-mail: ana.deha@gmail.com
Website: www.deha.com.br

United Kingdom & Ireland
Cliodhna Mulhern
Flowstone
Lisardhalla Lodge
127 Ardmore Road
Derry-Londonderry
BT47 3TD N Ireland
Telephone: 44-0-7929328513
E-mail: cliodhna@flowstone.org.uk

USA
Linda Sarita Rocco
Yoga Inlet
734 Penn Avenue
West Reading, PA 19611
Telephone: 610-376-2881
E-mail: yogainlet@earthlink.net
Website: www.yogainlet.com

Sundari Diane Finlayson
Yama Studio
5710 Bellona Avenue, Suite 102
Baltimore, MD 21212
Telephone: 410-464-9000
E-mail: yamastudio@verizon.net

Nina Molin, M.D.
Ananda Health Center for Integrative Medicine
P.O. Box 82
Lenox, MA 01240
Telephone: 413-822-0852
E-mail: ninamolin@ananda-health.com
Website: www.ananda-health.com

Ambika Theresa McGhee
Lotus Center for Health & Healing
1292 Metropolitan Avenue, SE
Atlanta, GA 30316
Telephone: 404-561-8873
E-mail: tessmcghee@yahoo.com

Kirati Kelly Grey
15950 Old Well Road
Prescott, AZ 86305
Telephone: 928-443-1072
        928-713-9631
E-mail: kgreyus@yahoo.com

Laura Martin-Eagle
Moon Jewel Healing
2 East 7th Street
Lawrence, KS 66044
Telephone: 785-550-8931
E-mail: bemovedStudio@yahoo.com
Website: www.moonjewelhealing.com

Rosemary Didi Jordan
707 Hill Street
Santa Monica, CA 90405
Telephone: 310-581-8347
E-mail: chantdancing@yahoo.com

Mary Vaishnavi Roberson, Ph.D.
Ayurveda Center for Natural Healthcare
665 Emory Valley Road, Suite A
P.O. Box 6408
Oak Ridge, TN 37831
Telephone: 865-482-0981
E-mail: ayurvedacentertn@bellsouth.net
Website: www.ayurvedacentertn.com

Ailene Sunari Radcliffe
Ayurveda Center for Natural Healthcare
665 Emory Valley Road, Suite A
P.O. Box 6408
Oak Ridge, TN 37831
Telephone: 865-406-1143
E-mail: Tennessee226@comcast.net

Lila Linnea Lindberg Jepsen
Great Grains Conversations for Health
1658 Dauphin Avenue
Wyomissing, PA 19610-2314
Telephone: 610-372-7248
E-mail: linnealj@verizon.net

Yogamaya Doe Wails
2126 Penn Road
Lewes, DE 19958
Telephone: 302-644-1022
E-mail: doegeorge@earthlink.net

Marcia Meredith R.N., N.P.
Health Through Ayurveda
1552 Osceola Avenue
Saint Paul, MN 55105
Telephone: 651-503-0471
E-mail: marciameredith77@hotmail.com

Cary Dharani Twomey
Haymarket Pilates & Yoga Center
311 North Eighth Street #210
Lincoln, NE 68508
Telephone: 402-477-5101
E-mail: carytwomey@aol.com

Lindsey Mann & Todd Roderick
238 Second Avenue
Decatur, GA 30030
Telephone: 770-335-7292
            706-338-4835
E-mail: lindseyemann@gmail.com
        ashtangayogaatlanta@gmail.com

Shilpa Rao
1304 West Marlboro Drive
Chandler, AZ 85224
Telephone: 480-963-5683
E-mail: shilpakka@cox.net

Sangita Hilary Clark
379 Baltic Street
Brooklyn, NY 11201
Telephone: 347-228-4634
E-mail: hdreamerc@aol.com

Karen Ling Chestnut
204 Crighton Circle
Fort Washington, MD 20744
Telephone: 240-351-3335
E-mail: klccye@yahoo.com

Margo Bachman
The Heart of Wellness
P.O. Box 4352
Santa Fe, NM 87502
Telephone: 505-670-4506
E-mail: santosa_m@yahoo.com

Judith Daya Kubish
921 West Glendale Avenue
Glendale, WI 53209-6513
Telephone: 414-221-9293
E-mail: judithkubish@mcleodusa.net

Mary E. Mangus, D.C.
3102 Chesterfield Avenue
Charleston, WV 25304
Telephone: 304-346-6688
E-mail: mbmango@hotmail.com

Kathryn Shankari McKann
152 Hidden Trails Road
Port Townsend, WA 98368
Telephone: 360-379-9209
E-mail: unmutable@wildmail.com

Blanca Colón-Simon
1546 Citrus Avenue
Chico, CA 95926
Telephone: 530-893-4792
          530-345-6234
E-mail: blancuz@pacbell.net

Floriana Tullio
6658 Youree Drive, #180
P.O. Box 151
Shreveport, LA 71105
Telephone: 718-744-4256
E-mail: Flori12@hotmail.com

Chris Arcucci
Divine Play
P.O. Box 2175
Mammoth Lakes, CA 93546
Telephone: 760-934-9343
E-mail: chris@divineplay.us
Website: www.divineplay.us

Nitya Jess Oppenheimer
Healing Arts Center
215 Jay Street
Albany, NY 12210
Telephone: 518-463-2222
E-mail: healingarts@healthinform.info
www.healingarts-center.com

Note: For contact information updates on the Wise Earth Ayurveda® Directory of Practitioners go to www.wisearth.org

AYURVEDA HERBAL DISTRIBUTORS

<u>Australia</u>
Ayurveda Elements
17 Orchard Road
Chatswood
NSW Australia 2067
Telephone: 61-2-9904-7754
E-mail: info@ayurvedaelements.com

India
Punarnava Ayurveda
A-21, Parsn Galaxy
Nanjundapuram Road
Coimbatore 641 036 India
Telephone: 91 422 2311521, 4308081
E-mail: kavita@punarnava.com
Website: www.punarnava-ayurveda.com

USA
Banyan Botanicals
6705 Eagle Rock Avenue NE
Albuquerque, NM 87113
Telephone: 541-488-9525
　　　　　800-953-6424
E-mail: info@banyanbotanicals.com
Website: www.banyanbotanicals.com

RESOURCES FOR MEHNDI HENNA KITS

Contra-indications: Do **not** use black henna. (A chemical called PPD, present in black henna, can cause chemical burns on your skin.)

Mehndi World
52/6, VIP Road
(Near Big Bazaar)
Phase 2, Flat 708
Kolkata 700 059 India
Telephone: 91-9331005999
E-mail: rashmi@mehndiworld.com
Website: www.mehndiworld.com

Earth Henna
Lakaye Studio
6025 Santa Monica Boulevard, Suite 202
Los Angeles, CA 90038
Telephone: 323-460-7333
E-mail: info@earthhenna.com
Website: www.earthhenna.com

INDEX

ABOUT THE AUTHOR

Considered an embodiment of the Spiritual Mother, Sri Swamini Mayatitananda, affectionately called "Mother," is an extraordinary teacher who has transformed thousands of lives with her healing presence—filling a significant void in the world culture as a nurturer, healer, and educator. A most courageous and extraordinary human being, Mayatitananda is a cancer survivor who has gone through the rigorous training to become a *Swamini* in the Vedic ancestry of her birth, and is one of few female monks (*Sannyasini*) to be ordained in the pre-eminent *Veda Vyasa* tradition. She is an expert in Ayurveda, and as a cancer survivor, she is living proof that intensive inner work, meditation, and faith in our own rhythmic power to heal ourselves can have profound curative results.

In 1981, Mother founded the first school for Ayurveda education in the U.S., the Wise Earth School of Ayurveda, which continues to flourish today. The Wise Earth Ayurveda® Inner Medicine healing practices are a unique body of holistic education developed by Mother to promote conscious self care education that is in accord with the greater rhythms of the cosmos.

She is also the founder of Mother Om Mission (MOM), a charitable organization that provides Inner Medicine healing education and services to some of the world's poorest, at-risk communities in New York's inner cities, and Guyana, SA. With MOM, she works in the trenches with the community by mobilizing a volunteer leadership force directly from these at-risk communities. By educating and empowering their members rather than bringing in privileged instructors from sophisticated communities to do the work, Mother takes a radical, grassroots approach that creates results.

Mother has created a unique niche in the world forum as a pre-eminent featured speaker—lauded by the Secretary General of the United Nations Millennium Peace Summit as a "compassionate Mother whose ancient wisdom can be applied to heal the present world crises." She has been presenting Wise Earth Ayurveda for humanity's healing and world peace for 25 years at conferences worldwide, and has been a featured speaker at the Global Peace Congress of Women's Spiritual Leaders in Geneva, Switzerland. She has taught hundreds of workshops at Wise Earth Monastery and at retreat centers around the world on Inner Medicine healing, teaching others how to use their own infinite Inner Medicine resources to heal themselves.

Mayatitananda is the best-selling author of the following books, under the name Maya Tiwari: *Ayurveda: A Life of Balance; Ayurveda Secrets of Healing;* and *The Path of Practice: A Woman's Book of Healing with Food, Breath, and Sound.*